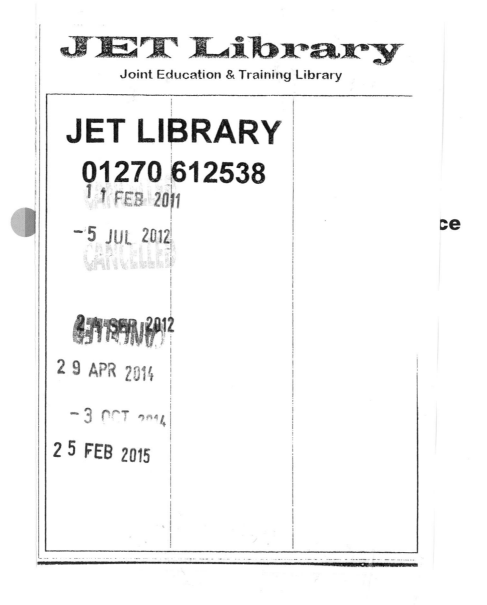

For Elsevier:

Commissioning Editor: *Mairi McCubbin*
Development Editor: *Sheila Black*
Project Manager: *K Anand Kumar*
Designer: *Charles Gray*
Illustration Manager: *Merlyn Harvey*

Advancing Skills in Midwifery Practice

Edited by

Jayne E. Marshall MA PhD PGCEA RGN RM ADM
Midwife Teacher, Post-graduate Education Centre,
Academic Division of Midwifery, School of Nursing, Midwifery and Physiotherapy,
Faculty of Medicine and Health Sciences, University of Nottingham,
Nottingham University Hospitals NHS Trust, Nottingham, UK

Maureen D. Raynor MA PGCEA RMN RN RM ADM
Midwife Teacher and Supervisor of Midwives, Post-graduate Education Centre,
Academic Division of Midwifery, School of Nursing, Midwifery and Physiotherapy,
Faculty of Medicine and Health Sciences, University of Nottingham,
Nottingham University Hospitals NHS Trust, Nottingham, UK

Foreword by

Paul Lewis
Professor and Associate Dean – Midwifery, Rehabilitation and Health Sciences,
Bournemouth University, Bournemouth, UK

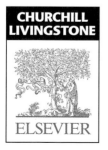

CHURCHILL LIVINGSTONE

ELSEVIER

Edinburgh   London   New York   Oxford   Philadelphia   St Louis   Sydney   Toronto   2010

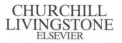

First published 2010

ISBN 978-0-7020-3006-2

British Library Cataloguing in Publication Data
A catalogue record for this book is available from the British Library

Library of Congress Cataloging in Publication Data
A catalog record for this book is available from the Library of Congress

Notice
Knowledge and best practice in this field are constantly changing. As new research and experience broaden our knowledge, changes in practice, treatment and drug therapy may become necessary or appropriate. Readers are advised to check the most current information provided (i) on procedures featured or (ii) by the manufacturer of each product to be administered, to verify the recommended dose or formula, the method and duration of administration, and contraindications. It is the responsibility of the practitioner, relying on their own experience and knowledge of the patient, to make diagnoses, to determine dosages and the best treatment for each individual patient, and to take all appropriate safety precautions. To the fullest extent of the law, neither the Publisher nor the Editors assume any liability for any injury and/or damage to persons or property arising out or related to any use of the material contained in this book.

The Publisher

 your source for books, journals and multimedia in the health sciences
www.elsevierhealth.com

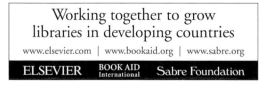

Working together to grow
libraries in developing countries

www.elsevier.com | www.bookaid.org | www.sabre.org

ELSEVIER   BOOK AID International   Sabre Foundation

The Publisher's policy is to use **paper manufactured from sustainable forests**

Printed in China

Contents

Contributors vii

Foreword ix

Preface xi

1   Introduction 1

2   The midwife's professional responsibilities in developing competence in
    new skills 7

3   Complementary therapies in midwifery: a focus on moxibustion for
    breech presentation 19

4   Ultrasonography in midwifery practice 29

5   Reducing unnecessary caesarean section by external cephalic version 47

6   Peripheral intravenous cannulation 57

7   Midwives undertaking ventouse births 67

8   Forceps-assisted birth 77

9   Facilitating vaginal breech birth at term 89

10 Perineal management and repair 103

11 Haemodynamic assessment and monitoring in maternity care 121

12 Physiological examination of the neonate 135

13 Infant massage 147

14 Postnatal physiological examination of the mother 161

15 Working in new ways to advance midwifery skills in practice 173

Index 181

Contributors

Robina Aslam MSc PGCEA ADM RGN RM
Midwife Teacher, Academic Division of Midwifery,
School of Nursing, Midwifery and Physiotherapy,
Faculty of Medicine and Health Sciences, University of
Nottingham; Lincoln County Hospital NHS Trust,
Lincoln; IAIM Instructor, UK
13 Infant massage

Debra Bick BA(Hons) MMedSc PhD RM
Professor of Evidence-Based Midwifery Practice,
Florence Nightingale School of Nursing and Midwifery,
King's College London, London, UK
14 Postnatal physiological examination of the mother

Abigail Cairns BA(Hons) DM
Midwife, Gloucester Royal Hospital, Gloucestershire
Hospitals NHS Trust, Gloucester, UK
*5 Reducing unnecessary caesarean section by external
cephalic version*

Carole England BSc(Hons) CertEd(FE) ENB405 RGN RM
Midwife Teacher, Academic Division of Midwifery,
School of Nursing, Midwifery and Physiotherapy,
Faculty of Medicine and Health Sciences, University of
Nottingham; Royal Derby Hospital NHS Trust,
Derby, UK
12 Physiological examination of the neonate

Christine Kettle DM PhD SCM SRN
Professor of Women's Health, Academic Unit of
Obstetrics and Gynaecology, Staffordshire University,
University Hospital of North Staffordshire,
Stoke-on-Trent, UK
10 Perineal management and repair

Jayne E. Marshall MA PhD PGCEA RGN RM ADM
Midwife Teacher, Post-graduate Education Centre,
Academic Division of Midwifery, School of Nursing,
Midwifery and Physiotherapy, Faculty of Medicine and
Health Sciences, University of Nottingham; Nottingham
University Hospitals NHS Trust, Nottingham, UK
1 Introduction
*2 The midwife's professional responsibilities in developing
competence in new skills*
8 Forceps-assisted birth
9 Facilitating vaginal breech birth at term

Carol McCormick BSc(Hons) PGDL RN RM ADM
Consultant Midwife and Supervisor of Midwives,
Labour Suite/Maternity Unit, Nottingham University
Hospitals NHS Trust, Nottingham, UK
*5 Reducing unnecessary caesarean section by external
cephalic version*

Maureen D. Raynor MA PGCEA RMN RN RM ADM
Midwife Teacher and Supervisor of Midwives,
Post-graduate Education Centre, Academic Division
of Midwifery, School of Nursing, Midwifery and
Physiotherapy, Faculty of Medicine and Health Sciences,
University of Nottingham; Nottingham University Hospitals
NHS Trust, Nottingham, UK
6 Peripheral intravenous cannulation
8 Forceps-assisted birth
10 Perineal management and repair
*15 Working in new ways to advance midwifery skills in
practice*

John Regan BSc(Hons) PGCertMedUS (Obs&Gyn) RGN RM
Midwife Sonographer, Radiology Department, Withybush
General Hospital, Haverfordwest, UK
4 Ultrasonography in midwifery practice

Louise C. Stayt BSc(Hons) MSc RN
Senior Lecturer in Professional Practice Skills, School of
Health and Social Care, Oxford Brookes University,
Swindon, UK
*11 Haemodynamic assessment and monitoring in mater-
nity care*

Vicky Tinsley BSc MA RN RM
Assistant Director for Maternity Services, Wiltshire Primary
Care Trust (Bath Clinical Area), Bath, UK
7 Midwives undertaking ventouse births

Denise Tiran MSc PGCEA RM RGN ADM
Director, Expectancy Ltd; Visiting Lecturer, University of
Greenwich, Greenwich, UK
*3 Complementary therapies in midwifery: a focus on
moxibustion for breech presentation*

Jean Wills BSc(Hons) PGDipAMP PGDipResMeth DPSN RM RN
Clinical Midwifery Manager, Labour Ward, Aberdeen
Maternity Hospital, Aberdeen, UK
8 Forceps-assisted birth

Foreword

The changing nature of society alongside rapid and significant advances in science and technology has led to increasing expectations being placed upon all Health and Social Care practitioners; nowhere is this felt more keenly than within the context of midwifery practice. The once-treasured permanence of our received skills and knowledge seems increasingly irrelevant as the continuing and irreversible progress of change appears to diminish and deny the previously cherished wisdom of the midwife, seeking to divide and differentiate our long-established and traditional roles.

Yet midwives and midwifery are themselves a part of the process of change and contemporary practice demands more of us than has ever been documented in our previous histories. Women and their families continue to seek out our advice and skills and, as always, it is the midwife's responsibility to respond in a manner that safely, effectively and efficiently addresses their needs and concerns within the context of current knowledge, rational expectations and established values.

Few would question that the role of the midwife is founded on the principles of 'normality', but the debate on what a midwife is and is not has in many respects served to contain and confine our work as practitioners and limit our usefulness to women and their families. Our enquiries, alongside our skills, knowledge and understanding, must go beyond initial learning. In the modernisation of the workforce, we must discover ways in which midwives can respond more effectively and flexibly in their efforts to support women and still continue to nurture the physiological process of pregnancy and childbirth, even when that process itself is in question, under increasing scrutiny and open to challenge.

All too often, our profession has confused *advancing skills* with the move to a medical model of care. In doing so, we fail to interpret the art and science of midwifery in a manner which remains meaningful to mothers and keeps pace with new ideas, new science and new technologies.

I felt immensely privileged when asked to write the Foreword to this book and had little doubt that, like previous publications by Marshall and Raynor, it would be a much welcomed and well-read addition to an increasing body of midwifery knowledge. It is in fact more than this.

Advancing Skills in Midwifery Practice draws together an eclectic mix of experience and expertise, which, while firmly rooted in the art of midwifery, also ably demonstrates the knowledge, skills and science needed to underpin and inform practice beyond initial registration. It will, I believe, become a seminal text that alters and affirms our understanding about what it means to be an advanced practitioner. In effect, it signposts the standards and requirements that will be expected of our future, continuing professional development as midwives and enable us to better address the demands of contemporary practice in a continually modernising healthcare system.

In each chapter there is a detailed and distinct knowledge base that provides important insights into the contributions that midwives and midwifery can make to the health and wellbeing of mothers and their families. It gives clarity and voice to the elements of advancing practice skills, in which autonomy, expertise, experience, decision-making, research and reflection culminate in the delivery of woman-centred, evidence-based, midwife-led care.

Advancing Skills in Midwifery Practice was a delight to read, informative, educational and challenging in equal measure. Above all, it gave me hope that through such exemplars, the future development and increasing diversity of midwifery roles could and would enhance the already valuable contribution of midwives to those in their care.

Like many other books, *Advancing Skills in Midwifery Practice* not only informs but also describes, empowers and enriches the work of the midwife. It has much to offer us as clinicians, but it should also enable educators, managers and leaders of our profession to envisage and engage with the possibilities, opportunities and benefits that advanced skills in midwifery practice might bring to our maternity services at the local, national and global level.

I believe this book will have an impact well beyond the shores of the United Kingdom and not only for midwives. It has resonance for all those engaged in the delivery of women's health and maternity services. It links closely to the quality-of-care agenda, in which continuity and choice remain hallmarks of good practice; and the central role of the midwife remains in keeping birth normal, but with the scope and skills to deal with events that differ or diverge from normality.

I have found it difficult to put into words the pleasure, excitement and enthusiasm I have felt whilst reading this book. It has re-ignited old dreams and a wish that I were 30 years younger and once again starting out in a profession that I have loved for more years than I care to remember. However, as this book attests and tantalisingly reminds us, it has the possibility to be a very different profession: one in which midwives can make the most of their advancing skills and expertise in the interests of women. That our much-vaunted autonomy as practitioners will find rich ground in our increasing scope of practice, and that as a profession, midwifery will regain the pre-eminence it once held, using its position wisely in the interest of those we serve, the women, children and families of the world.

Paul Lewis

This book aims to build on *Skills for Midwifery Practice* by Ruth Johnson and Wendy Taylor, following a format that is already familiar to a large proportion of midwives from their initial midwifery preparation. The text is grounded in safe practice with contemporary evidence cited throughout, and is intended to support midwives with their continuing professional development needs and fulfilment of the statutory Post-registration and Practice (PREP) requirements (Nursing and Midwifery Council [NMC 2008]). To be deemed competent to practise a skill safely, however, they will also need to fulfil the specific theoretical and practical requirements of the relevant training body.

Whilst the book is aimed primarily at registered midwives wishing to advance their knowledge and clinical skills beyond initial registration, the principles and philosophy are transferable across professional boundaries and other health professionals should also find the content of value. In addition, midwives undertaking Masters level studies, as well as student midwives in the latter stages of undergraduate pre-registration midwifery education programmes, will find the text useful when examining the diversity of the midwife's role and professional responsibilities that has emerged as a result of changing healthcare and maternity care demands.

Reference

Nottingham, 2009

Jayne E. Marshall
Maureen D. Raynor

Nursing and Midwifery Council, 2008. The PREP Handbook, NMC, London.

Chapter One

Introduction

Jayne E. Marshall

CONTENTS

Introduction 1
Advanced practice or advancing skills? . . 2
How to use the book 2
References 4

Introduction

Within contemporary midwifery practice, midwives are experiencing the need to undertake further education and training. The impetus of which is to develop/advance their clinical skills in order to meet the demands of the providers and consumers of the maternity services. Not only has government policy affected the way the childbearing woman should be part of the decision-making process and have access to a choice of care options to enhance her childbirth experiences (Department of Health [DH] 1993a, 1997, 1998a, 1999, 2000, 2003, 2007a, 2007b), but also the introduction of the Calman Report (DH 1993b), the European Working Directive (DH 1998b) and the guidance on junior doctors' working patterns (DH The National Assembly for Wales, the National Health Service [NHS] Confederation and the British Medical Association 2002) have created a gap in obstetric and paediatric cover necessitating a change in the delivery of care. Furthermore, the recent Darzi Report (DH 2008a) that sets out a vision for a NHS with quality at its heart, reinforces that workforce planning, education and

NB: From March 2009 onwards Health Care Commission name has changed to Care Quality Commission (CQC, www.cqc.org.uk).

training needs to change to enable health professionals, such as the midwife, to respond more effectively and flexibly to this dynamic health-care environment. Such a vision includes focusing on the current and emerging roles that health professionals may occupy, in order to deliver quality care based on the various needs of the local population. In addition, the Department of Health (2008b) in its follow-on publication *Framing the nursing and midwifery contribution: driving up the quality of care*, identifies a variety of work streams and activities that intend to form an integrated strategy so that health professionals can maximise their contribution to high-quality health care and improved health outcomes. One of which is to develop nurses and midwives so they can extend their clinical skills and roles, transform service through multiprofessional, clinically led commissioning and develop entrepreneurial approaches to provide health-care services that meet local needs.

Although some midwives have already begun developing their clinical skills in order to fill the void in obstetric and paediatric cover, it is vital that they do not lose sight of the fundamental role of the midwife that is embedded in normal physiological processes. It is, therefore, important that midwives are fully aware of their professional responsibilities when developing their role and advancing their clinical skills. It is also imperative that comprehensive education and training programmes are in place to ensure that not only are the midwives' continuing professional development needs being met, but also the health and well being of the childbearing woman and her baby/family remain at the forefront of care (DH 2008, Nursing and Midwifery Council [NMC] 2004, 2008a, 2008b).

Advanced practice or advancing skills?

It is acknowledged that there is a need for all midwives to advance their own practice in order to ensure that childbearing women and their babies/families receive care of the best quality. However, as there has been much critical discussion within the midwifery profession about the use of the term *advanced practice*, the editors had the challenge of selecting the most appropriate title for the text to reflect its philosophy.

The work of Benner (2001) advocates that practitioners acquire five levels of competence during their development in clinical practice: *novice*, *advanced beginner*, *competent*, *proficient* with the final level being that of *expert*. Furthermore, Benner (2001) equates the level of expert to that of advanced practice, suggestive of reaching the end point of one's development and not necessarily of further developing their knowledge and competence. It is for this reason that the NMC have expressed concern for some time about nurses who also hold job titles that imply an advanced level of knowledge and competence, but do not necessarily possess such knowledge and competence.

McGee (1992) highlighted that one of the complexities of advanced practitioners is that they should function academically intuitively on a higher level than a proficient health professional. This was further elaborated following a national consultation in 2005, where the NMC agreed that *advanced nurse practitioner* should be a *registrable* qualification and that a further sub-part of the nurses' register be opened. The government's White Paper: *Trust, Assurance and Safety: the Regulation of Health Professionals in the 21st Century* (DH 2007c) recommends that further discussions be held with the NMC regarding agreeing the next steps on advanced nursing practice. The midwifery profession, on the other hand, has been more cynical, believing that such terms as *advanced* are misleading to the public in relation to the sphere of the midwife's role and her responsibilities.

In Eire, the National Council for the Professional Development of Nursing and Midwifery (2008) set up a framework for the establishment and accreditation of advanced practitioners in both nursing and midwifery, in which the post holder is expected to be educated to masters/higher degree level with at least 7 years' post-registration experience: equivalent to an Assistant Director of Nursing/Midwifery grade practitioner. Begley et al (2007) relate that the content of the Master of Science course to prepare Ireland's first advanced midwife practitioners (AMP) has an emphasis in normal midwifery, is practice-led and encourages reflective evidence-based, woman-centred care. It is, therefore, expected the AMP, like her nursing counterpart, will be a visionary clinical leader committed to developing midwifery practice beyond the current sphere of practice. The four concepts of advanced midwifery practice identified by the National Council for the Professional Development of Nursing and Midwifery (2008), namely *autonomy in clinical practice, expert practice, professional and clinical leadership* and *research*, bear similarities with the key functions expected of the role of consultant midwife (DH 1999).

Although midwives can and do develop their sphere of practice through undertaking appropriate education and training in specialist areas such as ventouse births and ultrasonography, this does not mean they have advanced their *midwifery* practice, which has a defined sphere (NMC 2004). Work undertaken by Sookhoo and Butler (1999) emphasised that advanced practice in midwifery is not synonymous with extending the role of the midwife, and is not about achieving psychomotor skills and knowledge identified in medicine and obstetrics, rather it is about developing *midwifery* in order to enhance the quality of midwifery care that is woman-centred rather than organization-focused.

Whilst the term *advanced* is suggestive of a person already being at a higher stage of development or progress than other similar individuals, in comparison the term *advancing* implies an ongoing process of development/progression such as is expected of all registered midwives in whatever area of midwifery they practice. For these reasons the book was finally given the title *Advancing Skills in Midwifery Practice*, the justification for including all the skills in the text being that they each aim to enhance the quality and continuity of care that the childbearing woman and her baby/family receive from midwives.

How to use the book

In order to achieve the aims of the book, a broad variety of skills that midwives are currently undertaking in contemporary midwifery practice have been included. As each chapter focuses on a specific skill, it is expected the midwife will examine individual chapters that are of particular interest to her own individual clinical practice and professional development. In Chapter 2, a theoretical framework is provided in which the reader can examine the inherent responsibilities before contemplating developing competence in any new skill.

Building on numerous existing texts on complementary therapies, Chapter 3 examines the evidence and use of moxibustion for breech presentation as a means of improving choices to women regarding birth outcome. Also highlighted is the importance of midwives providing evidence of adequate and appropriate training related to the procedures being implemented, and of being involved in the monitoring of standards, and the evaluation and audit of service provision. Chapter 4 provides a basic understanding of routine ultrasonography in each of the three trimesters of pregnancy and the relevance of various diagnostic images and measurements. As with Chapter 3, this chapter should not be seen as a replacement for training via a recognised ultrasound course, as midwives should only undertake an ultrasound examination if deemed competent to do so following such training.

In order to improve choices to eligible women who present with a breech, the Royal College of Obstetricians and Gynaecologists [RCOG] (2006) recommend that robust training packages should be in place to train more health professionals in External Cephalic Versions (ECV). Chapter 5, therefore, outlines the rationale for midwives to undertake the procedure and reduce the incidence of Lower Segment Caesarean Sections (LSCS) at term. The rationale is further strengthened by the inclusion of a personal narrative from the perspective of a woman who had experienced a home birth following a successful ECV by a midwife.

Chapter 6 examines the legal and professional issues relating to peripheral intravenous cannulation (PIVC) building on the technique and procedure outlined in a number of earlier texts such as that by Johnson and Taylor (2006). Particular attention is drawn to the importance of the midwife's record keeping, in that the documentation should provide evidence of all communication, care provided, decision making, adherence to infection control policies and the rationale for the midwife undertaking PIVC.

In an effort to reduce the number of transfers into hospital from midwife-led units for assisted births due to the decline of general practitioner (GP) presence in intrapartum care and in order to address recent health reforms (DH 2007a, 2007b, 2004a, 2004b), Chapter 7 discusses the development of the Midwife Ventouse Practitioner (MVP) with specific reference to the practice in the Wiltshire Primary Care Trust. This chapter clearly indicates that midwives should only utilise the ventouse when they have exhausted all their skills in supporting women to give birth spontaneously. In addition, the development of good practice guidelines and clinical governance reporting structures that embrace the general principles of risk management, should also be in place to support the MVP. Chapter 8 continues exploring assisted birth procedures by presenting the case for midwives developing their skills in forceps births and it discusses how the practice was successfully implemented within the Grampian region of Scotland.

The knowledge and skills required to effectively facilitate planned vaginal breech births at term in both home and hospital settings is re-examined in Chapter 9 as a further means of improving choices available to childbearing women. As Allison (1996) reflects, this was a skill once associated with the role of the midwife and according to Burvill (2005) is still a part of normal midwifery practice in many parts of the world. The over-riding aim of this chapter is, therefore, to empower midwives and instil confidence. This is necessary to re-develop/advance midwifery skills in this area, recognising those situations where a physiological vaginal breech can be contemplated and successfully achieved with the baby being born aided by gravity and propulsion, and *NOT* traction: adopting the principle of *Hands off the Breech*.

Chapter 10 focuses on advancing the skills required by midwives to assess, clarify and repair more complex perineal trauma and reviews the contemporary evidence underpinning methods and suturing materials for the repair of episiotomy second, third and fourth degree tears. In addition, aspects of female genital mutilation (FGM) are addressed, further highlighting the importance of multi and interprofessional working to reduce maternal morbidity as well as working within a legal framework that may include liaison with child-protection agencies and women's advocacy and empowerment services. The necessary knowledge and skills midwives need to effectively assess and monitor the haemodynamic status of the childbearing woman are examined in Chapter 11. Whilst it is clearly accepted that careful documentation of observations is important, early recognition of complications, correct diagnosis and prompt treatment interventions is vitally important to preserve the health and well being of the pregnant woman and her unborn child, as well as reducing the risks of long-term morbidity.

Focusing on some of the aspects that are commonly challenging to midwife examiners, Chapter 12 discusses midwives undertaking the physiological examination of the neonate. This detail includes the examination of the baby's heart, eyes and hips, highlighting the need for simple, but subtle skills, and the need to undertake a specific training and assessment programme to ensure competence in knowledge and skill. Similarly, Chapter 13 does not provide the midwife with the specialist practical skills to teach or perform infant massage, as this can only be achieved by completing a course from a recognised institution, such as the International Association of Infant Massage (IAIM). The purpose of the chapter is to enable the midwife to appreciate what is offered by infant massage and consider her professional and legal responsibilities, such as the consent of minors and child-protection issues, should she decide to advance her skills in this area.

The importance of providing care and support tailored to the individual need of the woman during the postnatal period to reduce major maternal morbidity is explored in Chapter 14. As Lewis (2007) has highlighted, the growing concerns of obesity on maternal mortality/morbidity and the National Institute for Health and Clinical Excellence [NICE] (2008) has issued guidance on improved surveillance of perinatal mental health, particular emphasis has been placed on these issues and the importance of the public health role of the midwife within this chapter. The book concludes with Chapter 15, which summarises and draws together the key themes from each of the preceding chapters, making links between each one and the embracing of the philosophy of advancing skills in midwifery practice.

All chapters are written by health professionals with considerable knowledge and experience in the specific subject, thus ensuring the evidence is both robust and credible, and the content is contemporary and of the highest quality. At the beginning of each chapter are listed the necessary pre-requisites that each midwife should possess before considering developing the competence in the skill. Professional, legal and ethical considerations are explored as well as further training requirements. Every chapter is fully referenced with a further annotated reading list to inform the reader of other relevant texts on the subject. In some instances, relevant website addresses and details of professional bodies/organizations are also provided. Where appropriate there are practice examples and activities to further challenge the reader, as well as figures, diagrams and photographs to simplify the text and assist with explanations and reflection on practice. At the end of each chapter is a list of Key Practice Points that serves in providing a quick reference guide for the reader.

Although the term *midwife* is used throughout the book, it is appreciated this may also apply to other health professionals wishing to develop some of the skills addressed in the text. Similarly, whilst the midwife is commonly referred to in the female gender, it is assumed the reader will acknowledge that such references equally apply to male midwives.

References

Allison, J., 1996. Delivered at home, Chapman and Hall, London.

Begley, C.M., O'Boyle, C., Carroll, M., Devane, D., 2007. Educating advanced midwife practitioners: a collaborative venture. J. Nurs. Manag. 15 (6), 574–584.

Benner, P.E., 2001. From novice to expert: excellence and power in clinical nursing practice, commemorative ed. Prentice Hall, New Jersey.

Burvill, S., 2005. Managing breech presentation in the absence of obstetric assistance. In: Woodward, V., Bates, K., Young, N. (Eds.), Managing childbirth emergencies in community settings. Palgrave Macmillan, Basingstoke, pp. 111–139.

Department of Health, 1993a. Changing childbirth part 1: report of the Expert Maternity Group, HMSO, London.

Department of Health, 1993b. Hospital doctors: training for the future (Calman Report), HMSO, London.

Department of Health, 1997. The new NHS: modern-dependable, HMSO, London.

Department of Health, 1998a. A first class service: quality in the new NHS, HMSO, London.

Department of Health, 1998b. European working time directive, HMSO, London.

Department of Health, 1999. Making a difference: strengthening the nursing, midwifery and health visiting contribution to health and healthcare, HMSO, London.

Department of Health, 2000. The NHS plan, HMSO, London.

Department of Health, 2003. Building on the best: choice, responsiveness and equity in the NHS, The Stationary Office, London.

Department of Health, 2004a. The national services framework for children, young people and maternity services, HMSO, London.

Department of Health, 2004b. The NHS knowledge and skills framework (NHS KSF) and the development review process, HMSO, London.

Department of Health, 2007a. Maternity matters: choice, access and continuity of care in a safe service, HMSO, London.

Department of Health, 2007b. Our health, our care, our say: a new direction for community services, HMSO, London.

Department of Health, 2007c. Trust assurance and safety: the regulation of health professionals in the 21st century, The Stationary Office, London.

Department of Health, 2008a. High quality care for all: NHS next stage review final report (Darzi report), HMSO, London.

Department of Health, 2008b. Framing the nursing and midwifery contribution: driving up the quality of care, HMSO, London.

Department of Health The National Assembly for Wales, the NHS Confederation and the British Medical Association, 2002. Guidance on working patterns for junior doctors, HMSO, London.

Johnson, R., Taylor, W., 2006. Skills for midwifery practice, Elsevier, Churchill Livingstone, Edinburgh.

Lewis, G. (Ed.), 2007. The confidential enquiry into maternal and child health (CEMACH) saving mothers' lives: reviewing maternal deaths to make motherhood safer: 2003–2005, The seventh report of the confidential enquiries into maternal deaths in the United Kingdom. CEMACH, London.

McGee, P., 1992. What is an advanced practitioner? Br. J. Nurs. 1 (1), 5–6.

National Council for the Professional Development of Nursing and Midwifery, 2008. Framework for the establishment of advanced nurse practitioner and advanced midwife practitioner posts, fourth ed. NCNM, Dublin.

National Institute for Health and Clinical Excellence, 2008. Antenatal care: routine care of the healthy pregnant woman, NICE, London.

Nursing and Midwifery Council, 2004. Midwives rules and standards, NMC, London.

Nursing and Midwifery Council, 2008a. The code: standards of conduct, performance and ethics for nurses and midwives, NMC, London.

Nursing and Midwifery Council, 2008b. The PREP Handbook, NMC, London.

Royal College of Obstetricians and Gynaecologists, 2006. External cephalic version and reducing the incidence of breech presentation guideline no 20, RCOG, London.

Sookhoo, M.L., Butler, M.S., 1999. An analysis of the concept of advanced midwifery practice. British Journal of Midwifery 7 (11), 690–693.

NB: From July 1st onwards CEMACH name has changed to CMACE: Centre for Maternal and Child Enquries http://www.cmace.org.uk

Chapter Two

2

The midwife's professional responsibilities in developing competence in new skills

Jayne E. Marshall

CONTENTS

Introduction 7
A framework of responsibility 8
Professional responsibility 9
  Standards for education/training 9
  Maintaining and developing
  competence beyond registration 10
  Statutory supervision 11
Legal responsibility 11
  Negligence 11
  Consent 12
  Record keeping 12
Ethical responsibility 12
  Respect for autonomy and justice . . . 13
  Beneficence and non-maleficence . . . 13
Employer responsibility 14
  NHS Knowledge and Skills Framework
  (NHS KSF) 14
  Quality and clinical governance 14
  Risk management and vicarious
  liability 15
Conclusion 16
Key practice points 16
References 17
Useful websites 18

Introduction

There has been an unprecedented amount of socio-political influence in the United Kingdom (UK) since the 1990s, aimed at improving health-care choices and the overall quality of health-care provision. As a consequence, this has provided health professionals with opportunities to develop/advance their role to meet such demands and challenges (Department of Health [DH] 1993a, 1998a, 1999, 2003, 2004a, 2007a, 2007b). The role of the midwife has, indeed, become increasingly complex with midwives working in many different and divergent ways in an attempt to improve the choices and experiences of childbearing women, as well as dismantle the medicalisation of childbirth that had been evident from the 1970s.

Whilst some midwives have developed skills that support a holistic/social model of midwifery care, embracing the physiological processes of childbearing, e.g. complementary therapies, water births, perineal suturing, others have become competent in skills traditionally associated with the role of other health professionals, e.g. ventouse births and physiological examination of the neonate. Following the Calman Report (DH 1993b) and the European Working Time Directive (DH 1998b) culminating in the reduction in junior doctors' hours, National Health Service (NHS) Trusts have had to adopt more collaborative ways of working between health professionals (DH 2001a) leading to a redefining of their employees' roles and responsibilities. To what extent the role of the midwife and that of the obstetrician/paediatrician can be differentiated will depend on the experience, depth of knowledge, skills and level of competence of the midwife. The only limitations upon the midwife's scope of practice in what activities she can undertake are where specific Acts of Parliament or regulations require a named professional, other than the midwife, to perform certain functions. An example of this would be the Abortion Act 1967 that dictates only a registered medical practitioner can terminate a pregnancy.

The recent Darzi Report (DH 2008a) focuses on the current and developing roles of health professionals and the need to respond more flexibly and effectively to deliver quality care based on the needs of the local population. Furthermore, the DH (2008b) in its publication *Framing the nursing and midwifery contribution: driving up the quality of care*, elucidates that a variety of work streams and activities, including developing and extending the clinical skills and roles of nurses and midwives, have been authorised to form an integrated strategy. This is in order that health professionals can maximise their contribution to high-quality health care and improved health outcomes.

Whether the midwife advances her *midwifery* skills or develops skills normally associated with those of her medical colleagues, the fundamental issue is that she is both competent and safe to undertake the skill. When determining the feasibility of developing competence in a new skill, the skill should be seen as integral to her role, be reflective of the context in which she works and be of benefit to mothers and babies. This chapter will explore the factors that affect midwives developing and maintaining advanced clinical skills and provides a framework for readers to reflect upon their professional responsibilities when developing competence in new skills. Activities are included for midwives to examine their current skills in clinical practice and to formulate an action plan should they decide to develop competence in a new skill as part of their ongoing continuing professional development.

A framework of responsibility

As Batey and Lewis (1982) state, responsibility denotes a charge or activity that an individual is willing to fulfill. If a midwife accepts the charge, activity or task, she is equally accepting the responsibility for carrying out that particular action. Mander (2004) affirms that responsibility is fundamentally anticipatory, as it precedes the action, in that it permits the midwife to assume authority for the action she is about to undertake on the basis of her own expert knowledge and experience. Consequently, at the centre of any debate relating to a midwife developing competence in a new skill is the issue of her being responsible and answerable for her own actions or omissions, which is ultimately the key to professional accountability. Although the concepts of accountability and

responsibility are often used interchangeably and synonymously, accountability cannot exist without responsibility having previously been granted, accepted and assumed. Whether that responsibility is accepted will depend on the individual in terms of their preparation through their education and experience. It is, therefore, acknowledged that a midwife cannot be held accountable for an action or have accountability imposed unless she is given and accepts the responsibility on the basis of her professional preparation.

Bergman's (1981) 'Preconditions to Accountability' and Kitson's (1993) 'Dimensions of Accountability' have provided models for the nursing profession to realise their accountability through exploring the different aspects affecting clinical practice that can also be transferred to midwifery practice. In both these models the concept of *responsibility* is clearly evident as a key component of professional accountability (Figures 2.1. and 2.2).

More recently with the multifaceted ways in which health professionals work, Caulfield (2005) has debated that there is a need for each individual nurse (and midwife) to be aware of the many different sources of accountability and the way each affects clinical practice can be a complex issue. She articulates an alternative framework of accountability that explores approaches based on four pillars which provide a collective sense of accountability for the nurse, namely: professional, legal, ethical and employment accountability (Caulfield 2005). For the purposes of this chapter, this framework has been adapted as these four pillars would also seem pertinent to explore the various approaches

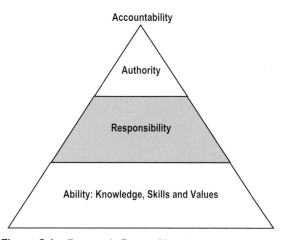

Figure 2.1 • Bergman's Preconditions to Accountability (from Bergman 1981).

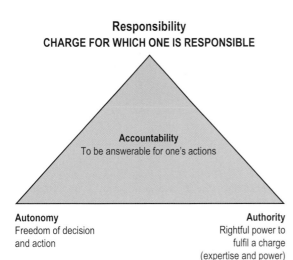

Responsibility
CHARGE FOR WHICH ONE IS RESPONSIBLE

Accountability
To be answerable for one's actions

Autonomy
Freedom of decision
and action

Authority
Rightful power to
fulfil a charge
(expertise and power)

Figure 2.2 • Kitson's Dimensions of Accountability (Kitson 1993).

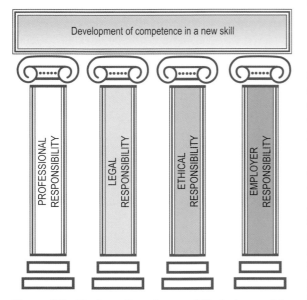

Development of competence in a new skill

PROFESSIONAL RESPONSIBILITY

LEGAL RESPONSIBILITY

ETHICAL RESPONSIBILITY

EMPLOYER RESPONSIBILITY

Figure 2.3 • The four pillars of responsibility that support the development of competence in a new skill (adapted from text in Caulfield 2005).

that provide a collective sense of *responsibility* for the midwife to address when developing competence in a new skill (Figure 2.3).

Professional responsibility

The key objective of the Nursing and Midwifery Council (NMC) as the regulatory body for the nursing and midwifery profession in the UK is to

> ### Box 2.1
>
> **Key functions of the Nursing and Midwifery Council**
> - Create and maintain a register of qualified nurses, midwives and specialist community public health nurses.
> - Set the requirements for evidence of good health and good character.
> - Create the standards of education and training to achieve the standards of proficiency for entry to the register.
> - Establish and review the standards of conduct, performance and ethics expected of registrants and provide appropriate guidance.
> - Remove a registrant from the register through the fitness to practise process.
> - Assess competence and impose conditions of practice orders.

safeguard the health and well being of persons using the services of its registrants, i.e. public protection. Consequently, the NMC is required to undertake a variety of functions according to the NMC Order 2001. These are listed in Box 2.1.

Standards for education/training

As regulator, the NMC sets the minimum standards for entry to the professional register that nurses and midwives must achieve in order to perform their duties both safely and effectively within their professional boundaries and, thus, be both fit for practice and purpose. Consequently, no midwife should undertake any activity for which they do not have the underpinning knowledge and expertise. The term *competent* has been defined by the NMC (2005a) in terms of a student, or a registrant, demonstrating capability in certain skills to a required standard at a particular point in time. Should advancements occur in midwifery practice that require the midwife to develop competence in new skills beyond those acquired in her initial training, consideration should be given as to whether these skills are fundamental to the role of *every* midwife, to then be integrated into all pre-registration education programmes. The Guidance Notes relating to Rule 6 Responsibility and Sphere of Practice of the *Midwives Rules and Standards* (NMC 2004, p. 19) clearly state that:

> *Developments in midwifery care often become an integral part of the role of the midwife and may be incorporated in the initial preparation of midwives. Other developments in midwifery and obstetric practice may require that you learn new skills, but these skills do not necessarily become part of the role of all midwives. In such circumstances, each employing authority should have a locally agreed guideline, which meets the NMC standards.*

Maintaining and developing competence beyond registration

Midwives are, therefore, responsible for maintaining and developing the competence they have achieved during initial and subsequent midwifery education. As a means of safeguarding the health and well being of the public, the Fitness to Practise Directorate of the NMC processes allegations of impairment of fitness to practise made against nurses and midwives on grounds that include lack of competence, misconduct and ill health. *The Code: Standards of conduct, performance and ethics for nurses and midwives* (NMC 2008a) guides the midwife in keeping her knowledge and skills up to date. This is to ensure that her practice and standard of midwifery care is always of the highest quality being reflective of local and national guidelines: a key requirement of self-regulation. *The Code* (NMC 2008a) outlines four key areas that a midwife should consider when developing new skills, these are:

- Have the knowledge and skills for safe and effective practice when working without direct supervision.
- Recognise and work within the limits of her competence.
- Maintain that her knowledge and skills are up to date throughout her working life.
- Undertake appropriate learning and practice activities that maintain and develop her competence and performance.

These key areas are further strengthened in the Post-Registration Education and Practice (PREP) requirements (NMC 2008b) that provide midwives with the flexibility to maintain and develop their knowledge and clinical practice in areas pertinent

to their individual role. Each practising midwife is responsible to fulfill the PREP standards for practice and continuing professional development (CPD) within a 3-year time frame in order to maintain their name on the NMC professional register. These standards are highlighted below in Box 2.2.

These standards may be met by a range of activities, taking the form of academic courses or modules, attendance at study days and conferences, in-service education sessions within their own place of work, visiting another area of midwifery practice or individually researching a specific area of interest. In addition, there should also be training mannequins for demonstration and simulation available in skills and competency centres or in the practice environment, as well as other resources such as DVDs, CD-ROMs and web-based learning packages. The emphasis is that the study should be of relevance to the midwife's professional practice, such that the midwife's supervisor of midwives and/or manager is convinced that the needs of the midwife, the organisation and the enhancement of midwifery care will be met by the activity. As time and finance may well be invested in the activity, the midwife should consider preparing a well-argued case for her continuing professional development when applying to her supervisor of midwives/manager for support.

Box 2.2

The Post-Registration Education and Practice (PREP) standards (NMC 2008b)
The PREP (practice) standard
You must:
- have worked in some capacity by virtue of your nursing or midwifery qualification during the previous 3 years for a **minimum of 450 hours**, or
- have successfully undertaken an approved return to practice course within the last 3 years.

The Continuing Professional Development (CPD) standard (PREP [CPD])
You must:
- undertake at least **35 hours** of learning activity relevant to your practice during the three years prior to your renewal of registration,
- maintain a personal professional profile of your learning activity, and
- comply with any request from the NMC to audit how you have met these requirements.

Statutory supervision

The NMC (2004) clearly states in Rule 12 that every practising midwife should have a named supervisor of midwives appointed by the local supervisory authority and that a supervisory meeting must be arranged at least once each year. The purpose of this meeting is to review the midwife's practice and discuss her personal and professional development needs. It is expected that a record of this meeting is made that may assist the midwife in securing support to develop her practice and, consequently, improve the quality of care that mothers and babies receive.

Activity 2.1

You are preparing to meet with your Supervisor of Midwives for the annual Supervisory Meeting. Consider your current role and any new skills you would wish to develop in order to advance your practice.
- List the skills.
- Justify your reasons for developing each of the skills to then present to your Supervisor of Midwives.

Legal responsibility

Law is the system by which a society determines the various rules and penalties that are used to provide a common framework by which each member of that particular society lives. In the UK, law covers every aspect of an individual's life, including health care, such that all health-care professionals must have an understanding of the law and how it relates to their practice. The key concepts in law that have significance to midwifery practice and the role of the midwife in relation to developing competence in new skills, relate to negligence and consent.

Negligence

Negligence is a civil tort that is based on case law principles and applies to health-care practice. Box 2.3 outlines the four principles that must be proven when claiming an act of negligence on the part of a midwife.

Box 2.3

Principles to be proven in a claim of negligence

- The midwife (defendant) owed a duty of care to the mother/baby (claimant).
- The midwife breached that duty of care by failing to act as a *reasonable* midwife.
- Injury resulted as a consequence of the midwife's breach of duty.
- There is compensation that can be paid as a result of the negligence.

Midwives have a responsibility for performing all procedures correctly and exercising professional judgment when deciding upon their actions/omissions. Each midwife, therefore, has a duty of care to ensure the care she provides to mothers and babies is of a *reasonable* standard that does not cause any actual harm to the recipients for which she would then become liable. The test to determine whether the duty of care has been breached is based on that of *the reasonable man* and the Bolam principle (Bolam v Friern Hospital Management Committee 1957). Where a midwife acts in such a way that would be supported by responsible midwifery opinion (expert witnesses) as being appropriate practice at the time of the alleged incident, it is unlikely the court will find her in breach of her duty of care and her actions, therefore, would not be considered to be negligent.

Where a midwife has developed competence in skills beyond those required in initial midwifery preparation, she will be judged by the law according to the standard expected by other midwives/health professionals who are also skilled in that particular aspect of practice. Consequently, the midwife will be deemed negligent if she does not maintain this standard should a mother or baby be harmed. It is worth noting that where student midwives or midwives undertaking further training in skill development are concerned, they will also be judged by the standards expected of an *experienced* midwife. This is as a result of the courts upholding that all members of society are entitled to receive health care that is deemed competent. It is thus important that where a student midwife/midwife is unclear about a procedure they act responsibly and seek advice and supervision from more experienced colleagues until they have been assessed as competent.

Consent

A midwife has a legal responsibility to only undertake midwifery care or any procedure that involves physical contact with the body of an individual, after consent has been obtained. Without consent, the touching of an individual's body will be considered as trespass to the person as the action is unlawful, with the midwife being liable for an action in battery. Consequently compensation can be claimed on behalf of the individual regardless of whether any harm resulted, or the midwife could face a criminal prosecution. Case law on consent has established three principles, all of which must all be satisfied for consent to be deemed lawful: these are identified in Box 2.4.

According to the law, the competent adult can refuse or withdraw their consent to any procedure at any time. The DH (2001b) produced a reference guide for health professionals whereby 12 key points relating to the law on consent were identified, of which all midwives should be familiar. Furthermore, the professional standards relating to consent are outlined in The Code (NMC 2008a) and are also based on the legal principles. It is thus the responsibility of all practising midwives to be fully conversant with issues relating to consent and how they not only relate to each individual mother and baby to whom they are providing care, but also the specific skill(s) they are aiming to develop. As with a student midwife, the midwife who is undertaking advanced skill development would be considered to be in a *learner* capacity, and should always ensure the woman is fully aware of her capabilities/limitations. This will provide the woman with the opportunity to make an autonomous informed choice to either give or decline consent to the midwife undertaking the procedure.

Record keeping

Good record keeping is the mark of a skilled and safe health professional. It is part of the midwife's duty of care owed to the individual woman, that clear, accurate, contemporaneous and comprehensive records are kept. Midwives have a specific statutory responsibility under Rule 9 of the *Midwives rules and standards* (NMC 2004) with additional advice provided by the NMC (2005b) *Guidelines for records and record keeping*. Maternity records relating to the care of the woman and baby are retained for 25 years to allow for any investigation which may be required as a result of an action brought under the Congenital Disabilities (Civil Liability) Act 1976 or as a result of any other complaint that needs to be investigated. Midwives need to be mindful of the quality of their record keeping as the more distant in the past that the events occurred, the more dependent will the witnesses be on the documentation that was kept at the time.

Actions or omissions relating to the discussions and decisions made with individual women about their midwifery care should be reflected by the midwife in her records, i.e. formal overt decision making (Marshall 2005). At local level, such records may be reviewed as evidence of the midwife's competence to audit the quality of care or investigate a complaint, as well as by a court of law, by the Care Quality Commission: the new health and social care regulator in England and by the NMC's Fitness to Practise Committee. It is, therefore, important that where the midwife is developing competence in a new skill, any limitations in her ability and judgment are acknowledged with evidence provided in the records that she has consulted appropriately experienced colleagues to support her decision making and consequential actions. It is good practice for the colleague supervising the midwife in developing competence in the skill, to countersign any entry that is made relating to that particular skill until the midwife has been deemed competent.

Ethical responsibility

Ethics is concerned with the basic principles and concepts that guide human beings in thought and action and which underpin their personal values. There are a number of ethical frameworks that can be applied to health-care practice and midwives

---

Box 2.4

Principles to be satisfied for consent to be lawful/valid

- The individual has the mental capacity to understand what the proposed procedure involves and give consent.
- Sufficient information should be given to the individual regarding the material risks, any alternatives and the nature and consequences of the proposed procedure/treatment.
- Consent should be freely given without any duress.

Box 2.5

Four ethical principles (Beauchamp & Childress 2004)

- *Respect for autonomy:* self-governance, liberty, rights and individual choices.
- *Justice:* fairness, equal distribution of benefits and burdens.
- *Beneficence:* promoting the welfare of individuals, doing good.
- *Non-maleficence:* (*primum non nocere*) above all, inflict no harm.

have a responsibility to understand the key concepts in ethics to enable them to analyze and reason why a particular issue in their practice may raise conflict, concern or a difference of opinion. Although application of such a framework can be invaluable for justifying decision making in midwifery practice, including the development of competence in new skills, there is no single answer to any ethical dilemma, as there is with legal issues.

Within the framework for moral reasoning outlined by Beauchamp and Childress (2004), are four ethical principles as detailed in Box 2.5.

When midwives are considering developing competence in new skills they have a responsibility to assess what impact these principles will have on themselves, their colleagues, the mothers and babies to whom they provide care and the organisation in which they work.

Respect for autonomy and justice

Society bestows *autonomy* upon those individuals who have the capacity to make decisions for themselves. However, public policy considerations are the principle used to guarantee that the ethics of society are of greater importance than the rights of the individual. Consequently, this places a limit on the extent to which autonomy can be respected, resulting in situations where autonomy of the individual may conflict with that of the wider society. Whilst midwives may determine what course of continuing professional development/skill advancement they wish to pursue, these tend to be considered by managers alongside the incurred costs to the organisation in terms of the resources available, such as the time and financial costs involved. This should not be seen as a deterrent for midwives to advance their skills. The role and responsibility of the manager is to

ensure that there is *justice*, such that there is fairness when apportioning continuing professional development resources among all staff members. Being an autonomous person also means the midwife should respect the decisions of others in order that some compromise may be reached, i.e. the midwife agreeing to part–fund and/or attend part of the course in her own time so as to advance her clinical skills. Midwives can also apply for a bursary or scholarship from various outside agencies to help with meeting the financial costs of the continuing professional development activity. The Royal College of Midwives (RCM) has a comprehensive list of agencies they are affiliated to for this purpose. See www.rcm.org.uk/college/rcm-news/bursariesandscholarships.

Beneficence and non-maleficence

When the ethical principle of *beneficence* is applied to health-care practice it tends to be in conjunction with the ethical principle of *non-maleficence*. It is expected that the practice of every midwife should be based on promoting the welfare of mother and baby without inflicting any intentional harm. This also applies to midwives intending to advance their clinical skills. The midwife should be clear in determining what benefit the skill will have on her own practice as well as the organisation in which she works and, more importantly, the mothers and babies to whom she is providing care.

It is well recognised that where midwives provide continuity of care or midwife-led care and social support, women are highly satisfied with the care they receive (DH 2007a, Hodnett et al 2007, Redshaw et al 2007). Midwives who are competent in skills such as perineal repair, the physiological examination of the neonate, vaginal breech birth and uncomplicated ventouse or forceps births, can improve the continuity of midwifery care mothers and babies receive by avoiding the unnecessary fragmentation of transferring the care to medical colleagues. However, the context in which these skills are to be utilised should be considered when determining where the midwife should advance her practice. To be competent in the skill of ventouse or forceps births would be of more benefit to the midwife working in a birth centre/midwife-led unit than the midwife working in a hospital, where there is obstetric cover to undertake the birth. In this context, the midwife ventouse practitioner is able to maintain continuity of care with the mother, alongside some degree of normality without necessitating a transfer to an obstetric unit. Consequently, both the mother and midwife benefits from the midwife having advanced her skills. However, as stated earlier, it is the responsibility of all midwives to maintain their advanced skills and always ensure their practice is safe, based on sound evidence so that no harm is likely to befall the mother or baby.

Employer responsibility

The relationship between an employer and employee is complex and brings the fourth and final pillar of responsibility into focus; however, this section will concentrate only on those issues pertaining to midwives advancing their skills, namely the NHS Knowledge and Skills Framework (NHS KSF) (DH 2004b), quality and clinical governance, risk management and vicarious liability.

NHS Knowledge and Skills Framework

The NHS Knowledge and Skills Framework (KSF) (DH 2004b) was developed through a partnership approach between management and staff representatives. Its aim is to provide a fair and objective framework that can help guide the development of *all* NHS employees. However, it is also designed to provide the basis of pay progression. Managers are expected to use this framework alongside current and emerging competence frameworks when working with individual members of staff to review their work, identify the knowledge and skills needed for their particular post and, subsequently, plan their training and development. As a consequence, the local university is ever responsive to the needs of the NHS Trusts within the area, and in collaboration continues to develop new modules and skill development activities to help prepare midwives for the challenges and ever dynamic midwifery service of the 21st century. Each course and module that is offered has been mapped against the NHS KSF so that the employer is aware of the level of competence that is intended to prepare the midwives for their respective role.

Quality and clinical governance

As an employer, each individual NHS Trust has a statutory duty for ensuring that its employees deliver quality of care to the public and that systems are in place for clinical governance (DH 1997, 1998a). This means that there should be a direct link from those working in the clinical areas to the Chief Executive at the pinnacle of the organisation, increasing accountability and prompting health professionals to be more critical of their practice. To improve quality of care, national standards have been set for NHS Trusts to take note of and to incorporate them within the development of their clinical guidelines and policies based on best available evidence.

A midwife should not only be aware of the national standard, but also the difference between clinical guidelines and NHS Trust policies. Clinical guidelines do not aim to regulate every single step of clinical practice, but to provide the parameters to direct midwives towards safe, confident practice that allows for flexibility, women's choices and preferences. Policies on the other hand, do not offer the same flexibility and form part of the employment relationship with the midwife and employer. They may be used as part of any disciplinary process where an issue arises about whether the midwife followed the content of the policy correctly. Whilst the employer has a responsibility to ensure that policies are regularly reviewed and updated, the individual midwife also has a responsibility to effectively utilise her knowledge of change management theory (Broome 1990, Lewin 1951, Wright 1989) to advocate that policies reflect a holistic midwife-led and woman-focused model of care rather than a medico-technocratic model (Davis-Floyd & Sargent 1997, Machin & Scamell 1997). Recent publications from the DH (2008a, 2008b) provide midwives with the opportunity to campaign for changes that improve the quality of care for mothers and babies, by influencing, managing and leading change.

Where midwives plan to advance their practice in skills commonly undertaken by medical staff, it is important that NHS Trust policy clearly defines the midwife's role and responsibilities in such a skill. If this detail is not apparent, the employer would not be held responsible should any harm be inflicted on the mother or baby as a consequence of the midwife's actions contravening Trust policy. Similarly, where a midwife who is competent to practise an advanced skill moves to another NHS Trust, she would only be able to continue undertaking such a skill if the NHS Trust policy of her new employer permits her to do so.

Risk management and vicarious liability

Each NHS Trust has a responsibility to ensure there is a *risk-management* process in place that identifies and examines unforeseen outcomes occurring during pregnancy and childbirth that can then be utilised in the prevention of similar instances. Risk management can be divided into two main areas: *health and safety risk* and *clinical risk*, both of which should be considered by the employer when midwives are developing competence in new skills.

The health and safety of employees is an important aspect of an employer's responsibility and, ultimately, their accountability, which is set out in the statutory framework of the Health and Safety at Work Act of 1974. An employer, therefore, has to provide safe systems that include information, training and supervision as is necessary to ensure the health and safety at work of employees. In areas where midwives are advancing their skills, this would include the use of complementary therapies such as aromatherapy oils and moxa sticks, as well as the introduction of new equipment to undertake assisted births. An employer may be sued by an employee where the actions or omissions of the employer lead to injury that may result in a fine imposed by the Health and Safety Commission, or in certain circumstances, criminal sanctions may be imposed. The Health and Safety Commission is responsible to the Secretary of State for Work and Pensions and one of its functions is to ensure that the public is overall protected against risks to health or safety arising from work activities.

When a midwife is developing competence in a new skill, there will be certain parameters within which she will need to work and be assessed as competent in order to minimise clinical risk and also fulfill the requirements of the education and training programme. Some NHS Trusts may recognise that each midwife has individual needs and will become competent at her own pace whereas others may specify the exact number of times the skill should be undertaken before the midwife is judged to be competent. It is, however, useful if a minimum number of attempts is stipulated as a guide for the midwife and assessor. Some midwives may achieve competence in the skill after a limited number of attempts whilst others may lack the confidence and need to practice the skill a number of times before determining they are competent.

Not only may an employer be held responsible for negligence against the employee, but also for negligence caused by the employee. It is thus important that the employer ensures that all employees are competent as they can be directly liable in negligence for allowing an inexperienced employee to undertake skills for which they are not competent to perform without supervision. It is usual that in the case of an employed midwife, that her employer would be sued in the event of her being negligent as the employer is more likely to be able to pay the compensation due as a result of the harm incurred. Public policy dictates that the doctrine of *vicarious liability* applies in order that an innocent victim obtains compensation for injuries caused by an employee. However, for vicarious liability to be established, the elements in Box 2.6 must be determined.

Providing a midwife undertook an approved education and training programme to develop competence in a new skill, has followed clinical guidelines and risk-management procedures, and has evidence that she has maintained that skill, it is highly unlikely her employer would refuse to accept responsibility for her practice should there be a case of alleged negligence. Thus, the employer is responsible to protect midwives via indemnity cover for clinical negligence liabilities through the Clinical Negligence Scheme for Trusts (CNST): a statutory indemnity scheme managed by the NHS Litigation Authority. However, if a midwife does something considered to be negligent that is outside of her contractual duty, or practices beyond her skills and competence then she may find herself vulnerable.

At present, independent midwives are not covered by CNST and, thus, will need to provide their

---

Box 2.6

Elements in vicarious liability

- *There must be NEGLIGENCE:* a duty of care has been breached and as a reasonably foreseeable consequence, has caused harm or some other failure by the employee.
- *The negligent act or omission or failure must have been by an EMPLOYEE.*
- *The negligent employee must have been acting in the COURSE OF THEIR EMPLOYMENT:* on duty.

own indemnity insurance to support any alleged claims of negligence and the quest for compensation. Should the independent midwife have an agreement with the local NHS Trust to come into the hospital and continue caring for the mother, the NHS Trust would only be vicariously liable for her actions if she has a contract of employment for the time she works on the Trust's premises. However, through the DH social enterprise scheme looking to contract in with Primary Care Trusts (PCT)/NHS Trusts to cover independent midwives, vicarious liability is likely to be afforded to these midwives in the near future (DH 2007c). As with every midwife, it is vitally important that independent midwives are also fully conversant with current evidence and maintain their knowledge and clinical skills. With the support of their supervisor of midwives, independent midwives can engage in activities that will not only minimise clinical risk, so that they continue to demonstrate safe and competent practice, but also further advance their clinical skills.

Activity 2.2

Having developed an interest in external cephalic version as a means of improving the normal vaginal birth rate, you wish to develop competence in the skill with the aim of incorporating it into midwifery practice within the maternity unit in which you work.

- Consider the four pillars of responsibility and the specific issues you would need to address in relation to developing this new skill.
- Devise an action plan to present to your manager supporting your request.
- Detail as to how you would anticipate acquiring the competence and maintaining the skill.
- Consider in what format you would provide the evidence of your competence and ongoing professional development in this aspect of practice.

Conclusion

This first chapter has provided a workable framework of responsibility for midwives to utilise when considering the many factors affecting the development and advancement of clinical skills: namely professional, legal, ethical and employer responsibility. Midwives have an ideal opportunity to respond to the Darzi

Report (DH 2008a) by examining how they can develop their roles to effectively meet the needs of childbearing women and their families in the 21st century with support from their colleagues, managers and supervisors of midwives. Whether the midwife advances her *midwifery* skills or develops skills normally associated with those of her medical colleagues, the fundamental issue is that she is both competent and safe to undertake the skill.

Key practice points

When midwives plan to develop competence in new skills/advance their clinical practice they should consider the following:

- Central to new skill development is that the midwife remains responsible and answerable for her own actions or omissions.
- The skill should be integral to the midwife's role, be reflective of the context in which she works and ultimately be of benefit to mothers and babies.
- The *four pillars of responsibility* regarding *professional, legal, ethical* and *employer responsibilities* can provide a workable framework for the midwife to use in planning her continuing professional development.
- The supervisor of midwives can play a supportive role to midwives in ensuring any development/ advancement of skills is pertinent to their area of practice and continuing professional development needs.
- Having developed competence in skills beyond those required in initial midwifery preparation, a midwife will be judged by the law according to the standard expected by other midwives/health professionals who are also skilled in that particular aspect of practice.
- NHS Trust policy should clearly define the midwife's role and responsibilities in skills that have been commonly undertaken by medical staff.
- In cases of alleged negligence, a midwife will not be protected by the employer's vicarious liability if she has acted outside of her contractual duty, or practises beyond her skills and competence.
- Midwives should be familiar with risk management processes that include minimising clinical risk and following health and safety procedures when developing competence in new skills.
- All members of society are legally entitled to receive health care that is deemed **competent:** including from those who are in a learner capacity.

References

Abortion Act: An act to amend and clarify the law relating to termination of pregnancy by registered medical practitioners, 1967. c 87. HMSO, London.

Batey, M., Lewis, F., 1982. Clarifying autonomy and accountability in nursing service: part 1. J. Nurs. Adm. 12 (9), 13–18.

Beauchamp, T., Childress, J., 2004. Principles of biomedical ethics, fifth ed. Oxford University Press, Oxford.

Bergman, R., 1981. Accountability: definitions and dimensions. Int. Nurs. Rev. 28 (2), 53–59.

Bolam v Friern Hospital Management Committee QBD, [1957]. 2 All ER 118.

Broome, A., 1990. Managing change, Macmillan, London.

Caulfield, H., 2005. Vital notes for nurses: accountability, Blackwell Publishing, Oxford.

Congenital Disabilities (Civil Liability) Act, 1976. c 28 HMSO, London.

Davis-Floyd, R.E., Sargent, C.F., 1997. Childbirth and authoritative knowledge: cross-cultural perspectives, University of California Press, Berkeley.

Department of Health, 1993a. Changing childbirth part 1: report of the expert maternity group, HMSO, London.

Department of Health, 1993b. Hospital doctors: training for the future (Calman report), HMSO, London.

Department of Health, 1997. The new NHS: modern-dependable, HMSO, London.

Department of Health, 1998a. A first class service: quality in the new NHS, HMSO, London.

Department of Health, 1998b. European working time directive, HMSO, London.

Department of Health, 1999. Making a difference: strengthening the nursing, midwifery and health visiting contribution to health and healthcare, HMSO, London.

Department of Health, 2001a. Working together, learning together: a framework for lifelong learning in the NHS, HMSO, London.

Department of Health, 2001b. Reference guide to consent for examination or treatment, HMSO, London.

Department of Health, 2003. Building on the best: choice, responsiveness and equity in the NHS, The Stationary Office, London.

Department of Health, 2004a. National Service Framework for children, young people and maternity services, HMSO, London.

Department of Health, 2004b. The NHS Knowledge and Skills Framework (NHS KSF) and the development review process, HMSO, London.

Department of Health, 2007a. Maternity matters: choice, access and continuity of care in a safe service, HMSO, London.

Department of Health, 2007b. Our health, our care, our say: a new direction for community services, HMSO, London.

Department of Health, 2007c. Welcoming social enterprise into health and social care: a resource pack for social enterprise providers and commissioners, HMSO, London.

Department of Health, 2008a. High quality care for all: NHS next stage review final report (Darzi report), HMSO, London.

Department of Health, 2008b. Framing the nursing and midwifery contribution: driving up the quality of care, HMSO, London.

Hodnett, E.D., Gates, S., Hofmeyr, G.J., Sakala, C., 2007. Continuous support for women during childbirth, Cochrane Database Syst. Rev. Issue 2. Art. No: CD003766. DOI: 10.1002/14651858.CD003766.pub2.

Kitson, A., 1993. Accountable for quality. Nurs. Stand. 8 (1), 4–6.

Lewin, K., 1951. Field theory in social science, Harper and Row, New York.

Machin, D., Scamell, M., 1997. The experience of labour: Using ethnography to explore the irresistible nature of the bio-medical metaphor during labour. Midwifery 13 (2), 78–84.

Mander, R., 2004. Where does the buck stop? Accountability in midwifery. In: Tilley, S., Watson, R. (Eds.), Accountability in nursing and midwifery. Blackwell Science Ltd, Oxford, pp. 132–142.

Marshall, J.E., 2005. Autonomy and the midwife. In: Raynor, M.D., Marshall, J.E., Sullivan, A. (Eds.), Decision making in midwifery practice. Elsevier, Churchill Livingstone, Edinburgh, pp. 9–21.

Nursing and Midwifery Council, 2004. Midwives rules and standards, NMC, London.

Nursing and Midwifery Council, 2005a. Consultation on a review of pre-registration midwifery education, NMC, London.

Nursing and Midwifery Council, 2005b. Guidelines for records and record keeping, NMC, London.

Nursing and Midwifery Council, 2008a. The code: standards of conduct, performance and ethics for nurses and midwives, NMC, London.

Nursing and Midwifery Council, 2008b. The PREP handbook, NMC, London.

Redshaw, M., Rowe, R., Hockley, C., Brocklehurst, P., 2007. Recorded delivery: a national survey of women's experience of maternity care 2006, National Perinatal Epidemiology Unit, Oxford.

The Health and Safety at Work Act, 1974. The Stationary Office, London.

The Nursing and Midwifery Order, 2001. Statutory Instrument 2002 No 253, The Stationary Office, London.

Wright, S.G., 1989. Changing nursing practice, Edward Arnold, London.

Useful websites

For information on professional guidance, national standards and guidelines, skills for health and competence framework and publications and bursaries/scholarships to support midwives' clinical practice and advancement of skill development are included below. In addition, other websites provide useful information on women's satisfaction surveys and the National Patient Safety Agency (NPSA) that contributes to improvement in health care by enabling the NHS to learn lessons from clinical incidents relating to issues of safety.

www.cqc.org.uk
www.dh.gov.uk
www.nice.org.uk

www.nmc–uk.org
www.npeu.ox.ac.uk
www.npsa.nhs.uk
www.rcm.org.uk
www.rcog.org.uk
www.skillsforhealth.org.uk

Chapter Three

Complementary therapies in midwifery: a focus on moxibustion for breech presentation

3

Denise Tiran

CONTENTS

Introduction and rationale 19

Professional responsibilities
of the midwife 20

Mechanism of action 21

   Mechanism of action of moxibustion . . 22

Outline of the 'skill' 23

Contraindications and precautions 23

   Moxibustion: specific contraindications
   and precautions 24

Evidence-based practice 25

Conclusion 26

Key practice points 26

References 26

Further reading 27

Resources 28

Before reading this chapter, you should be familiar with:

- Breech presentation: the causes, predisposing factors, recognition, management and care.
- The skills to facilitate a vaginal breech birth (see Chapter 9).
- The advantages and disadvantages of external cephalic version (see Chapter 5) and caesarean section for breech presentation.
- The professional issues involved in implementing new techniques into midwifery practice.

Introduction and rationale

Many midwives choose to train in one or two complementary therapies as an adjunct to their normal practice. However, the subject of complementary medicine is vast, with numerous different therapies and it is not possible, in a single chapter, to cover the depth of information required to enable midwives to use or advise women on all the therapies and natural remedies without further study and the acquisition of skills relevant to each therapy. This chapter therefore discusses some of the general principles of complementary medicine in relation to midwifery practice, but focuses specifically on the increasingly popular technique of **moxibustion for breech presentation**. Other complementary therapies commonly used by midwives have been explored elsewhere and readers with an interest in specific therapies are referred to the Further reading and Resources lists at the end of the chapter.

Complementary therapies (CTs) are extremely popular with the general public, particularly pregnant women, for whom they facilitate choice and control (Dooley 2006, Williams & Mitchell 2007). CTs focus on holistic – or 'whole person' – care, in which individuals are seen as a combination of the three inter-related aspects of body, mind and soul, i.e. the bio-psycho-social elements. As a result of demand from mothers, midwives increasingly look to CTs to aid them in returning to being 'with woman', and there are many examples of UK maternity units that have successfully introduced different therapies into normal midwifery practice (McNabb et al 2006, McNeill et al 2006, Mousley 2005, Tiran 2003a). CTs offer a timely opportunity to facilitate normal birth in the light of increasing caesarean section rates; those such as reflexology, aromatherapy and yoga aid mental and physical relaxation, improving the balance between stress hormones and oxytocin, thus facilitating homeostasis in pregnancy, birth and the puerperium. Some, such as massage, acupuncture and osteopathy offer non-pharmacological options for dealing with antenatal and postnatal symptoms such as backache, nausea and breast feeding problems; others, including aromatherapy, hypnosis and Bach flower remedies, increase maternal choices for managing pain and aiding progress in labour. For midwives, CTs provide a range of additional tools, notably those which enable them to support and empower mothers. It could be argued that CTs also empower midwives, possibly increasing staff recruitment and retention, as occurred in Oxford following introduction of a comprehensive intrapartum aromatherapy service (Burns et al 2000).

However, it must be recognised that 'complementary medicine' constitutes not one single entity, but indeed several hundred different therapies, some of which are well established as *complementary* to health care in the UK, such as osteopathy, aromatherapy and acupuncture; others are considered *alternative*, e.g. reiki and Indian Ayurvedic medicine, and a still larger group would be deemed to be 'fringe', including dowsing and crystal therapy. It is, therefore, impossible to consider 'complementary therapies' as a single 'set of skills' to be learned by midwives, since whilst individual therapies may share a similar philosophy, each has its own theoretical basis, clinical and technical skills, mechanism of action, mode of delivery and, in some cases, a growing body of supportive evidence. Midwives may wish to develop the requisite knowledge and skills to use specific therapies in their practice but should be wary of 'cherry picking' snippets from other therapies which they then offer to mothers as 'informed' advice, for example, being trained to use aromatherapy in labour, but advising women on the herbal remedy, raspberry leaf, in pregnancy without adequate knowledge. Whilst a 'fusion' approach may be appropriate, in which aspects of several therapies are combined for 'woman-centred' care, and this has been discussed elsewhere by Tiran (2003b, 2004a, 2006a), inappropriate use by poorly informed midwives

could potentially be disastrous. Conversely, certain aspects of CTs can be incorporated as extensions to the midwife's role, without compromising care, although it is important to acquire an understanding of the philosophy of the therapy from which the technique is extracted.

An example of this is the use of the increasingly popular **moxibustion**, a technique in which moxa sticks, made from the compressed dried herb mugwort, are used as a heat source, applied over specific acupuncture points on the feet to turn a breech-presenting fetus to cephalic. The technique of moxibustion is simply learnt, but it is the underpinning knowledge which denotes the skill of the practitioner, requiring the midwife to apply principles to conventional obstetrics. Despite concerns over the number of caesareans specifically for breech presentation, the Royal College of Obstetricians and Gynaecologists (RCOG) advocates external cephalic version (ECV), proceeding to caesarean if unsuccessful, but dismisses the value and safety of moxibustion as apparently unsubstantiated (RCOG 2006). However, moxibustion offers women an additional option for managing breech presentation, which may avoid unnecessary caesarean, and which is potentially more successful than ECV (Cardini et al 1991, Cardini & Huang 1998, Kanakura et al 2001). Moxibustion is inexpensive and, when used appropriately, is at least as safe as, if not safer than, ECV (Bensoussan et al 2000). It can be taught to the mother by the midwife and performed by the mother at home, either as an alternative to or prior to ECV, or following an unsuccessful attempt at version, but does not preclude medical intervention later if it fails to convert the presentation to cephalic.

Professional responsibilities of the midwife

UK midwives are permitted by the Nursing and Midwifery Council (NMC) to extend their skills and knowledge if it is in the best interests of the mother and baby, on condition that they are adequately and appropriately trained and can justify their actions (NMC 2004). It is *not* essential to possess a formal therapy qualification but midwives must understand the mechanism of action, indications, precautions and potential dangers of each chosen therapy. It is possible, for example, to develop the skills of moxibustion for breech, or to gain a working knowledge of specific aromatherapy oils for pain relief in labour, whereas the complex nature of reflexology or acupuncture may indicate the acquisition of more comprehensive skills with relevant underpinning theory. However, it *is* vital that midwives apply the principles of CTs to maternity care – and it is this aspect in which some midwives are sadly lacking, believing that a formal therapy qualification automatically equips them adequately to treat expectant mothers within their NHS practice. Unfortunately, many CTs courses do not include comprehensive study of pregnancy; those that do fail to consider the application of theory to clinical practice within an institutional setting such as the NHS. This places the responsibility for applying generic principles on the individual midwife, which can be difficult without appropriate education and mentoring. For example, the use of aromatherapy vaporisers in a hospital ward setting, in which all women inhale the aromatic vapours, is contraindicated because the essential oil chemicals may be inappropriate for some mothers and should be individually prescribed. With moxibustion, consideration should be addressed to the situation of fire alarms prior to commencing the procedure within the maternity unit.

The development of evidence-based policies and/ or written parameters to guide and inform practice is advisable to protect mothers, babies *and* midwives, even if a policy applies only to a single named midwife, for example where one midwife provides a moxibustion or acupuncture service. The normal parameters of professional practice also apply, including the provision of sufficient information to enable mothers to give 'informed consent' to CTs, adequate contemporaneously maintained records and evaluation of treatments given. Where a unit has an established CTs service, midwives' enthusiasm for the benefits and enjoyment of many of the relaxing therapies must not be at the expense of acknowledging that some mothers may not wish to receive CTs and have the right to decline them. Provision of CTs must not, of course, be at the expense of normal midwifery priorities.

The requirement for all health care professionals to produce evidence of continuing professional development (CPD) also means that midwives have a duty to maintain competence in respect of both their conventional and their complementary practice. Furthermore, CTs use must, where possible,

be based on currently available evidence, but it is of concern that many midwives do not work within this remit. There are examples of maternity units known to this author, whose long-established CTs services have resulted in complacency amongst midwives who are enthusiastic about the benefits of CTs, but who conveniently decline to consider the possible risks (Tiran 2004b, 2006b) perhaps because lack of CPD means that they are unaware of advances which have changed practice in their particular therapy. Indeed, it has been suggested that, due to the huge increase in interest amongst midwives (and nurses), the NMC may need to intervene and consider more constructive regulatory monitoring of registrants' use of CTs when integrated into NHS care (Tiran 2007). CTs services should also be evaluated and audited in the same way as other aspects of maternity care; indeed, audit may provide rudimentary statistics to support the case for continuation of local services and suggestions for more formal research studies. Supervision of a midwife's use of CTs should be included within the annual supervisory review, although the increased use of CTs amongst midwives suggests a need for supervisors to have a basic appreciation of the relevant issues (Tiran 2007). Similarly, managers who permit their staff to introduce CTs into the unit should be aware of issues related to health and safety, risk management and evidence-based practice. For professional indemnity insurance purposes, midwives should have permission of their employing authority to incorporate CTs into their practice; failure to gain this permission could invalidate the midwife's right to vicarious liability insurance cover in respect of both her use of CTs *and* her normal midwifery care.

Mechanism of action

Mechanisms of action vary considerably between different CTs, although most can be classified into a few groupings with common themes. Each therapy induces various physiological and/or psychological effects, for many of which there is an increasing body of research evidence. Some therapies work in several ways, for example aromatherapy administered via massage, constitutes a touch therapy, producing physio-psychological relaxation, while absorption of the oils into the bloodstream acts pharmacologically, eliciting various physiological – and potentially adverse – effects; in addition, communication of the aromas via the olfactory system to the limbic system in the brain produces a psychological response, often referred to as the mind-body effect. Some therapies are manipulative, such as chiropractic, some manual therapies have underlying theory in which various points on the body link one area to another, for example, acupuncture and reflexology. Still other therapies focus more on the mind-body approach, including hypnosis and stress management. Others, such as homeopathy and Bach flower remedies, do not work pharmacologically but are thought to be forms of energy or vibrational medicine, in which subtle energies are released which impact on the individual's 'vital force', the innate energy within each of us. Certain Eastern therapies, including traditional Chinese medicine, Indian Ayurveda and Japanese shiatsu, also harness this life force, termed respectively *Qi*, *prana* and *Ki*.

Mechanism of action of moxibustion

Moxibustion is a component of Traditional Chinese Medicine (TCM), performed using moxa sticks which burn with a slow but intensive heat which is easily absorbed into the body via specific acupuncture points, with less risk of burning the external skin than would be the case with a different type of heat source. The traditional moxa stick is comprised of compressed dried mugwort (*Artemesia vulgaris)*, but 'smokeless' sticks are also available, in which charcoal has been impregnated with moxa; these are slightly more expensive but eliminate the risk of setting off institutional fire alarms.

TCM is based on the principle that the body has energy lines – meridians – linking one part of the body to another, conveying the individual's *life force* as a form of energy (*Qi*, pronounced 'chi'). There are 14 major and 365 minor meridians in a branching network throughout the body. Along each meridian there are focus points (tsubos/acupoints), thought to be closely linked to anatomical trigger points (Baldry 2004); over 2000 tsubos have been identified, although only about 200 are commonly in use today. In optimum health, energy flows around the body unhindered, but physical, mental or spiritual disease or distress causes blockages or excesses of energy at certain tsubos along the meridians. Various methods are used to correct these *Qi* imbalances, including the insertion of needles

(acupuncture) or stimulation with thumb pressure (acupressure or shiatsu) via specific acupoints, Chinese herbal medicine, special massage called *tuina*, cupping (a technique in which small suction cups are placed over the skin to draw out excess energy) or moxibustion (heat) to stimulate *Qi* in cases where there is deficient energy.

'Heat', in TCM terms, refers to one element of the state of balance (which includes the eight opposing principles of hot-cold, Yin-Yang, empty-full and excessive-deficient) which is needed for optimum health; 'heat' is not related solely to thermal temperature. A person in optimum health is well balanced, although most of us have a tendency to be slightly more biased to one set of principles than the other. Someone who is primarily 'Yang' is positive, warm, expressive and active, but excessive Yang energy causes her to become overactive with excessive heat and loss of control, an example of this being the peri-menopausal woman suffering menorrhagia and hot flushes. Yin energy is more cold, negative, introspective, quiet and passive; Yin imbalance would lead to a sluggish or static constitution, with an accumulation of waste, such as constipation. Warming of a tsubo with moxa is thought to initiate a local inflammatory response which is then transmitted along the meridian and around the body.

Moxibustion is used to treat a variety of conditions; for breech presentation, it is applied to the Bladder 67 or 'Zhiyin' acupoint on the outer edge at the base of the little toe nails. The Bladder meridian starts in the eye socket (this first point being called Bladder 1), passes up and over the head, down the back either side of the spine, around the kidneys and through the bladder, and continues down the legs, around the outer edges of the ankle bones, along the feet, ending at the Bladder 67 point on the little (fifth) toes (see Figure 3.1). The Bladder meridian is

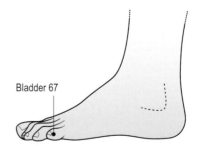

Figure 3.1 ● Position of bladder 67 acupoint for moxibustion.

closely linked to the Kidney meridian, which is said to govern reproduction and, because the bladder is in close proximity to the uterus, Bladder Qi influences uterine function. Bladder meridian deficiency may contribute to infertility or cause dysmenorrhoea. In pregnancy, Kidney deficiency (Yin) can affect uterine and fetal tone, resulting in the fetus being unable to maintain a cephalic presentation or, indeed, a longitudinal lie. Thus, Kidney deficiency can be corrected by working on the Bladder meridian, which in turn, affects the uterus. The Bladder 67 point used for moxibustion is specifically useful as it is known to promote *downwards cephalic movement* (the point can also be useful in labour, in conjunction with other points, to encourage descent). In physiological terms, moxibustion is thought to work by enhancing the immune system as a result of the moxa heat raising stress hormone levels, then increasing circulating natural killer cells and cytokines. The stress hormones also increase prostaglandin 2α production, which promotes myometrial contractility. This, combined with a slight but noticeable rise in the fetal heart rate facilitates conversion from breech to cephalic presentation – basically, the fetus moves itself around in a minimally enlarged uterine cavity.

Outline of the 'skill'

Moxibustion is performed for 15 minutes, twice daily for up to ten treatments, or until the fetus has turned. It is considered most effective if commenced at around 34 weeks' gestation, although it has been used from 28 weeks' gestation or even as late as term. The presentation must be confirmed as still being breech before the first treatment and the maternal and fetal conditions must be assessed in accordance with the contraindications and precautions. The mother can be shown the technique so that she can take the moxa sticks home and undertake the procedure herself (with help from her partner). During the actual procedure she should be comfortably reclining in a chair, having previously emptied her bladder and with clothing loosened. She should be warned that the fetus may become active during the procedure and for up to 24 hours afterwards but that she should contact her midwife if she has any undue concerns about fetal movements, although there is some recent evidence to demonstrate that fetal heart rate

may, in fact, reduce during both moxibustion and acupuncture (Neri et al 2004). The use of a leaflet may reinforce the information given at her initial appointment, including advice about lighting and extinguishing the moxa sticks and the optimum place to undertake the moxibustion, especially if the mother has chosen to use traditional moxa sticks which may be unpleasantly smoky in a confined space. She should be encouraged to continue the technique for up to ten treatments (5 days) unless she feels that the fetus has turned, in which case she should seek confirmation, as continuation of the procedure is thought to increase the risk that the fetus may revert to a breech presentation. In TCM terms this may seem overly cautious and there is some ongoing debate on the subject, since stimulation of the Bladder 67 tsubo promotes *downwards cephalic movement*; therefore, continuation of the treatment is unlikely to make the fetus revert, and, indeed, may encourage further engagement of the fetal head (Dharmananda 2004).

Contraindications and precautions

The commonest misconception amongst both mothers and professionals is that because CTs are natural they are also safer than conventional medical, surgical or pharmacological interventions, but this is not true. *Any* modality with the capacity to effect physiological or psychological changes can be positive or negative depending on how it is used, and midwives must understand both the benefits and possible hazards of any CTs that they use in their practice. They must also work within existing professional boundaries; for example, whilst there is evidence that acupuncture or reflexology may initiate contractions (Gaudernack et al 2006, Harper et al 2006, Tiran 2006a), a potentially useful intervention for post-dates pregnancy, it would be inappropriate for these therapies to be used prior to term, as a form of 'labour priming' merely because the mother was impatient to have her baby. Similarly, some modes of administration may be inappropriate within an institutional setting, e.g. inhalation of essential oils via a vaporiser with a naked flame would contravene fire regulations. In respect of moxibustion, breech presentation may be viewed by some as a complication of pregnancy and, therefore, more within the remit of obstetrics than midwifery, so good inter-professional communication is vital.

Midwives should devise guidelines for practice which specify the gestation at which a therapy is or is not appropriate, and identify any medical, obstetric or other relevant contraindications or precautions, such as antepartum haemorrhage, threatened preterm labour, multiple pregnancy, diabetes, or cardiac or thyroid disease. In the opinion of this author, pregnant women with epilepsy should *never* be treated with CTs – not even massage – since their condition may become unstable during pregnancy and the deep relaxation effect of reduced cortisol and increased endorphins may initiate an unanticipated fit. However, whilst epilepsy is an absolute contraindication, other medical conditions such as diabetes may be a precaution, with decisions based on whether the condition is pre-existing or gestational, and on materno-fetal well being. Furthermore, whilst there may be anecdotal evidence that certain aspects of CTs or natural remedies could effectively treat complications, the midwife needs to balance the risks and benefits of using them to the individual mother's situation and the availability of proven conventional methods of management, for example treatment of postpartum haemorrhage with unproven homeopathic remedies rather than the accepted use of oxytocic drugs would be unacceptable.

Moxibustion: specific contraindications and precautions

(see Box 3.1)

The exclusion criteria for performing moxibustion are similar to those for ECV. Major medical or obstetric complications are definite contraindications, since expert obstetric management will be required and it would be ethically wrong to expose the mother and baby to what remains, essentially, an experimental procedure within conventional maternity care in the UK. Moxibustion should not be performed if the woman is pyrexial, although this is disputed by some authorities (Dharmananda 2004); in women with hypertension and pre-eclampsia, moxibustion is contraindicated as the moxa heat may increase maternal blood pressure. The heat may also accelerate the onset or establishment of labour contractions in mothers with a

Box 3.1

Moxibustion contraindications

- Unstable lie.
- Multiple pregnancy.
- Antepartum haemorrhage.
- Placenta praevia.
- Asthma or other severe respiratory disease.
- Diabetes.
- Abnormal liquor volume.
- Pyrexia.
- Preterm labour in this or previous pregnancy.
- Premature ruptured membranes.
- Known cephalopelvic disproportion.
- Intrauterine fetal death or distress.
- Maternal preference.
- Hypertension/pre-eclampsia.
- Previous caesarean/uterine scar.
- Caesarean planned for medical reasons.
- Established labour.
- Cephalic presentation.

history of threatened or actual preterm labour in this or a previous pregnancy (Roemer 2006). Asthmatics may be affected by the smoke of original moxa sticks and should be persuaded to avoid moxibustion – it may be appropriate to refer them for acupuncture instead. There would obviously be no reason to convert to cephalic presentation in the event of known cephalo-pelvic disproprortion, or if caesarean section is planned for some other medical indication, while the risks of fetal entanglement preclude its use in multiple pregnancy. If there is an unstable lie moxibustion may theoretically be attempted towards term, with planned induction to follow if the presentation turns to cephalic, to prevent it from reverting to a less favourable lie or presentation. However, there is no evidence in the UK to support this and current practice advocates avoiding moxibustion in these cases. Polyhydramnios is considered a precaution, any success with moxibustion possibly requiring progression to controlled induction, whereas insufficient amniotic fluid constitutes a contraindication. Moxibustion in the case of intrauterine death is inappropriate since fetal atonia is unlikely to maintain a converted breech in the cephalic presentation.

A previous caesarean section or the presence of a uterine scar from other surgery is considered a contraindication to moxibustion in contemporary Western obstetrics, as this presents a weak point on the uterus, although this is a contentious issue disputed by acupuncturists who are not midwives or doctors, as they believe that no harm will occur from attempting the technique. However, given that the author is currently debating the introduction of a 'new' procedure into conventional obstetrics, and one for which the limited evidence is somewhat inaccessible, it would seem professionally expedient to continue to include previous caesarean as a contraindication in the same way as it is for ECV.

Evidence-based practice

It has been claimed that there is insufficient evidence of either safety or effectiveness of CTs to warrant their use by pregnant women (National Collaborating Centre 2003), although this has been challenged by Tiran (2005). It is true that the number of randomised controlled trials (RCTs) is limited, although it can be difficult to locate them, especially in relation to TCM and moxibustion, on which studies may be published in non-English-language journals. Despite the lack of formal trials, it is estimated that over half of expectant mothers self-administer natural remedies (Refuerzo et al 2005) and it is of growing concern to this author that many women with breech presentation resort to the Internet for information, which is not always accurate or complete, even purchasing moxa sticks and commencing the procedure independently and without informing their midwife (personal experience).

Early Chinese studies on the *effectiveness* of moxibustion for breech presentation demonstrate success rates of between 80.9% and 90.3% (Cooperative Research Group 1984); later work achieved 92% cephalic version; however, the inclusion of women between 28 and 33 weeks' gestation may have contributed to the high success rate and the number of reversions to breech was not specified (Cardini et al 1991, Cardini & Huang 1998, Kanakura et al 2001). A study on 33 women between 30 and 38 weeks' gestation achieved a 66.6% rate of conversion to cephalic presentation, now generally considered to be the overall success rate and

suggested 34 weeks as the optimum gestation for the procedure to be performed (Cardini & Huang 1998). Experience suggests that, as might be expected, the procedure is less successful when the legs are extended. In another RCT by the same team, 260 primigravidae with breech presentation after 33 weeks' gestation, 130 were randomised to receive moxibustion for between 7 and 14 days; the other 130 acted as control, receiving no intervention (Cardini & Marcolongo 1993). The moxa group achieved the higher rate of cephalic births at term, despite the potential for both spontaneous cephalic version in the control group and reversion to breech in those successfully turned by moxa. Women in whom moxa was not successful were offered ECV after 35 weeks. Interestingly, most of these studies were conducted in China, where ECV and moxibustion are both commonplace options for breech management. A subsequent RCT undertaken in Italy by the same team (Cardini et al 2005) found that success rates for moxibustion were considerably less successful, and caused them to debate the cultural philosophy in which CTs are used, postulating that the expectation and acceptance of moxa and/or ECV by Chinese women provoked a positive response which could be argued to be placebo. Some work has been undertaken in which moxa is compared with, or sometimes used concurrently with acupuncture, with moxa achieving as much as 80% success (Neri et al 2004, Neri et al 2007).

With regard to *safety*, reports of adverse events following moxa are rare, although this may be due to a difference in reporting practices and a greater use of ECV in the West. Minor adverse reactions such as burns have been reported, but these accounts mostly related to ill patients, whereas healthy pregnant women normally have good manual dexterity or can seek help to carry out the procedure (Bensoussan et al 2000). No signs of fetal distress or abnormal uterine action were found in a single-blinded study by Neri et al (2002), although there is one earlier case study (Engel et al 1992) of a primigravida in whom cephalic presentation with moxibustion at term had been successful, but in whom feto-maternal blood transfusion was found during emergency CS for fetal distress. However, unlike the potential of ECV to force an unwilling fetus to turn to cephalic, moxibustion will only stimulate fetal activity, which may have increased spontaneously, and it is difficult to attribute the above case solely to the use of moxibustion. Ewies and Olah's review (2002) suggests that moxa is a safe, painless, inexpensive and easily administered option, but highlights the small sample sizes of most studies, with lack of randomization. A large-scale, multi-centre trial by acupuncturists is currently underway (Grabowska 2006), although the majority of practitioners are not midwives.

Conclusion

CTs are increasingly becoming a standard component of the practice of some midwives, but it must be remembered that they constitute an extension to the midwife's role and, therefore, demand adequate preparatory education and a quality of practice comparable with that of other elements of midwifery care. Moxibustion offers an extra choice for mothers and a new tool for midwives to manage breech presentation, which is potentially more successful than ECV, less fraught with complications than caesarean section and vaginal breech birth.

Key practice points

- **Education** – midwives must have evidence of adequate and appropriate training, related to implementing the procedure into (NHS) midwifery practice; annual updating and ongoing CPD.
- **Professional accountability** – midwives must be able to justify their actions and their decisions regarding the advice on or treatment with moxibustion.
- **Ethico-legal issues** – midwives should be aware of informed consent, the mother's right to refuse, her record keeping and equity of moxibustion service provision.
- **Evidence-based practice** – midwives must keep up to date with contemporary research on moxibustion effectiveness and safety, and work within currently accepted boundaries.
- **Practical issues** – midwives must be aware of health and safety issues and the environment in which moxibustion is performed.
- **Monitoring of standards** – evaluation and audit of the moxibustion service effectiveness, success rates and maternal and staff satisfaction should be undertaken to inform its continued use.

References

Baldry, P.E., 2004. Acupuncture, trigger points and musculoskeletal pain, third ed. Elsevier, Edinburgh.

Bensoussan, A., Myers, S.P., Carlton, A.L., 2000. Risks associated with the practice of traditional Chinese medicine: an Australian study. Arch. Fam. Med. 9 (10), 1071–1078.

Burns, E., Blamey, C., Ersser, S.J., Lloyd, A.J., Barnetson, L., 2000. The use of aromatherapy in intrapartum midwifery practice an observational study. Complement. Ther. Nurs. Midwifery 6 (1), 33–34.

Cardini, F., Basevi, V., Valentini, A., Martellato, A., 1991. Moxibustion and breech presentation: preliminary results. Am. J. Chin. Med. XIX (2), 105.

Cardini, F., Marcolongo, A., 1993. Moxibustion for correction of breech presentation: a clinical study with retrospective control. Am. J. Chin. Med. 21 (2), 133–138.

Cardini, F., Huang, W., 1998. Moxibustion for correction of breech presentation: a randomised controlled trial. JAMA 280 (18), 1580–1584.

Cardini, F., Lombardo, P., Regalia, A.L., Regaldo, G., Zanini, A., Negri, M.G., et al., 2005. A randomised controlled trial of moxibustion for breech presentation. Br. J. Obstet. Gynaecol. 112 (6), 743–747.

Cooperative Research Group of Moxibustion Version of Jangxi Province, 1984.

Dharmananda, S., 2004. Moxibustion: practical considerations for modern use of an ancient technique, Available online: www.itmonline.org/arts/moxibustion. Accessed February 2008.

Dooley, M., 2006. Complementary therapy and obstetrics and gynaecology: a time to integrate. Curr. Opin. Obstet. Gynaecol. 18 (6), 648–652.

Engel, K., Gerke-Engel, G., Gerhard, I., Bastert, G., 1992. Fetomaternal macrotransfusion after successful internal version from breech presentation by moxibustion

Geburtshilfe Frauenheilkd 52 (4), 241–243.

Ewies, A., Olah, K., 2002. Moxibustion in breech version – a descriptive review. Acupunct. Med. 20 (1), 26–29.

Gaudernack, L.C., Forbord, S., Hole, E., 2006. Acupuncture administered after spontaneous rupture of membranes at term significantly reduces the length of birth and use of oxytocin. A randomized controlled trial. Acta Obstet. Gynecol. Scand. 85 (11), 1348–1353.

Grabowska, C., 2006. Turning the breech using moxibustion. RCM Midwives 9 (12), 484–485.

Harper, T.C., Coeytaux, R.R., Chen, W., Campbell, K., Kaufman, J.S., Moise, K.J., et al., 2006. A randomized controlled trial of acupuncture for initiation of labor in nulliparous women. J. Matern. Fetal Neonatal Med. 19 (8), 465–470.

Kanakura, Y., Kmetani, K., Nagata, T., Niwa, K., Kamatsuki, H., Shinzato, Y., et al., 2001. Moxibustion treatment of breech presentation. Am. J. Chin. Med. 29 (1), 37–45.

McNabb, M.T., Kimber, L., Haines, A., McCourt, C., 2006. Does regular massage from late pregnancy to birth decrease maternal pain perception during labour and birth? – A feasibility study to investigate a programme of massage, controlled breathing and visualization, from 36 weeks of pregnancy until birth. Complement Ther. Clin. Pract. 12 (3), 222–223.

McNeill, J.A., Alderdice, F.A., McMurray, F., 2006. A retrospective cohort study exploring the relationship between antenatal reflexology and intranatal outcomes. Complement Ther. Clin. Pract. 12 (2), 119–125.

Mousley, S., 2005. Audit of an aromatherapy service in a maternity unit. Complement Ther. Clin. Pract. 11 (3), 205–110.

National Collaborating Centre for Women's and Children's Health, 2003. Antenatal care: Routine care for the healthy pregnant woman. RCOG Press, London.

Neri, I., Fazzio, M., Menghini, S., Volpe, A., Facchinetti, F., 2002. Non-stress test changes during acupuncture plus moxibustion on BL67 point in breech presentation. J. Soc. Gynecol. Investig. 9 (3), 158–162.

Neri, I., Airola, G., Contu, G., Allais, G., Facchinetti, F., Benedetto, C., 2004. Acupuncture plus moxibustion to resolve breech presentation: a randomized controlled study. J. Matern. Fetal Neonatal Med. 15 (4), 247–252.

Neri, I., De Pace, V., Venturini, P., Facchinetti, F., 2007. Effects of three different stimulations (acupuncture, moxibustion, acupuncture plus moxibustion) of BL.67 acupoint at small toe on fetal behavior of breech presentation. Am. J. Chin. Med. 35 (1), 27–33.

Nursing and Midwifery Council, 2004. Midwives' Rules and Standards. NMC, London.

RCOG, 2006. Guideline no 20a External Cephalic Version and Reducing the Incidence of Breech Presentation. Available online: www.rcog.org.uk/resources. Accessed February 2008.

Refuerzo, J.S., Blackwell, S.C., Sokol, R.J., et al., 2005. Use of over-the-counter medications and herbal remedies in pregnancy. Am. J. Perinatol. 22 (6), 321–324.

Roemer, A.T., 2006. Medical acupuncture in pregnancy. Thieme, Germany.

Tiran, D., 2003a. Implementing complementary therapies into midwifery practice. Complement. Ther. Nurs. Midwifery 9 (1), 10–13.

Tiran, D., 2003b. Nausea and vomiting in pregnancy: an integrated approach to care. Elsevier, London.

Tiran, D., 2004a. Breech presentation: offering women additional choices. Complement. Ther. Nurs. Midwifery 10 (4), 57–59.

Tiran, D., 2004b. Viewpoint – midwives' enthusiasm for complementary therapies: a cause for concern? Complement. Ther. Nurs. Midwifery 10 (2), 77–79.

Tiran, D., 2005. Complementary therapies in maternity care: NICE guidelines do not promote clinical excellence. Complement. Ther. Clin. Pract. 11 (2), 50–52.

Tiran, D., 2006a. Late for a very important date: complementary therapies for post-dates pregnancy. Pract. Midwife 9 (2), 2–6.

Tiran, D., 2006b. Complementary therapies in pregnancy: midwives' and obstetricians' appreciation of risk. Complement. Ther. Clin. Pract. 12 (2), 126–131.

Tiran, D., 2007. Complementary therapies: time to regulate? Pract. Midwife 10 (3), 14–19.

Williams, J., Mitchell, M., 2007. Midwifery managers' views about the use of complementary therapies in the maternity services. Complement. Ther. Clin. Pract. 13 (2),129–123.

Further reading

Tiran, D., 2009. Reflexology in pregnancy and childbirth. Elsevier, Edinburgh (in preparation, manuscript due Nov 2008).
Explores the increasingly popular therapy of reflexology and its direct application to midwifery practice.

Tiran, D., 2009. Complementary therapies in labour and delivery. In: Walsh, D., Downe, S. 2008 (Eds.), Essential Midwifery Skills: Intrapartum Care. Wiley, London (in preparation, manuscript submitted).
Explores the uses of various complementary therapies to normalise birth, including a debate on the evidence-base and safety.

Tiran, D., 2005. Downloadable information leaflets for expectant mothers (CD). Expectancy Ltd, London.
A CD of eighteen single-sheet downloadable information leaflets which could be distributed to mothers, but which also provide basic information for midwives; includes assorted references.

Tiran, D., 2005. Implementing aromatherapy in maternity care: a manual for midwives and managers. Expectancy Ltd, London.
A manual designed to facilitate the process of implementing complementary therapies into midwifery practice, with particular reference to aromatherapy.

Tiran, D., Mack (Eds.), 2000. Complementary therapies for pregnancy and childbirth, second ed. Balliere Tindall, London.
A multi-contributed book in which several different complementary therapies are discussed in relation to pregnancy, childbirth and the puerperium.

Resources

Journals

Complementary Therapies in Clinical Practice. Elsevier, London.

Complementary Therapies in Medicine. Elsevier, London.

Websites

www.expectancy.co.uk Expectant Parent's Complementary Therapies Consultancy – courses, study days, educational resources, information and advice for professionals and mothers

www.nccam.nih.gov/camonpubmed Database of complementary medicine research abstracts; includes Medline, Cinahl and other conventional and complementary therapies databases

Chapter Four

4

Ultrasonography in midwifery practice

John Regan

CONTENTS

Introduction 29
Safety of ultrasound 30
Self-regulation 30
Basic ultrasound technology 31
Early pregnancy ultrasound 32
Multiple pregnancies in the first trimester 33
First trimester screening for
chromosome abnormalities 34
    Cystic hygroma 35
Second trimester ultrasound 35
Fetal measurements used in the
second trimester 35
    Head circumference 36
    Abdominal circumference 36
    Femur length 36
The second trimester fetal anomaly
ultrasound scan 36
Normal head shape and internal
structures 37
    Cerebral ventricles 37
    Cerebellum 38
    Choriod plexus cysts 38
    Nuchal pad/fold 38
    Head and face 38
    Fetal spine 38
Abdominal shape and content 39
    Fetal urinary tract 39
Examination of the fetal heart 40
Fetal limbs 40
Placental location 41
Monitoring for twin-to-twin transfusion
syndrome 41

Cervical length 42
Third trimester ultrasound 42
    Fetal growth 42
    Obtaining an umbilical artery Doppler
    waveform 43
    Large for gestational age 44
Key practice points 44
References 44
Further reading 45

Before reading this chapter, you should be familiar with:
- Ultrasound technology and the physics of ultrasound.
- Recommendations of NICE antenatal care guidelines (NICE 2008).
- Recommendations of national screening committees for antenatal ultrasound screening.
- The responsibilities of the midwife in maintaining competencies in the development and acquisition of new skills.

Introduction

This chapter will provide a basic understanding of routine ultrasound in the three trimesters of pregnancy. It is not intended to provide a comprehensive guide to all obstetric ultrasound nor should it be seen as a replacement for training via a recognised ultrasound course. Diagnostic ultrasound has had a significant impact on the practice of modern medicine, particularly in the field of fetal medicine and obstetrics. Ultrasound appears to have gained acceptance because it is comfortable for women, easy to use, produces instant results and does not appear to be associated with hazardous side effects. Traditionally radiographers have extended their roles to become sonographers. Now, with ultrasound being provided as a routine part of pregnancy care for most women, more midwives are advancing/extending their skills and becoming midwife-sonographers.

Safety of ultrasound

When ultrasound was first developed and introduced, it was assumed that the possible hazards and bio effects would be kept under constant review. Recent research has led to the belief that ultrasound has been continually evaluated and has proved to be safe (Newnham et al 2004). However the growing trend to apply ultrasound techniques such as colour Doppler, colour flow imaging, harmonic imaging and three/four dimensional imaging, at earlier stages of fetal development, have been accompanied by the potential use of substantial increases in acoustic power output.

The likelihood of diagnostic ultrasound producing harmful effects is thought to be linked to the amount of acoustic exposure released by an ultrasound machine. Ultrasound bio effects can occur through three mechanisms, heating, cavitation and micro streaming. It is considered that a temperature rise of 4° centigrade or more, sustained for more than 5 minutes, may cause irreversible damage to the developing embryo and fetal brain (Barnett 2001). The majority of conclusions related to the safety of ultrasound have been drawn from animal studies. Studies relating to the bio effects on humans from ultrasound have been limited. Two studies in the early 1990s implied that women having repeated routine ultrasound scans in pregnancy gave birth to low-birth-weight babies with an increased incidence of left handedness (Newnham et al 1993, Salveson et al 1993). Beech (1999) and Wagner (1999), in their critical reviews of ultrasound use, suggest that from the evidence produced it is safe to conclude that prenatal ultrasound scans do carry risks for the unborn fetus. However, it should be acknowledged that Newnham et al

(1993) set out to test the hypothesis that frequent ultrasound examinations would improve pregnancy outcome, and not that they would cause harm. Consequently, the findings in this study may not be as reliable as experimental studies in supporting causality. Recently, Newnham et al (2004) have followed up their earlier work and could not demonstrate any long-term damaging effects in the children who were exposed to ultrasound in the uterus. Whilst most of the findings support the assumption that ultrasound is safe and causes no harm, some studies acknowledge that, at present, no definite conclusions can be drawn.

Self-regulation

It is unlikely that conclusive research relating to the safety of fetal ultrasound will ever be undertaken, either because ultrasound technology is advancing so quickly or because there is a lack of interest in such studies. It is important that midwives, who undertake ultrasound examinations of the fetus, introduce a form of self-regulation for themselves. Midwives should consider a number of points as outlined in Box 4.1.

Midwife sonographers should aim to ensure they maximise the benefits of the ultrasound examination while reducing unnecessary exposure to the fetus. The British Medical Ultrasound Society

---

Box 4.1

Issues of self-regulation for midwives to consider

- Are you appropriately trained to perform the examination that has been requested?

  If you are not trained to undertake an examination, do not do it. Inappropriate use of ultrasound by untrained health professionals is potentially one of its most harmful effects.

- Is the ultrasound procedure necessary?

  Ultrasound requests are often received when pregnant women bleed in the third trimester and an abruption is questioned.

  An ultrasound examination cannot always confirm or rule out an abruption; therefore its use as a diagnostic tool in this clinical situation is debatable.

Box 4.2

Recommendations for safety and exposure time

- **Exposure time**
  Minimising the examination time to as short as necessary to achieve the diagnostic result.

- **Stationary probe**
  The probe should be kept moving and should be removed from the woman when real time imaging has been stopped e.g. when taking measurements.

- **Thermal index (TI) and Mechanical index (MI)**
  These displays provide the sonographer with information about the potential risks from temperature rises within tissues and the likelihood of cavitation. In obstetric ultrasound usually two forms of TI are displayed on the ultrasound machine: thermal index in soft tissue (TIS) and thermal index in bone (TIB). BMUS (2000) suggest that when on screen TI and MI are displayed, their guidelines should be followed. For example if the TI is 0.7 then the maximum exposure time for the fetus should be sixty minutes.

(BMUS 2000) make a number of recommendations to aid sonographers to implement ALARA (as low as reasonably achievable). This form of self-regulation places the emphasis for safety and exposure levels with the sonographer. A summary of the recommendations are outlined in Box 4.2.

Basic ultrasound technology

Ultrasound images are produced by the generation of sound waves, the reception of returning echoes and the interpretation of returning echoes. Sound waves are produced by a transducer. The transducer is a piezoelectric crystal that converts power from one source (electricity) into another form (sound waves). Sound waves are produced at high frequencies that are unheard by the human ear, this is ultrasound. The piezoelectric crystal also works in reverse. The returning echoes are converted by the crystals into electrical signals from which the ultrasound images are produced (Chudleigh & Thaliganathan 2004). The pattern produced by the returning echoes is converted into information by a digital scan converter, which relays the information via a grey scale into an image on a television monitor.

To produce an ultrasound image on the screen the ultrasound machine needs to know the direction of the returning echo, how strong the echo is and how long it took the echo to be received, from when the ultrasound wave was first transmitted. There are a number of factors that affect the returning echoes, which include attenuation, absorption, reflection and refraction. The intensity and amplitude of a sound wave will decrease as it travels, the wave becoming weaker the deeper it travels into the body. There is a tendency for higher frequencies to be attenuated more quickly. Absorption gives rise to the loss of energy from the beam, which is converted into heat that remains in the tissues. Higher frequencies will give rise to greater absorption, therefore, impairing the penetration ability of the sound wave. Thus, lower frequencies are needed for increased penetration, whilst higher frequencies are preferred when penetration is not necessary. Reflection occurs at tissue interfaces where there is difference in acoustic impedance. The larger the acoustic difference the more reflected the sound wave. These reflected echoes return to the ultrasound machine and form the basis of the ultrasound image.

Ultrasound machines have various controls, which allow the sonographer to maximise the interpretation of the returning echoes, thus obtaining the best quality image possible. *Gain* is the term used to describe the amplification of the reflected ultrasound waves. The echoes that are reflected from tissues, which are further away from the transducer need more amplification than those that come from tissues closer to the probe and, thus, ultrasound units have separate gain controls. Gain should be set so fluid-filled structures appear black. Dense structures such as bone should appear bright white. The dynamic range control determines the range of echoes, which will be displayed on the screen. It can be adjusted either to display or reduce low-level echoes returning to the probe. The depth control alters the depth of the beam during real-time scanning. The focus control allows the ultrasound beam to be adjusted so that it is focused at a particular depth, thus improving resolution. Focus should be set at the level of interest or just below it. Zoom allows the sonographer to enlarge an area of interest for easier examination. The cineloop function enables sonographers to review past images in the previous frames: an action replay of the captured images.

Early pregnancy ultrasound

Although ultrasound imaging has been used extensively in the first trimester for a number of years, the practice and use has mainly gone unchallenged since this has been limited to confirming dates and number of gestational sacs. The advent of new technology and the introduction of screening programmes to detect and eliminate fetuses that are considered unwanted so early in the pregnancy begins to raise many issues, including ethical considerations, psychological effects and safety. These issues are further highlighted when considering relevant research, which has suggested that routine ultrasound offers no benefits in terms of morbidity and mortality rates (Ewigman et al 1993). Bricker et al (2000) in their systemic review of ultrasound in pregnancy, appear to support this conclusion and imply that the only benefit gained from early ultrasound is the reduction in post-term pregnancy induction rates.

The identification of an intrauterine gestation sac is usually the first ultrasound confirmation of a pregnancy. Pregnancy dating has traditionally been calculated from the first day of the last menstrual period (LMP). This method assumes that conception occurred two weeks after the LMP, which is often not the case. Current national recommendations advice is that all pregnant women should be offered an early pregnancy scan, at approximately 10 to 13 weeks' gestation, to assess gestational age and detect multiple pregnancies (National Institute for Health and Clinical Excellence [NICE] 2008). During the first 12 weeks of pregnancy, various ultrasound methods and examinations have been used to calculate gestational age. These include, mean sac diameter (MSD) and crown rump length (CRL) (Chudleigh & Thaliganathan 2004).

First-trimester ultrasound can be performed using the abdominal approach or transvaginal approach. An intrauterine gestation sac can usually be reliably seen at approximately 5 weeks' gestation, via transvaginal ultrasound (TVS), and nearer 6 weeks via transabdominal ultrasound (TA). In very early pregnancy, usually before 8 weeks' gestation, the transvaginal method is preferred, as the greater resolution obtained using the higher frequency transducer, produces a higher quality image. The woman is usually scanned in the supine position with her legs placed in the lithotomy position. A transvaginal probe, covered with a protective latex

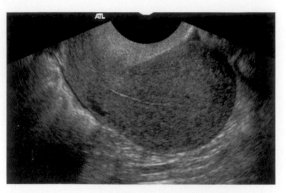

Figure 4.1 • Transvaginal ultrasound showing the longitudinal view of the uterus. The uterus is retroverted.

sheath, is lubricated with gel and inserted into the vagina. When the uterus has been located it should be scanned and examined in the longitudinal plane, taking note of uterine position, anomalies and contents (Figure 4.1). The probe should be moved from right to left (or vice versa) so a complete sweep of the uterus, in the longitudinal plane is performed. Once the uterus has been examined in the longitudinal plane, the probe should be rotated through 90°, to obtain an image of the uterus in the transverse plane. The probe should be moved from head to foot so the uterus is evaluated in the transverse plane. After the uterus has been examined in both planes, then the ovaries should be assessed. To examine the ovaries the transducer is usually kept in the same position as used for examining the transverse plane of the uterus. The transducer is angled to the left or right, depending on which ovary is being examined. The easiest way to try and locate the ovaries is to locate the iliac vessels first and the ovaries are usually found anterior to the vessels.

As pregnancy progresses and fetal structures become visible, the transabdominal method is usually preferred. Using the abdominal approach, the women will usually need a partially filled bladder (although not over distended) to allow for visualization of the pelvic anatomy. The technique is the same as for transvaginal scanning. Using a transabdominal probe, usually three to five megahertz, the uterus should be located and examined in both longitudinal and transverse planes. The ovaries should also be examined. Once the uterus and ovaries have been fully examined in this way, the focus can then shift to the gestation sac and its contents. The gestation sac is usually eccentrically placed and lies towards the fundus of the uterus.

There is an echogenic ring around the gestation sac, which is approximately 2 mm thick and appears brighter than the myometrium. When identifying a gestation sac in early pregnancy, the above features are important in confirming an intrauterine pregnancy. To calculate the gestational age, if a fetus is not visible, then the MSD should be calculated and used. To obtain the correct view to calculate the MSD, a longitudinal section of the uterus should be obtained showing the maximum anterior/posterior and longitudinal diameters of the gestation sac. The sac should be measured by placing the on-screen callipers on the inner margins, taking care not to include the echogenic ring. The probe should then be rotated 90° to obtain a transverse section of the uterus and the gestation sac should be measured across the maximum transverse diameter. The sum of the three diameters, divided by three, equates to the MSD. The MSD plus 30 days, gives an approximate gestational age in days.

For example sac measurements of:

10 mm + 16 mm + 10 mm = 36

36 ÷ 3 = 12

12 + 30 = 42 days.

Many ultrasound machines will now automatically calculate the approximate gestational age from the sac measurements.

As pregnancy progresses, first a yolk sac is seen and then what is commonly referred to as a fetal pole is noted. The yolk sac is seen as a bright round ring within the gestation sac. The fetal pole is a mass of cells, which is usually visualised after the 6th week of pregnancy. The fetal pole is seen separately from the yolk sac and usually grows at a rate of 1 mm a day. Fetal cardiac activity is usually visible once a fetal pole is more than 4 mm in length (Judge 2004). The length of the fetus is obtained by taking a measurement of the CRL. The CRL is the measurement from the top of the fetal head to the rump (Figure 4.2). If performed correctly, the CRL has been shown to be the most accurate method of estimating gestational age (Chudleigh & Thaliganathan 2004). However, obtaining an accurate CRL can be challenging since any degree of flexion of the fetal spine will result in an underestimation of the CRL. The measurement of the CRL is usually taken in millimetres and then cross-referenced with a gestational age chart. Most ultrasound machines will have charts already programmed into

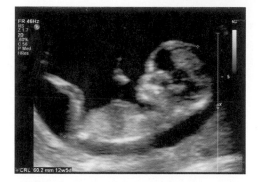

Figure 4.2 • Crown rump length at 12 weeks and 5 days' gestation.

their software; however, it is important for midwives to be aware of which chart is being used, since variations in charts and measurements do exist. National screening committees for antenatal care will usually offer guidance on the appropriate charts to use. Once the pregnancy progresses beyond 13 weeks the fetal position tends to be flexed. Thus CRL becomes inaccurate as a method for dating a pregnancy, so the head circumference (HC) should be used.

Multiple pregnancies in the first trimester

Multiple pregnancies have increased in recent years, probably as a result of more assisted reproduction techniques being readily available (Nicolaides 2004). It is estimated that twins account for approximately 1% of all pregnancies, with two-thirds being dizygotic and one-third monozygotic (Nicolaides 2004). Dizygotic twins result after the ovulation and fertilisation of two eggs. These twins are not identical. They will be in their own gestation sacs, each having their own placenta, chorion and amnion. They are usually referred to as dichorionic diamniotic (DC/DA) twin pregnancies. Monozygotic twins result from the ovulation, fertilisation and division of one egg. These twins will be identical. There are generally three types of monozygotic twin pregnancies. The time of egg division will determine the type of pregnancy (Chudleigh & Thaliganathan 2004). Table 4.1 explains the different types of monozygotic twins and their chorionicity. If egg division tries to occur after day 12, the twins will be conjoined.

Table 4.1 Different types of monozygotic twins and their chorionicity

Classification	Monozygotic twins		
	Dichorionic diamniotic (DC/DA)	Monochorionic diamniotic (MC/DA)	Monochorionic Monoamniotic (MC/MA)
Time at which egg division occurs	1–3 days	3–9 days	9–12 days
Number of gestation sacs	2	1 chorionic sac with dividing membrane	1
Number of placentas	2	1	1
Number of chorions	2	1	1
Number of amnions	2	2	1

Ultrasound evaluation of twin pregnancies in the first trimester is important, since it allows for chorionicity to be established. Determining chorionicity and amnionicity is clinically important since it allows health care practitioners to plan appropriate antenatal care and counsel couples about potential complications such as twin-to-twin transfusion syndrome (TTTS). Establishing the chorionicity and amnionicity is usually performed after 8 weeks' gestation and preferably between 11 and 14 weeks. The ultrasound identification of two separate gestation sacs with a thick dividing membrane and two placentas is confirmation of a DC/DA twin pregnancy. The dividing septum is thickest and easily identified at the base of the membrane and is commonly referred to as the 'lambda' sign (Figure 4.3).

The presence of a single placenta and a thin dividing membrane, often difficult to visualise and the absence of the lambda sign is diagnostic of a

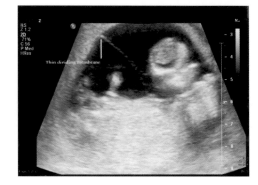

Figure 4.4 • Dividing membrane of a monochorionic diamniotic (MC/DA) twin pregnancy – T sign.

MC/DA pregnancy. The dividing membrane is made up of just the amnions and appears as a 'T' sign when inserting into the shared placenta (Figure 4.4). The presence of one placenta and the absence of a dividing membrane is confirmation of a MC/MA pregnancy.

First trimester screening for chromosome abnormalities

In the early 1990s prenatal screening for Down's syndrome by a combination of fetal nuchal translucency, measured by ultrasound at 11 to 14 weeks, and consideration of maternal age, was first considered by Nicolaides (Nicolaides et al 1992). Observations made more than 100 years ago noted that the skin of people with Down's syndrome appeared too large for their bodies. In the 1990s Nicolaides et al (1992) reported that the excess skin could be

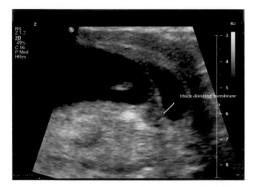

Figure 4.3 • Dividing membrane of a dichorionic diamniotic (DC/DA) twin pregnancy – Lambda sign.

seen with ultrasound as an increased nuchal translu-cency (NT) at the back of the fetal neck: becoming the basis for the screening programme. This method of screening has been reported to detect approxi-mately 75% of fetuses affected with Down's syn-drome. With the introduction of maternal serum biochemistry analysis, combined with maternal age and fetal NT measurement in the first trimester, the detection rate is reported to be 85–90% (Nico-laides 2004). Although there is no disputing that using this screening programme will detect a large proportion of affected fetuses, the benefits and advantages of detecting such abnormalities so early in the pregnancy continues to be the subject of fur-ther research. Current national guidance suggests that Down's syndrome screening should be offered at the end of the first trimester, thus NT measure-ment, with maternal biochemistry analysis, is the method of choice (NICE 2008).

During the process of confirming viability, estab-lishing gestation and screening for chromosome abnormalities in the first trimester, it is also possible to detect other fetal abnormalities. The majority of fetal abnormalities will not be detected until the fetal anomaly scan is performed at 20 weeks' gestation; however, there are a range of abnormalities which will be evident during the first trimester ultrasound scan. It is important when establishing consent for the first trimester scan, that women understand that some abnormalities may be evident. It is also a vital part of the consent process that women are informed that confirmation of certain abnormalities, may have to wait until the second trimester.

Cystic hygroma

A cystic hygroma is seen as excessive swelling, usually at the back of the fetal neck, although it may be seen in other areas around the body (Jeanty 1991). The swelling results from an interruption of the lymphatic vessels and the extent of the cystic hygroma may vary (Figure 4.5A). Cystic hygromas can be associated with chromosome abnormalities, particularly Turn-er's syndrome and Down's syndrome, so the finding usually prompts the offer of diagnostic invasive test-ing after counselling. If chromosome analysis is nor-mal, then it is necessary to screen for structural abnormalities during the second trimester anomaly scan, as cystic hygromas are reported to be associated with defects of the cardiovascular system, pulmo-nary system and haematological system (Nicolaides

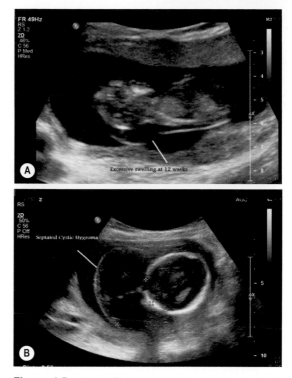

Figure 4.5 • (A and B) Increased oedema at the back of the fetal neck at 12 weeks. At 17 weeks the swelling has developed into a cystic hygroma.

2004). As a result a cystic hygroma usually, but not always, indicates a poor prognosis (Figure 4.5B).

Second trimester ultrasound

The majority of second trimester ultrasound exam-inations involve screening and diagnosing fetal abnormalities. National guidelines advocate that all pregnant women be offered a second trimester ultrasound examination to detect fetal abnormal-ities (NICE 2008). It is recommended that this examination be performed between 18 and 20 weeks' gestation, when the majority of fetal anat-omy can be evaluated.

Fetal measurements used in the second trimester

The Biparietal diameter is no longer recommended for estimation of fetal age or fetal growth (BMUS 2008).

Head circumference

To measure the head circumference (HC), a transverse view of the fetal head demonstrating an oval-shaped head, cavum septum pellucidum (CSP) and the choriod plexus within the posterior horn of the lateral ventricles should be obtained (Figure 4.6). Measurement of the HC is performed by taking the measurements of the BPD and the occipital frontal diameter (OFD) and then using the equation:

$$\frac{\pi(\textbf{BPD} + \textbf{OFD})}{2} = \textbf{HC}$$

To measure the BPD the on-screen callipers should be placed on the outer borders of the parietal edges (outer to outer). To measure the OFD the callipers should be placed on the outer edges of the occipital and frontal bones (outer to outer). The majority of ultrasound machines will derive the HC automatically from the BPD/OFD, using the above equation.

Abdominal circumference

The correct section to obtain an abdominal circumference (AC) measurement is seen in Figure 4.7. The fetal abdomen should be demonstrated in cross section showing one section of vertebrae, a short length of umbilical vein and the fetal stomach. Once the correct section is imaged, the AC measurement is obtained in the same way as for the HC. The transverse abdominal diameter (TAD) and the anterior posterior abdominal diameter (APAD) are used to calculate the AC. To measure the APAD, the on-screen callipers are placed on the outer borders of

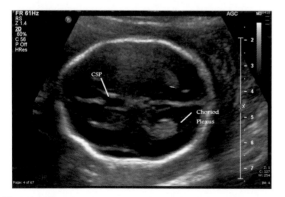

Figure 4.6 ● Cross section of the fetal head demonstrating the section needed to measure the head circumference.

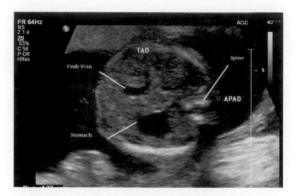

Figure 4.7 ● Cross section of the fetal abdomen demonstrating the section needed to measure the abdominal circumference. Transverse abdominal diameter (TAD), anterior posterior abdominal diameter (APAD).

the fetal abdomen at the spine to the abdominal wall. The TAD is measured by placing the callipers on the outer borders of the fetal body across the transverse section of the abdomen, as seen in Figure 4.7. The majority of ultrasound machines will automatically calculate the AC from the two measurements.

Femur length

Measurement of the femur length (FL) is obtained by measuring the 'U' shape at each end of the femur. The femur should be in the horizontal plane, with both ends clearly visible.

The second trimester fetal anomaly ultrasound scan

The Royal College of Obstetricians and Gynaecologists [RCOG] (2000), in their supplement to ultrasound screening for fetal abnormalities, state that the 20-week anomaly scan is to reassure a woman that her baby appears to have no obvious structural abnormalities. For the majority of women this will be the case. For some women the detection of structural abnormalities will allow for termination of the pregnancy. For other women, the ultrasound will heighten their anxiety because of the uncertainty surrounding the significance of certain ultrasound findings. Ultrasound markers have been described as non-permanent structural changes in the fetus, which appear to have little long-term significance in the absence of serious underlying pathology (Antenatal Screening Wales 2004). Although there may be a link between the presence of numerous ultrasound markers and aneuploidy, in the majority of circumstances the risk will be small. The following text outlines the minimum standard recommended for the fetal anomaly ultrasound scan. Some common ultrasound markers are described to aid midwives in their recognition; however, it is recommended that midwives follow national screening guidelines in reporting their significance.

The minimum standard set out by the RCOG (2000) for performing the 20-week fetal anomaly scan is the standard that tends to be adopted by the majority of obstetric units. Box 4.3 outlines the minimum standard.

Extended views include imaging the face and lips and examination of the cardiac outflow tracts. Midwives should be aware of how the normal views of each structure should look and any deviation from the norm should prompt referral for further evaluation.

When commencing the fetal anomaly scan, the midwife sonographer should start the examination by distinguishing between the right and left side of the fetus. The midwife should first determine which part of the fetus is presenting, e.g. cephalic, breech, and then determine the fetal lie and the position of the fetal spine. The maternal left will be on the right of the ultrasound display monitor. Once fetal position has been established, the anatomy should be examined.

Normal head shape and internal structures

Normal head shape is usually assessed from the view obtained for taking the HC measurement. The normal fetal skull is oval shape and rounded at the back and front (see Figure 4.6). Deviation from the characteristic rugby ball shape is usually fairly obvious. Figure 4.8 shows a lemon-shaped fetal skull. This finding is often associated with neural tube defects such as spina bifida. The cavum septum pellucidum (CSP) is seen in the fetal skull as two parallel echoes either side of the midline. The CSP interrupts the midline and occupies the front third of the fetal skull (as in Figure 4.6). Examination of the CSP can be undertaken from the same view obtained for taking the HC measurement. The presence of a normal CSP rules out a number of abnormalities such as agenesis of the corpus collosum and major degrees of holoprosenchaly.

Cerebral ventricles

The contents of the fetal brain are mainly made up of tissue, blood and cerebrospinal fluid (CSF). CSF is produced by the choriod plexus and circulates through the ventricular system, the brain and the spine (Proud 1997). Enlargement of the ventricular system can result from a build up of CSF, which can occur from over production, blockage or lack of absorption. The ventricles are bilateral and contain the choriod plexus. Examination of the cerebral ventricles usually involves visualising and measuring the lateral ventricles. This can be undertaken from the section used for taking the HC.

Box 4.3

Minimum standard for 20 weeks fetal anomaly scan

- Head shape and internal structures.
- Spine.
- Abdominal shape and contents at the level of the stomach.
- Abdominal shape and contents at the level of the kidneys and umbilicus.
- Renal pelvis (AP measurement < 5 mm).
- Longitudinal view of the abdomen/thorax.
- Four chamber view.
- Arms (three long bones and hand).
- Legs (three long bones and feet).

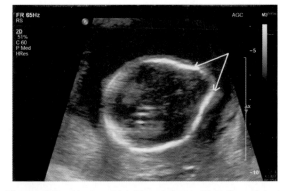

Figure 4.8 • Abnormal fetal head shape. Note the pointed sinciput demonstrated by the arrows.

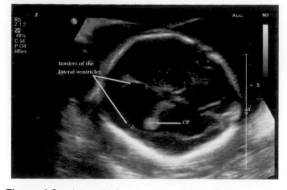

Figure 4.9 • A ventricular measurement of 20.6 mm indicating hydrocephalus. Note the chorioid plexus dangling due to the excessive cerebrospinal fluid.

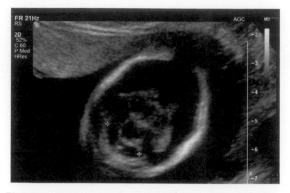

Figure 4.10 • Abnormal cerebellum. Note the transcerebellum diameter is 15.2 mm at 20 weeks' gestation.

Chudleigh and Thaliganathan (2004) suggest that the measurement of the lateral ventricle is taken from the medial edge of the medial border to the outer edge of the lateral border. Others have suggested that the lateral ventricle is measured by placing the calipers on the edges of the inner borders (Pilu et al 1999). Midwives should follow local guidelines on which method should be used. A measurement of less than 10 mm is considered within normal limits. Measurements of 10 to 15 mm are described as mild to moderate ventricularmegaly, and a measurement of 16 mm or above is described as hydrocephalus (Figure 4.9).

Cerebellum

Moving/rotating the transducer slightly from the view needed to obtain the HC (lateral ventricle view), will image the cerebellum. It appears as two circular hemispheres that are bilaterally symmetrical. Measurement of the trans cerebellum diameter (TCD) is performed by measuring the widest point between the two hemispheres, from the outer border of one to the outer border of the other. The diameter in millimetres should correspond to the gestation in weeks. A small cerebellum may indicate problems such as Dandy Walker Malformation. An abnormally shaped cerebellum, usually described as banana shaped, is indicative of spina bifida (Figure 4.10).

Choriod plexus cysts

Choriod plexus cysts (CPC) are fluid-filled spaces within the choriod plexus and are seen in approximately 1–2% of normal pregnancies. There has been much debate and controversy regarding CPCs in recent years, but current evidence suggests that neither their size nor number affect the risk of chromosomal abnormalities (Walkinshaw 2001). If CPCs are seen and no other structural problems are identified, the chance of aneuploidy is low. It is suggested that midwives follow national guidance on the reporting of CPCs.

Nuchal pad/fold

Oedema of the soft tissues at the back of the fetal neck (occiput) can be associated with chromosome abnormalities such as Down's syndrome. Measurement of the nuchal pad (NP) can be obtained from the view used to examine and measure the TCD. The measurement is taken from the outer border of the fetal skull to the skin edge. A measurement of 6 mm or above is usually an indication for further counselling and follow-up.

Head and face

Examination of the fetal face is undertaken by obtaining a coronal section of the fetal face, imaging the orbits and soft tissues. Manipulating the probe slightly forward from this view will demonstrate the fetal nose and lips, as shown in Figure 4.11A. This extended view will detect cleft lip as seen in Figure 4.11B.

Fetal spine

Ultrasound examination of the fetal spine usually involves assessment of the spine in two planes – longitudinal and transverse. The majority of ultrasound departments also add the coronal views

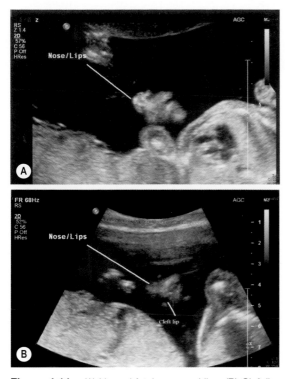

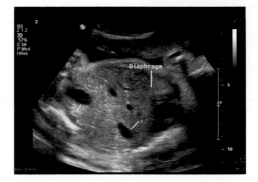

Figure 4.12 • Longitudinal section of the fetus demonstrating the fetal diaphragm (B – bladder, S – stomach).

Figure 4.11 • (A) Normal fetal nose and lips. (B) Cleft lip.

to their standards. The spine is easily visualised with ultrasound and is seen as three high level reflective echoes in the transverse section and two parallel rows of reflective echoes in the longitudinal section. Each of the vertebrae should be examined in the transverse section, ensuring that the cervical, thoracic and lumbar vertebrae form a triangular shape and the lower lumbar vertebrae form a 'u' shape. The spine should also be examined throughout its length in the longitudinal view. The spine should be symmetrical in both its vertebral sequence and curvature. The skin edge should be evident in both sections and the characteristic upward flick of the sacrum should be seen. Since the majority of women are now offered and accept a fetal anomaly ultrasound scan, it is not necessary to screen for neural tube defects by maternal serum alpha feto protein (NICE 2008).

Abdominal shape and content

To examine the abdominal shape and contents at the level of the stomach, a transverse view of the fetal abdomen should be obtained. The stomach should be seen on the left side of the fetus. Just below the stomach, the umbilical cord insertion should be seen. Clear views of the cord insertion allow exclusion of abdominal wall defects such as gastroschisis. It is necessary to demonstrate the two arteries and single vein within the cord. These can usually be seen in the section obtained for examining the cord insertion. Sliding the transducer downwards will image the structures of the lower abdomen. Rotating the transducer through 90° will demonstrate the longitudinal image of the abdomen. Figure 4.12 shows the diaphragm and related structures. The diaphragm is a thin membrane that separates the thorax from the abdomen. In the routine examination of the diaphragm it is important to demonstrate an echo poor line separating the heart from the stomach in the longitudinal view. The chest cavity should contain no structures apart from the great vessels and the heart. Congenital diaphragmatic hernia (CDH) can be difficult to diagnose with ultrasound. Suspicion of CDH is usually raised if a cystic structure is seen in the thorax, when examining the structures of the fetal heart.

Fetal urinary tract

The fetal bladder is usually easily visualised and is seen as an echo-free structure in the pelvis. If the bladder is not initially visible then waiting for it to fill (possibly 30–40 minutes) is advisable. Kidneys can be seen on each side of the lumbar spine. The echogenicity of the kidneys is similar to that of the fetal lungs. If the kidneys appear particularly bright (increased echogenicity) then this warrants further examination and evaluation, as it may be an indication of polycystic kidneys.

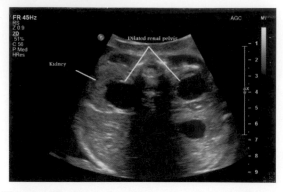

FR 45Hz
RS
Z 0 9
20
51%
C 56
P Med
HRes

Dilated renal pelvis

Kidney

Figure 4.13 • Bilateral, pelvi calycaceal dilation (PCD).

The fetal renal pelvis is seen as an echo-free space at the centre of the kidney. Since antenatal diagnosis of pelvi calycaceal dilation (PCD) is useful to ensure appropriate and early treatment, any dilation is measured. The anterior/posterior diameter is measured from inner border to inner border (Figure 4.13). A measurement of 5 mm or more is an indication for further evaluation of the fetal kidneys later in the pregnancy, at 28–32 weeks. A measurement of greater than 10 mm can be an indication for referral to a fetal medicine centre for further assessment. The most common cause of PCD is reflux; however, obstruction and duplication of the kidneys, needs to be considered. In the absence of other structural abnormalities, there does not appear to be enough evidence to support offering invasive testing for chromosome abnormalities.

Examination of the fetal heart

Cardiovascular defects are one of the commonest groups of major congenital anomalies. The optimum standard for examining the fetal heart is the views of the four chambers and the outflow tracts. Most advocate examining the heart in a series of sequential views from upper abdomen to upper medisternum. During this sweep of the heart, five views are obtained which can be examined for normality (Jones et al 2002, Yagel et al 2001). The views are illustrated and explained in Box 4.4.

Becoming familiar with this regimented approach to examining the fetal heart, during the anomaly scan, should ensure that deviation from the normal standard are noted such that prompt referral for further cardiac evaluation is initiated.

Box 4.4

The five views of the fetal heart

1. **Abdominal situs** – the right and left side of the fetus is first established. The stomach should be on the left, below the fetal heart, the aorta should be towards the front and slightly to the left of the fetal spine. The inferior vena cava should also be in front of the spine, to the right.
2. **Four-chamber view** – the fetal heart should occupy approximately one-third of the chest. The apex of the heart should be 45° to the left. The right ventricle appears slightly thicker than the left, due to the presence of the moderator band. The atria should be of similar size. Both atria ventricular valves should be seen to open. The mitral valve (left) appears slightly higher than the tricuspid valve (right). This 'offset' can be seen when examining the crux of the heart (Figure 4.14A). Once an adequate four-chamber view has been obtained, the transducer should be moved towards the fetal head to obtain views of the outflow tracts.
3. **Left ventricular outflow tract (LVOT)** – the aorta arises from the left ventricle and leaves the heart and heads towards the right shoulder. The ventricular septum and anterior wall of the aorta are seen as a continuous line (Figure 4.14B).
4. **Right ventricular outflow tract (RVOT)** – the pulmonary artery arises from the right ventricle and heads towards the fetal spine. It can be seen crossing over the aorta as it heads towards the spine (Figure 4.14C).
5. **Three-vessel view** – the three vessels, which are seen in this view, are the transverse aortic arch, ductural arch and the superior vena cava.

Fetal limbs

Examination of the fetal limbs involves inspection of the long bones of the arms and legs. The femur is usually the only long bone to be measured; however, subjective assessment of all the long bones is undertaken. To obtain an image of the humerus, the midwife sonographer should obtain a cross sectional/transverse view of the fetal abdomen and then move the transducer slowly towards the fetal head until the humerus begins to come into view. When the humerus is visible the probe should be rotated until the whole of the humerus is visible. If a measurement is needed this can be done in the same way as for the femur. Examination of the

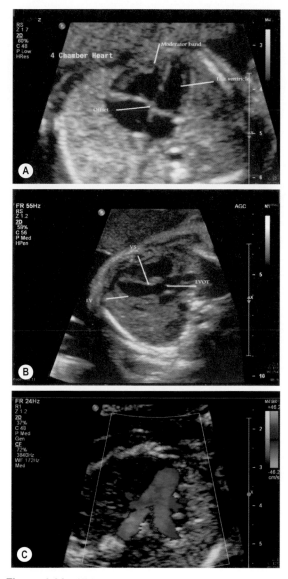

Figure 4.14 • (A) Normal four chamber view. (B) Normal Left ventricle outflow tract (LVOT). VS – ventricular septum, LV – left ventricle. (C) Colour flow imaging demonstrating the right ventricular outflow tract.

demonstrate the femur. When the femur is visible the probe should be rotated until the full length of the femur can be seen. Examination of the tibia and fibula is similar to that of the radius and ulna. Both bones should be examined ensuring that they are straight and of a similar length. The presence and position of the foot should be noted, although it is not necessary to count the toes.

Placental location

Placental location is undertaken during the fetal anomaly scan, at 20 weeks. Placenta praevia has been defined as a placenta that inserts wholly or partially into the lower segment of the uterus (RCOG 2005a). Previously placenta praevia was classified into grades, ranging from I to IV and then, more recently, into major or minor placenta praevia. Major being a placenta that covers the internal os (partially or wholly) and minor being a placenta located in the lower segment of the uterus that does not cover the internal cervical os. Historically the reporting of a low-lying placenta at 20 weeks has always necessitated a rescan in the third trimester to ensure that the placenta had migrated away from the internal os. With the introduction of the NICE guidelines in 2003 (updated 2008), it has become necessary to only rescan those placentae, which cover the internal os at 20 weeks. A rescan in the third trimester is usually performed at 32 weeks. The use of transvaginal ultrasound (TVS) is not con-traindicated in placenta praevia and TVS may be necessary to confirm or refute the diagnosis.

Monitoring for twin-to-twin transfusion syndrome

Twin-to-twin transfusion syndrome (TTTS) occurs in monochorionic twin pregnancies as a result of pla-cental vascular anastamoses, which allows fetofetal transfusion (Nicholaides 2004). The fetofetal trans-fusion results in a shunting of blood from one twin (the donor) to the other (the recipient). As a result the donor twin becomes hypovolaemic, hypotensive and anaemic. The recipient twin becomes hypervo-laemic. The reported incidence varies from 15 to 30%. Ultrasound surveillance of monochorionic twin pregnancies aims to try and detect TTTS. Sur-veillance usually begins at 16 weeks and continues

lower arm involves assessment of both the radius and ulna. As with the examination of the humerus, the full length of the bones should be viewed. Both bones should be straight, with the ulna being slightly longer than the radius. The presence and position of the hands should be noted, although it is not neces-sary to count all the fingers.

From the cross sectional view of the fetal abdo-men, sliding the probe towards the fetal legs, will

every 2 weeks until birth. Since the donor twin becomes hypovolaemic and hypotensive, a reduction in the blood supply leads to reduced urine output and consequently, oligohydraminos. The bladder in the donor twin is usually not visible or very small and because most of the blood and nutrients are diverted to the recipient twin, the donor becomes growth restricted. Because of hypervolaemia, the recipient produces more urine and thus, polyhydraminos. The fetal bladder may also be very large/prominent. TTTS can have a very high perinatal mortality rate and, therefore, treatment and management is undertaken at fetal medicine centres.

Cervical length

In developed countries a major cause of perinatal mortality and morbidity is preterm birth. In the United Kingdom (UK) as stated in Perinatal Mortality 2006, it is estimated that approximately 77% of neonatal deaths and 67% of stillbirths occur in preterm infants (Confidential Enquiry into Maternal and Child Health [CEMACH] 2008). Consequently, ultrasound examination of the cervix is becoming an increasing practice for the prediction and management of preterm labour. While a link between cervical length and preterm labour has been acknowledged, using the results from TVS to prevent preterm birth is proving more difficult. Current evidence does not support the notion of a normal or abnormal cervical length. Although many suggest that a cervical length of less than 25 mm in the second trimester is an optimum threshold for predicting premature labour (Owen et al 2001), a cervical length of over 25 mm does not rule out preterm labour. Recent recommendations do not advocate screening for preterm labour in low risk women.

When performing ultrasound of the cervix it is best to perform the procedure transvaginally. Although the cervix can be visualised transabdominally, women are usually asked to fill their bladder, which causes pressure on the cervix, resulting in elongation of the cervical length. The woman should be asked to empty her bladder and lie in the dorsal lithotomy position. The transvaginal probe is covered with a sterile sheath and lubricated with sterile gel. The probe is inserted into the vagina and advanced into the anterior vaginal fornix until a saggital view of the cervix is seen. The image should be

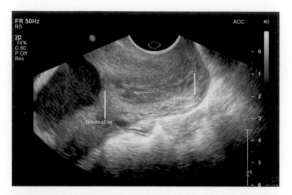

Figure 4.15 • Transvaginal measurement of the cervix.

magnified so that the saggital view of the cervix fills most of the screen. The cervical length measurement is from the internal os to the external os (Figure 4.15). Three measurements are obtained and the shortest reported. It is also important to note any changes in the cervix during the ultrasound examination, for example, funnelling of the cervix.

Third trimester ultrasound

In the third trimester ultrasound is used to assess a number of fetal and maternal conditions including those outlined in Box 4.5:

Fetal growth

Throughout pregnancy, various methods are used to assess fetal growth, including abdominal palpation, measurement of symphysis fundal height and ultrasound. The use of routine third trimester ultrasound has not been proved to be of benefit and consequently referral for a fetal growth scan in the

---

Box 4.5

Third trimester ultrasound assessment

- Placental location – ultrasound scan at 32 weeks if the placenta covers the internal os at 20 weeks.
- Fetal growth – assessing for fetal growth restriction and monitoring growth velocity in pregnancies considered to be at risk.
- Monitoring previously diagnosed fetal anomalies.
- Surveillance of multiple pregnancies.

third trimester, is usually as a result of a suspicion of small for gestational age (SGA). SGA has been defined as a fetus that fails to achieve a certain biometric or estimated weight by a specific gestational age (RCOG 2002). Ultrasound assessment of fetal growth involves measuring the HC, AC and FL. These measurements can then be used to estimate the weight of the fetus (EFW). It is common to use the tenth centile (AC and EFW) as the threshold for defining the SGA fetus; however, using this threshold will mean that at least 10% of the population will be defined as carrying a fetus that is SGA. The majority of these fetuses will be constitutionally small, that is, they are normal and healthy, but small. These fetuses do not appear to have a higher incidence of mortality or morbidity. On the other hand a small proportion will show fetal growth restriction (FGR).

Differentiating between a fetus that is SGA from one which is growth restricted, can be difficult but biophysical tests such as umbilical and uterine artery Doppler combined with a practice of measuring growth velocity rather than a single ultrasound assessment, may aid diagnosis. For example a fetus whose first ultrasound scan shows an AC and EFW that plots on the tenth centile with normal liquor volume and normal umbilical artery Doppler wave forms/indices should have a second ultrasound scan for growth velocity (usually after a period of at least 2 weeks). If the follow-up scan shows that the growth has continued along the tenth centile and the liquor and umbilical artery Dopplers remain normal, then the fetus is likely to be constitutionally small rather than growth restricted, providing the fetal anomaly scan was normal. A fetus that is growth restricted is likely to show evidence of poor growth velocity and also abnormal biophysical tests, such as reduced amniotic fluid volume and abnormal uterine/umbilical artery Dopplers. It is advisable that when monitoring fetal growth the AC and EFW should be used. Causes of FGR include chromosome abnormalities, structural abnormalities, fetal infection and placental insufficiency. Since placental insufficiency is a leading cause of FGR, evaluation of down stream placental vascular resistance can be obtained by measuring Doppler velocities in the fetal umbilical arteries. Resistance to blood flow usually decreases with increasing gestation due to the development of the placental bed throughout pregnancy. With placental insufficiency, impedance to flow is usually seen when a large proportion of the placental bed has been destroyed.

Obtaining an umbilical artery Doppler waveform

Umbilical artery Doppler studies should be obtained using a free loop of cord, preferably towards the placental insertion as the resistance indices are lower here than at the fetal end. The cord should be perpendicular to the probe and the sample gate should be placed over one of the umbilical arteries. It may be necessary to increase the size of the sample gate to ensure that a recording of the umbilical vein is achieved (Figure 4.16A). It will also be necessary to adjust the beam/vessel angle to ensure velocity measurements are accurate.

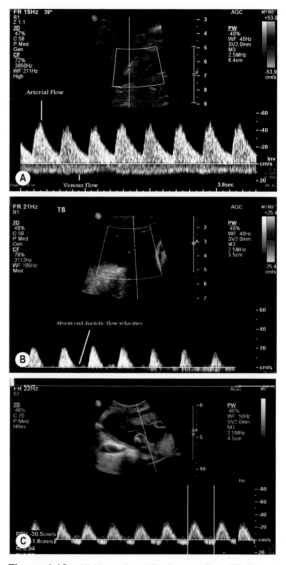

Figure 4.16 • (A) Normal umbilical artery flow. (B) Absent end diastolic flow. (C) Reversed end diastolic flow.

The Doppler waveform demonstrated should show the umbilical artery in forward flow and the umbilical vein in reverse flow. It is important to try and sample the umbilical artery during periods of fetal apnoea, since fetal breathing causes fluctuations in the signal received (Chudleigh & Thaliganathan 2004). The Doppler waveform is measured from the beginning of systole, to the beginning of the next systole. Several indices have been used to quantify the umbilical Doppler waveform, the most common being the resistance index (RI) and pulsatility index (PI). The Doppler waveform should also be described in terms of end diastolic flow: for example, positive end diastolic flow, absent end diastolic flow and reverse end diastolic flow (Figures 4.16A, B and C). Loss of end diastolic frequencies, with associated FGR, suggests that the fetus has an 85% chance of hypoxia. Reversed end diastolic frequencies, in a fetus that is growth restricted, indicates a tenfold increase in perinatal mortality (Chudleigh & Thaliganathan 2004). Reversed end diastolic flow is usually an indication for immediate birth.

Midwives need to be aware that while umbilical artery Doppler studies are of proven benefit in the management of high-risk pregnancies due to FGR, their value in all high-risk pregnancies, e.g. those complicated by maternal diabetes, is not well established. Metabolic abnormalities may cause acidaemia without hypoxia, as a result the fetus of a woman with diabetes may be compromised, but umbilical artery Doppler indices can be normal, unless FGR is also present (Nicolaides et al 2002).

Large for gestational age

The scanning of a woman for a suspected large for gestational age (LGA) fetus in the absence of maternal diabetes and other risk factors is debatable. Despite current evidence and recommendations, some health care professionals believe they can predict and prevent shoulder dystocia and use ultrasound estimation of fetal weight to aid their management of a suspected LGA fetus (RCOG 2005b). While ultrasound may be able to give an estimation of fetal weight, the size of a fetus is not a reliable predictor of shoulder dystocia, since nearly half of all cases of shoulder dystocia occur in infants with a birth weight of less than 4 kg. There is also some evidence to suggest that ultrasound assessment of fetal weight in suspected LGA increases the caesarean section rate without improving clinical outcome (Weiner et al 2002). Recent clinical guidance has recognised the inappropriate use of ultrasound in the management of suspected LGA unborn babies and has recommended that in the low-risk population, ultrasound estimation of fetal size for suspected LGA, should not be undertaken (NICE 2008).

Key practice points

- While ultrasound itself may be safe, its inappropriate use by untrained health professionals may be one of its most harmful hazards.
- Midwives should only undertake an examination if deemed competent to do so, having undertaken appropriate training in ultrasonography.
- Midwives should practice a form of self-regulation and apply the principles of ALARA.
- Routine use of ultrasound should be limited to the early pregnancy ultrasound scan and the 18–20-week fetal anomaly ultrasound scan.
- Routine use of ultrasound in the third trimester is not recommended.
- Ultrasound estimation of fetal size for suspected large-for-gestational-age should not be undertaken in the low-risk population.
- All findings should be recorded in the woman's records and discussed with the woman/referral made to other agencies if necessary.

References

Antenatal Screening Wales, 2004. Specific antenatal ultrasound findings: guidelines for health professionals in Wales. Velindre NHS Trust, Wales.

Barnett, S., 2001. Intracranial temperature elevation from diagnostic ultrasound. Ultrasound Med. Biol. 27 (7), 883–888.

Beech, B.L., 1999. Ultrasound: weighing the propaganda against the facts. Midwifery Today 51, 31–33.

Bricker, L., Garcia, J., Henderson, J., Mugford, M., Neilson, J., Roberts, T., et al., 2000. Ultrasound screening in pregnancy: a systemic review of the clinical effectiveness, cost-effectiveness and women's views. Health. Technol. Assess. 4 (16) (Executive summary).

British Medical Ultrasound Society, 2000. Guidelines for the safe use of diagnostic ultrasound equipment, Available online: http://www.bmus.org/ultras–safety/us–safety03.asp

British Medical Ultrasound Society, 2008. Fetal size and dating: charts recommended for clinical obstetric practice, Available online: http://www.bmus.org/publications

Chudleigh, T., Thilaganathan, B., 2004. Obstetric ultrasound: How, why and when? Churchill Livingstone, Edinburgh.

Confidential Enquiry into Maternal and Child Health, 2008. Perinatal mortality 2006, England, Wales and Northern Ireland. CEMACH, London.

Ewigman, B.G., Crane, J.P., Frigoletto, F.D., LeFevre, M.L., Bain, R.P., McNellis, D., et al., 1993. Effect of prenatal ultrasound screening on perinatal outcome. RADIUS Study Group. N. Engl. J. Med. 329 (12), 821–827.

Jeanty, P., 1991. Sonographic depiction of normal fetal anatomy. In Fleischer, A.C., Romero, R., Manning, F.A., Jeanty, P., Everette James, A. (Eds.), The principles and practice of ultrasonography in obstetrics and gynecology. Prentice Hall, Connecticut, pp. 77–92.

Jones, A., Cook, A., Simpson, J., 2002. Prenatal detection of congenital heart disease: identification of high risk groups and normal sonographic appearances. British Medical Ultrasound Society Bulletin 10 (1), 6–10.

Judge, N., 2004. First trimester sonography. In: Dogra, D., Rubens, D. (Eds.), Ultrasound Secrets. Hanley and Belfus, Philadelphia, pp 37–51.

National Institute for Health and Clinical Excellence, 2008. Antenatal care: routine care for the healthy pregnant woman. Clinical guidelines 62, National Collaborating Centre

for Womens and Childrens Health, NHS London.

Newnham, J.P., Evans, S.F., Michael, C.A., Stanley, F.J., Landau, L.I., 1993. Effects of frequent ultrasound during pregnancy: a randomised controlled trial. The Lancet 342 (8876), 887–891.

Newnham, J.P., Doherty, D.A., Kendall, G.E., Zubrick, S.R., Landau, L.L., Stanley, F.J., 2004. Effects of repeated prenatal ultrasound examinations on childhood outcome up to 8 years of age: follow up of a randomised controlled trial. The Lancet 364 (9450), 2038–2044.

Nicolaides, K.H., 2004. The $11–13^{+6}$ weeks scan, Fetal Medicine Foundation, London.

Nicolaides, K.H., Azar, G., Byrne, D., Mansur, C., Marks, K., 1992. Fetal nuchal translucency: ultrasound screening for chromosomal defects in first trimester of pregnancy. Br. Med. J. 304, 867–869.

Nicoliades, K.H., Rizzo, G., Hecher, K., Ximenes, R., 2002. Doppler in obstetrics, Fetal Medicine Foundation, London.

Owen, J., Yost, N., Berghella, V., Thom, E., Swain, M., Didly, G.A., et al., 2001. Mid-trimester endovaginal sonography in women at risk for spontaneous preterm birth. JAMA 286 (11), 1340–1348.

Pilu, G., Falco, P., Gabrielle, S., Perolo, A., Sandri, F., Bovicelli, L., 1999. The clinical significance of fetal isolated cerebral borderline ventriculomegaly; report of 31 cases and review of the literature. Ultrasound Obstet. Gynecol. 14, 320–326.

Proud, J., 1997. Understanding obstetric ultrasound, second ed. Books for Midwives Press, Cheshire.

Royal College of Obstetricians and Gynaecologists, 2000. Routine ultrasound scanning in pregnancy,

Protocol, standards and training. Supplement to ultrasound screening for fetal anomalies – Report of the RCOG working party. RCOG Press, London.

Royal College of Obstetricians and Gynaecologists, 2002. The investigation and management of the small-for-gestational-age fetus, Guideline no 31, November, RCOG Press, London.

Royal College of Obstetricians and Gynaecologists, 2005a. Placenta praevia and placenta praevia accreta: diagnosis and management, Guideline no 27, October, RCOG Press, London.

Royal College of Obstetricians and Gynaecologists, 2005b. Shoulder dystocia. Guideline no 42, December, RCOG Press, London.

Salvesen, K.A., Vatten, L.J., Eik-Nes, S.H., Hugdahl, K., Bakketeig, L.S., 1993. Routine ultrasonography in utero and subsequent handedness and neurological development. Br. Med. J. 307, 159–164.

Wagner, M., 1999. Ultrasound: more harm than good? Midwifery Today 50, 28–30.

Walkinshaw, S.A., 2001. Minor markers and aneuploidy. British Medical Ultrasound Society Bulletin 9 (1), 19–22.

Weiner, Z., Ben-Shlomo, I., Beck-Fruchter, R., Goldberg, Y., Shalev, E., 2002. Clinical and ultrasonographic weight estimation in large for gestational age fetus. Eur. J. Obstet. Gynecol. Reprod. Biol. 105 (1), 20–24.

Yagel, S., Cohen, S.M., Achiron, R., 2001. Examination of the fetal heart by five short axis views: a proposed screening method for comprehensive cardiac evaluation. Ultrasound Obstet. Gynecol. 17 (5), 267–369.

Further reading

Bates, J., 1997. Practical gynaecological ultrasound. Greenwich Medical Media, London.

Lees, C., Deane, C., Albaiges, G., 2003. Making sense of obstetric Doppler ultrasound. Arnold, London.

Zagzebski, J.A., 1996. The essentials of ultrasound physics. Mosby-Year Book Inc, St. Louis.

The above texts complement the contents of this chapter, providing midwives with an insight into the physics of ultrasound and assist them in

developing an understanding of coincidental gynaecological problems that may be identified during obstetric ultrasound scanning.

Chapter Five

5

Reducing unnecessary caesarean section by external cephalic version

Carol McCormick and Abigail Cairns

CONTENTS

Introduction 47
The significance of breech
presentation 48
Rationale for trying to avoid breech
presentation 48
    Avoiding planned caesarean section . . 48
Who should be offered an external
cephalic version? 49
What is the optimal gestation? 49
What influences the success of
external cephalic version? 49
Complications associated with external
cephalic version 50
The procedure 50
Is external cephalic version
cost effective? 51
Professional issues and challenges
when educating and training
midwives to perform external
cephalic version 51
Information for women 52
Some alternatives to external cephalic
version 52
Key practice points 53
Acknowledgement 53
External cephalic version: a mother's
perspective 53
References 55
Further reading 55
Useful websites 55

Before reading this chapter, you should be familiar with:
- Patient Group Directions (PGDs).
- Professional accountability and liability.
- How to develop the role of the midwife and the responsibilities of the midwife in maintaining competencies in the development and acquisition of new skills.
- Recommendations of Confidential Enquiries into Maternal and Child Health Report (CEMACH 2007) and previous Confidential Enquiries into Stillbirths and Deaths in Infancy (CESDI) reports.
- Legal and ethical decision-making frameworks in midwifery practice.
- Local NHS Trust clinical governance/risk-management procedures.
- The role of the supervisor of midwives.

Introduction

This chapter examines the rationale for the procedure of external cephalic version (ECV) and discusses why and how midwives and obstetricians should achieve competency at performing the skill. It concludes with Abigail Cairns poignant personal narrative of experiencing an ECV first hand when she unexpectedly discovered her baby was presenting by the breech at term with a home birth

Box 5.1

The fetus who presents by the breech adopts one of three presentations:

1. **Extended or frank breech:** the hips are flexed, knees extended and thighs are against the chest with the feet by the baby's ears.
2. **Flexed breech:** hips are flexed; thighs against the chest and knees are also flexed with the calves against the back of the thighs and feet just above the bottom.
3. **Footling breech:** as above, except the hips are not flexed as much and the feet are below the bottom.

planned. Box 5.1 highlights the three main presentations that the fetus can adopt.

The significance of breech presentation

Breech presentation occurs in 3–4% of all term births and a higher proportion of preterm births. It is more common where there has been a previous breech presentation (Cheng & Hannah 1993). Overall perinatal mortality and morbidity is higher in vaginal breech births (Hofmeyr & Hannah 2003) as breech presentation is associated with preterm labour and birth as well as fetal abnormalities. Whatever the mode of birth breech presentation is associated with increased risk of subsequent handicap. Following publication by Hannah et al (2000) most term, planned breech births were achieved by elective caesarean section rather than vaginal birth, as the trial concluded that elective caesarean section was safer for the fetus in terms of mortality and morbidity and of similar safety to the mother when compared with intention for the woman to birth vaginally. Vaginal breech birth carries risks to the neonate such as brachial plexus injuries, fracture of long bones, occipital diastases, severance of spinal cord and severe neurological damage (Danielian et al 1996). Absence of experienced practitioners at birth increases the risk of adverse outcomes, which means measures to reduce the incidence of breech presentation have become more important. These facts also emphasise the importance of practising skills when possible and the use of skill drills for labour ward staff to include hands-on simulated

breech birth (Crofts et al 2007). Chapter 9 further explores the acquisition of skills necessary for midwives to support women who choose to give birth vaginally when their baby is presenting by the breech.

Rationale for trying to avoid breech presentation

Non-cephalic presentation is one of the most common indications for elective caesarean section; however, it may also be one of the most preventable. Increasingly, it is recognised in the United Kingdom (UK), and is of international importance, that midwives and obstetricians should be actively trying to reduce the incidence of unnecessary elective caesarean section. Lewis (2007), in the Confidential Enquiry into Maternal and Child Health (CEMACH), concluded that, whilst acknowledging that for some mothers and their babies caesarean section may be the safest mode of birth, mothers must be advised that caesarean section is not without its own risk and can cause problems in current and future pregnancies. Women need to be made aware not only that caesarean section has increased risk of immediate morbidity such as bleeding, infection and deep vein thrombosis, but also that there are increasingly recognised long-term risks. The mother may suffer scar dehiscence in a subsequent pregnancy, and she has an increased risk of repeat caesarean section. As highlighted in the CEMACH report (Lewis 2007) the risk of placenta accreta and percreta also need to be taken into account when considering the risks and benefits of planned caesarean section. The report (Lewis 2007) recommends that women who have had a previous caesarean section should have placental localization in their current pregnancy to exclude placenta praevia, and, if present, further investigations to try to identify placental accrete, as deaths from this are on the increase.

Avoiding planned caesarean section

A safe alternative to planned caesarean section for breech presentation is ECV. This is the manual handling of the breech fetus through the maternal abdomen, moving the fetus from breech presentation to cephalic presentation. It is an art from the time of Aristotle (384–322 BC); the technique has been practised for thousands of years. The Royal College of Obstetricians and Gynaecologists [RCOG] (2006) recommendation is that an ECV should be offered to all women with an uncomplicated breech pregnancy at term, i.e. 37–42 weeks. Furthermore, the RCOG (2006) guideline on ECV identifies that it has been demonstrated how ECV carried out beyond 37 weeks' gestation is associated with reduction in non-cephalic births and reduction in caesarean section. A conservative estimate of the impact of performing ECV on 2% of the 750 000 pregnancies in the UK every year would be a reduction in the number of breech births by 5100 and a reduction in the number of caesarean sections by 2100. The rationale behind ECV is to reduce the incidence of breech presentation at term and, therefore, the associated risks, particularly of avoidable caesarean section.

Who should be offered an external cephalic version?

All women with a healthy physiological pregnancy other than breech presentation should be offered ECV, providing there are the facilities for caesarean section, scan, cardiotocography (CTG) and a trained practitioner available. Box 5.2 identifies the absolute contraindications to ECV and Box 5.3 outlines the relative contraindications where ECV might be considered to be more complicated and challenging.

Box 5.2

Absolute contraindications to external cephalic version

- Where caesarean birth is required for other reasons.
- Antepartum haemorrhage within the last 7 days.
- Abnormal cardiotocograph.
- Major uterine anomaly.
- Multiple pregnancy (except for birth of second twin).

What is the optimal gestation?

The Early ECV Pilot Trial (Hutton et al 2003) found that starting ECV earlier, at 34 or 35 weeks' gestation compared to 37–38, resulted in a clinically

---

Box 5.3

Relative contraindications where the risks of external cephalic version may be increased

- Small-for-gestational-age fetus with abnormal Doppler parameters.
- Proteinuric pre-eclampsia.
- Oligohydramnios.
- Major fetal anomalies.
- Scarred uterus (De Meeus et al 1998).

---

important decrease in the number of non-cephalic presentations at birth, i.e. 66/116 (56.9%) in the early ECV group and 77/116 (66.4%) in the delayed ECV group. These results are promising and suggest that there may be a real benefit to beginning the procedure early. However, the pilot study conducted by Hutton et al (2003) would suggest that early ECV does increase the risk of preterm birth and associated fetal outcomes. At the time of writing, a large collaborative ($n = 1460$ women with 730 per group) multi-centre randomised controlled trial of early ECV is being done to assess this approach further in terms of caesarean section rates and neonatal outcomes. Recruitment for the study began in December 2004 and results are expected during the course of 2009. Eighty study centres are involved internationally, including Nottingham University Hospitals NHS Trust where the author works. The study is funded by the Canadian Institute of Health Research and is jointly co-ordinated by the Maternal, Infant and Reproductive Health Research Unit in Toronto and McMaster University in Canada. Further information about the study including the trail protocol can be accessed at: http://clinicaltrials.gov/ct2/show/NCT00141687

What influences the success of external cephalic version?

The ECV practitioner is usually either a midwife or an obstetrician. The success rate is higher if the practitioner undertakes the procedure regularly thus maintaining competence and confidence in the skill. Currently, it is usual for the procedure to be offered after 36 completed weeks of pregnancy or later.

Box 5.4

Factors that influence the success rate of external cephalic version

- Race (higher success in black Africans).
- Parity (lower in primigravid women).
- Uterine tone (more successful in women with less tone).
- Liquor volume (decreased in lower liquor volume) (Haas & Magann 2005).
- Engagement of the breech and whether the head is easily palpable.
- Fetal position (extended breech more successful: see Box 5.1).
- Use of tocolytics (recommend terbutaline 0.25 mg subcutaneous 5–10 minutes prior to hands on the abdomen) (Impey & Pandit 2005).
- Maternal weight (more difficult in obese woman).
- Placental position (optimally fundal and/or posterior).

The successful version rates vary from 30% up to 80%. The factors that influence the success rate are detailed in Box 5.4.

A second attempt, particularly with a different practitioner and use of tocolytics, may lead to a small increase in overall success rates (Impey & Pandit 2005).

A low spontaneous version rate and the very low complication rate makes offering ECV from 36 weeks' gestation onwards the most common current practice. There is no upper time limit on the gestation for ECV and it has been reported as effective at 42 weeks of gestation. The author has even successfully performed ECVs in early labour, but it is recommended that the membranes should be intact to prevent cord or limb prolapse as the fetus is being turned.

Complications associated with external cephalic version

ECV should be performed where facilities for monitoring and immediate birth are available. ECV is rarely associated with complications; nevertheless, a few case reports exist of complications such as placental abruption, uterine rupture and fetomaternal haemorrhage. Trials suggest a 0.5% immediate emergency caesarean section rate and no excess perinatal morbidity or perinatal mortality (Collaris & Oei 2004, Vandenbussche & Oepkes 2005).

ECV does not appear to promote labour, but is associated with alterations in some fetal parameters. These include fetal bradycardia and a nonreactive cardiotocograph that are almost invariably transient (Hofmeyr & Sonnendecker 1983), alterations in umbilical artery and middle cerebral artery waveforms (Leung et al 2004) and an increase in amniotic fluid volume (Brost et al 1999). The significance of these features is unknown.

The procedure

The standard preoperative preparations for caesarean section are not required for women undergoing ECV. Starvation, anaesthetic premedication and intravenous access are not considered necessary due to the low complication rate. Despite the low complication rate, ECV should be performed with theatre facilities and access to immediate caesarean section.

The ECV practitioner needs to have the skill to perform ultrasound (see Chapter 4) enabling the fetal heart rate to be checked and visualization of the fetus before, during and after the procedure. Consent (usually written) is obtained from the woman. A 20-minute CTG should be performed before the procedure and only if normal should the procedure be carried out. A further CTG should be performed after an attempted ECV. The actual technique varies a little depending on personal preference. Various topical applications are used on the abdomen to prevent pulling of the maternal skin – most often talcum powder. The author has found ultrasound gel the best medium, which enables the fetal heart to be constantly heard during the procedure via cardiotocography. It also allows immediate use of the ultrasound scan probe if required.

Figure 5.1 provides a step-by-step approach to the procedure of ECV. One hand is used to remove the breech from the pelvis using a pincer grasp, a cupped hand or the flat heel of the hand. If the breech disengages the chance of success is high. While maintaining the elevated breech the other hand is placed on the fetal occiput. Seventy per cent of the pressure should be on the hand under the breech and 30% on the occiput. Most commonly a forward roll is the manoeuvre of choice. A backward roll may be considered if the forward roll is not successful or in an oblique lie when it is the shortest rotational move. Movements should be slow and steady rather than quick and jerky. There is a huge variation in the

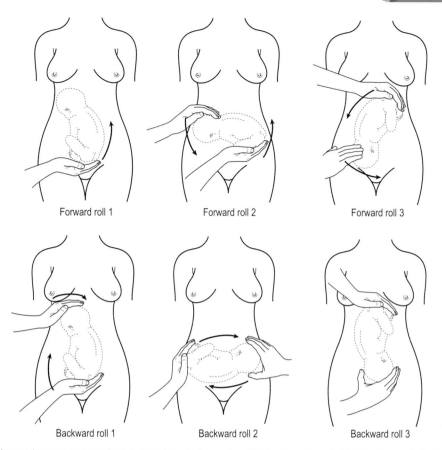

Forward roll 1   Forward roll 2   Forward roll 3

Backward roll 1   Backward roll 2   Backward roll 3

Figure 5.1 ● A step-by-step approach to external cephalic version (ECV). (From Clay et al 1993, with permission.)

amount of pressure needed to move the fetus, and most operators will try a forward roll a couple of times first then consider a backward roll before abandoning the attempt. ECV can be painful, with few women experiencing no discomfort and around 5% reporting high pain scores (Fok et al 2005). The procedure may need to be stopped because of this. Reported experience of pain is greater where the procedure fails. Following the attempt at ECV, whether successful or not, the fetal heart is checked and a CTG recommenced. As a prophylactic measure to prevent sensitization, Anti-D immunoglobulin is given to rhesus-negative women.

Is external cephalic version cost effective?

A UK study looked at the staff cost, capital cost, consumable cost and other costs of ECV service. The total expected cost of the care pathway when

ECV was offered and accepted (including the probability of adverse events) was considered and concluded by the authors to demonstrate very significant savings (James et al 2001).

Professional issues and challenges when educating and training midwives to perform external cephalic version

One of the major obstacles to introducing an ECV service is lack of formally trained personnel. Training to conduct ECV is slightly more protracted for a midwife than a doctor in the UK, as the average labour ward midwife does not have ultrasound training and cannot prescribe the tocolytic drugs. These issues can be easily overcome by undergoing a basic practical ultrasound training course with experience being concentrated on the mature fetus. This is an extremely useful skill to have available on the labour ward and will help with previously undiagnosed breech detection rate. Furthermore, a midwife will need to obtain the use of a specific Patient Group Direction (PGD) to give terbutaline for ECV procedures. Some additional training may also be considered necessary to take consent if the midwife is not used to taking formal written consent. To ensure competency supervised practice is recommended until the practitioner feels competent to deal not only with the procedure but also with any complications that may arise. Some hospitals that have previously only had obstetricians perform the procedure may also require a risk assessment to go to a hospital risk management/clinical governance committee prior to agreeing to provide vicarious liability to the midwife undertaking ECV. Midwives could also use the mechanism of statutory supervision to help them advance their knowledge, skills and proficiency in this area.

Information for women

Women need information and time to discuss the procedure of ECV both with health care professionals and with their own supporter/partner prior to the procedure. Suggested minimum information that women should be provided with is detailed in Box 5.5. Due to the fact that ECV is often successful, a policy of offering it to every woman with a breech fetus at 37 weeks should mean there will be fewer caesarean sections for breech presentation.

Some alternatives to external cephalic version

The woman should be encouraged to consider options prior to ECV if the procedure is not available, appropriate or successful. Prior to the procedure or following an unsuccessful ECV attempt women may wish to try turning techniques that can be done at home. Exercises that may or may not help are those adopting the knee-chest position. To do this, the pregnant woman kneels with her bottom in the air with hips flexed at slightly more than 90° (not letting the thighs press against the abdomen). Head, shoulders, and upper chest need to be lower that the pelvis. It is suggested if the woman is comfortable to maintain this position for

---

Box 5.5

Suggested minimum information that women should be provided with when considering external cephalic version

Women should be counselled that:

1. With a trained operator, about 50% of external cephalic version (ECV) attempts will be successful but this rate can be individualised for them using interpretation of the factors above.
2. In the UK the procedure will be done in hospital by a trained professional.
3. She may be at the hospital for up to 2 hours.
4. She will have an ultrasound scan.
5. A cardiotocograph will be undertaken and an injection will be given to relax the muscles of her uterus as this increases the success rate.
6. She should be aware that ECV is more likely to be successful if:
   a. This is not her first baby.
   b. There is plenty of amniotic fluid around her baby (Boucher et al 2003).
   c. Her baby has not yet descended into her pelvis and that:
   d. Spontaneous version to breech after successful ECV occurs in less than 5% of cases.
   e. There is a risk of 0.5% immediate emergency caesarean section following ECV is suggested (Impey & Pandit 2005) with no excess perinatal morbidity or perinatal mortality.
7. ECV can be uncomfortable and the procedure will be stopped if she wishes.

---

15 minutes every two waking hours. Alternatively, the woman may wish to try lying on her back with buttocks slightly elevated and hips and knees flexed. Then gently rolling from side to side for 10 minutes and repeat this manoeuvre three times a day.

Finally, women may wish to try moxibustion, which is a form of acupuncture currently being researched to see if it could help turn breech babies (Grabowska 2006). A lit moxa stick (a tightly packed dried herb) is held close to the skin near the outer toenail of the fifth toe which is acupuncture point B67 (Zhiyin point). The lit moxa is held very close to the skin for up to 20 minutes until vasodilatation occurs. This can be repeated twice a day. Version using moxa, according to some therapists has up to 80% success rate, but before trying it, woman should be advised to seek advice from a qualified acupuncturist via the British Acupuncture Council. Chapter 3 provides more detailed information about the use of moxibustion.

Key practice points

- All eligible women should be offered ECV.
- Efforts should be made to improve breech detection rates. Including easy access to ultrasound scan from 36 weeks' gestation (Nasser 2006).
- Expanding the inclusion criteria to offer ECV to women who have undergone one previous caesarean section will enhance the impact of ECV. There is evidence to suggest that ECV after one previous caesarean section is safe (DeMeeus et al 1998).
- Robust training packages for both midwives and obstetricians need to be implemented to train more health professionals thus ensuring the procedure is more readily available.

Acknowledgement (Carol McCormick)

I would like to thank my mentors Dr Lucy Kean and Dr Andrew Simm for kindly and patiently facilitating me in acquiring this skill.

External cephalic version: a mother's perspective (Abigail Cairns)

My experience suggests that midwives can play an important role in maintaining and promoting normal birth by their involvement with women at a time of crucial decision making.

At my 36 weeks appointment the midwife suspected I might be carrying breech, and we discussed the possibility of ECV. At the time I took the news and information fairly calmly. It wasn't until I got home and began to think about what it might mean for my birth options that I became really emotional. I realised how attached I was to the experience of birthing at home and I was determined to try anything that might enable me to achieve my birth plan. My attitude was that such a small intervention to prevent such a huge one (caesarean section) had

to be worth a try. I saw a different midwife at my next appointment who assured me that the baby was cephalic and I was elated at the prospect of my birth plan being back on track.

Then, in the typical rollercoaster ride that is pregnancy, the day before my due date at a routine antenatal appointment the doctor (who I was seeing for the first time in my pregnancy) again queried presentation, being unable to palpate anything in my pelvis. Being term, and planning a home birth I was referred immediately for a scan, at which point everything seemed to be gaining a rather alarming momentum. Neither hospital midwife nor consultant could accurately determine position on palpation, and it wasn't until the consultant scanned me that he determined that the baby was breech: to be precise OP, oblique, footling breech, just to be doubly awkward. All I heard was 'breech' and all my plans for a lovely home birth seemed to vanish in a puff of smoke.

My immediate reaction was to start madly processing my options now. I knew that with a breech it was unrealistic to expect a home birth, but felt it was really crucial to let everyone know that I was determined to avoid a caesarean section if at all possible. I hadn't registered the position of the baby properly, and realised later that there wouldn't have been a realistic chance of vaginal birth anyway, so ECV really was my only choice.

At the time all I remember is feeling really worried that I wouldn't be listened to properly and being quite anxious that I got my preferences across. The consultant had a great bedside manner and discussed my options in such a relaxed manner that I was reassured to some extent, but I was still somewhat sceptical of what his agenda or motivation might be – probably unfairly. He asked whether I had heard of the Term Breech Trial (Hannah 2000), and went on to explain the findings that recommend ECV and then caesarean section if that is unsuccessful. I knew there was some debate about this research, but being 9 months pregnant and anxious about my own care I couldn't for the life of me remember what they were. Here I was, sure of my preferences but adrift in a sea of research and protocol that I had no idea how to assess rationally. I felt utterly reliant on the consultant's information, and I was nervous about that.

I was aware that one of the midwives on the unit Carol (the lead author of this chapter) performed ECV too, and when I asked the doctor he was more than happy to see if she was available, which made me feel much more secure. He even went so far as to tell me that her rate of successful ECV was higher than his, which made me doubly confident in her care. Knowing I could talk to a midwife about this choice made me feel as though my preferences would be supported, and, indeed, I felt much less defensive when I was voicing my objection to routine caesarean section for breech, and my preference for a vaginal birth. To be totally fair, when I reflect back on the experience, the consultant also voiced his total support for my choices, but I think the essential difference was that I simply trusted midwives, and felt safe in Carol's hands.

The choices were simple – ECV or elective surgery; with the possibility of the ECV either failing or resulting in emergency surgery. Either way it was a simple choice between a relatively simple, minor intervention and major abdominal surgery with inherent risks for mother and baby. I opted for giving myself the best chance of achieving a normal birth and chose the ECV.

Carol discussed the risks and benefits with me and explained the procedure fully, and I was happy with what to expect. I was given an injection into my abdomen to help relax the uterine muscles, and then positioned on my back, slightly inclined towards one side and supported by a pillow behind my back – this she explained was to assist in the rotation of the baby. Obstetric jelly was squirted all over my tummy and Carol scanned me one more time to determine the exact position and axis of rotation. It wasn't exactly painful, more like an extremely firm massage. And, anyway, there was no way I was complaining; this was my one big chance to avoid a surgical birth and I was desperate for it to work. I was really anxious but put on a brave face as she tried numerous times, checking the baby's heart rate in between to assure herself it wasn't having an adverse reaction to the procedure. I remember feeling very red and hot which Carol commented on, and I think it was partly the physical nature of the ECV and partly the fact that I was so emotionally charged about the whole event. It was a make or break point in my pregnancy.

Carol explained that since the baby seemed to be tolerating the ECV really well she would have one last attempt and then call it a day if it didn't work this time. She placed my hands on my tummy to show me where the head was and where it needed to go, and as she started again I pushed with her, willing baby to turn with all my might. Then when she put the probe to my stomach and we saw his head nestled

down in my pelvis it was such an incredible relief. I was absolutely over the moon. Apparently it was one of the most difficult versions she had performed, but I was just content that it had worked.

I was delighted that he was head down now, but suddenly terrified of moving in case he turned. I didn't want to risk having a bath, I even wondered about going to bed that night in case lying flat made him turn around again. But I soon realised I was being ridiculous, had a long soak and got a good night's rest. The next morning we returned to the hospital to be scanned, were shown quickly into the room and it was confirmed that the baby was still cephalic. On leaving I thanked all the midwives and told them I hoped never to see them again in this pregnancy, which I think they took in the spirit in which it was meant, and then literally skipped all the way back to the car. Here we were, finally on the other side of what could have been such a huge turning point in my pregnancy, and we were back on track, back to the dreaming and mooning over plans for my lovely cosy home birth. Five days later my son Bede came into the world in the beautiful calm of a birthing pool in my dining room, in the presence of my sister and husband. Five minutes later my sister ran next door to fetch my 15-month-old daughter, mother, brother, nephew and brother-in-law to come and meet him, and they crowded in around the pool and welcomed the newest member of our family in calm and gentleness. It was the most incredible outcome and the most convincing argument I've got for ECV (see Figure 5.2).

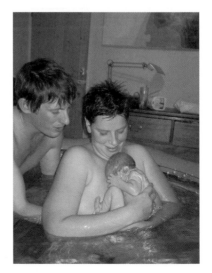

Figure 5.2 • Abigail birthing/welcoming her son Bede into the family.

References

Boucher, M., Bujold, E., Marquette, G.P., Vezina, Y., 2003. The relationship between amniotic fluid index and successful external cephalic version: a 14-year experience. Am. J. Obstet. Gynecol. 189, 751–754.

Brost, B.C., Scardo, J.A., Newman, R.B., Van Dorsten, J.P., 1999. Effect of fetal presentation on the amniotic fluid index. Am. J. Obstet. Gynecol. 181, 1222–1224.

Cheng, M., Hannah, M., 1993. Breech delivery at term: a critical review of literature. Obstet. Gynecol. 82, 605–618.

Clay, L.S., Criss, K., Jackson, U.C., 1993. External cephalic version. J. Nurse. Midwifery 38 (2 Suppl.), 72S–79S.

Collaris, R.J., Oei, S.G., 2004. External cephalic version:a safe procedure? A systematic review of version related risks. Acta. Obstet. Gynecol. Scand. 83, 511–518.

Crofts, J.F., Ellis, D., Draycott, T.J., 2007. Change in knowledge of midwives and obstetricians following obstetric emergency training: a randomised controlled trial of local hospital, simulation centre and teamwork training. BJOG 114 (12), 1534–1541.

Danielian, P.J., Wang, J., Hall, M.H., 1996. Long term outcome by method of delivery of fetuses in breech presentation at term: population based follow up. BMJ 312, 1451–1453.

De Meeus, J.B., Ellia, F., Magnim, G., 1998. ECV after previous LSCS 38 cases. Eur. J. Obstet. Gynecol. Reprod. Biol. 81, 65–68.

Fok, W.Y., Chan, L.W., Leung, T.Y., Lau, T.K., 2005. Maternal experience of pain during external cephalic version at term. Acta Obstet. Gynecol. Scand. 84, 748–751.

Grabowska, C., 2006. Turning the breech using moxibustion. RCM Midwives 9 (12), 484–485.

Haas, D.M., Magann, E.F., 2005. External cephalic version with an amniotic fluid index < or = 10: a systematic review. J. Mater.Fetal. Med 18, 249–252.

Hannah, M.E., Hannah, W.J., Hewson, S.A., Hodnett, E.D., Saigal, S., Willan, A.R. Term Breech Trial Collaborative Group, 2000. Planned caesarean section versus planned vaginal birth for breech presentation at term: a randomised multicentre trial. Lancet 356, 1375–1383.

Hofmeyr, G.J., Hannah, M.E., 2003. Planned caesarean section for term breech delivery. Cochrane Database of Systematic Reviews. Chichester, Wiley.

Hofmeyr, G.J., Sonnendecker, E.W., 1983. Cardiotocographic changes after external cephalic version. BJOG 90, 914–918.

Hutton, E.K., Kaufman, K., Hodnett, E., Amankwah, K., Hewson, S.A., McKay, D., et al., 2003. External cephalic version beginning at 34 weeks' gestation versus 37 weeks' gestation: a randomized multicenter trial. Am. J. Obstet. Gynecol. 189, 245–254.

Impey, L., Pandit, M., 2005. Tocolysis for repeat external cephalic version after a failed version for breech presentation at term: a randomised double-blind placebo controlled trial. BJOG 112, 627–631.

James, M., Hunt, K., Burr, R., Johanson, R., 2001. A decision analytical cost analysis of offering ECV in a UK district general hospital. Bio-Medical Central Health Service Research 1, 6. Accessible at: http://www.pubmedcentral.nih.gov

Leung, T.Y., Sahota, D.S., Fok, W.Y., Chan, L.W., Lau, T.K., 2004. External cephalic version induced fetal cerebral and umbilical blood flow changes are related to the amount of pressure exerted. BJOG 111, 430–435.

Lewis, G. (Ed.), 2007. The Confidential Enquiry into Maternal and Child Health (CEMACH). Saving Mothers' Lives: reviewing maternal deaths to make motherhood safer – 2003–2005. The Seventh Report on Confidential Enquiries into Maternal Deaths in the United Kingdom, CEMACH, London.

Nasser, N., Roberts, C.L., Cameron, C.A., Olive, C.E., 2006. Diagnostic accuracy of clinical examination for detection of non cephalic presentation in late pregnancy a cross sectional analytic study. BMJ 333, 578–580.

Royal College of Obstetricians and Gynaecologists, 2006. External cephalic version and reducing the incidence of breech presentation; Guideline No. 20. RCOG, London.

Vandenbussche, F.P., Oepkes, D., 2005. The effect of the term breech trial on medical intervention behaviour and neonatal outcome in The Netherlands: an analysis of 35,453 term breech infants. BJOG 112, 1163.

Further reading

Olof, A., Bixo, M., Högberg, U., 2005. Evidence-based changes in term breech delivery in Sweden. Acta. Obstet. Gynecol. Scand. 84, 584–587.

This text provides an international perspective on the management of breech presentation at term.

Useful websites

British Acupuncture Council: www.acupuncture.org.uk

Royal College of Obstetricians and Gynaecologists: www.rcog.org.uk

For reports on the Confidential Enquiries into Maternal and Child Health as well as the Confidential Enquiries into Stillbirths and Deaths in Infancy: www.cemach.org.uk

Chapter Six

Peripheral intravenous cannulation

Maureen D. Raynor

CONTENTS

Introduction 57
Peripheral intravenous cannulation:
redefining the role of the midwife 58
Legal and professional responsibilities
of the midwife 58
   Developing competency in new skills . . 58
   Education/training 59
   Accountability 60
   Legal responsibility 60
   Consent: informed or valid 61
   Negligence 61
   Proof of negligence 61
   Reasonable care 62
   Vicarious liability 62
   Record keeping 62
Conclusion 64
Key practice points 65
References 65
Further reading 66
Useful website 66

Before reading this chapter, you should be familiar with:
- Cannulation devices, optimal sites and procedure for intravenous peripheral cannulation.
- Risk-management procedures, including health and safety issues, e.g. prevention of infection and safe disposal of sharps.
- Ethico-legal frameworks.
- Statutory rules, standards and professional codes governing the midwife's practice.

- Prevention, recognition and management of anaphylaxis.
- The importance of evidence-based practice.
- The value of inter-professional working.
- Key recommendations from CEMACH on critical care skills (Lewis 2007).
- Local NHS Hospital Trust's policies/guidelines on intravenous cannulation as well as their Code of Practice on Medicine administration involving intravenous bolus injections and intravenous therapy.
- Patient Group Directions (PGDs).

Introduction

Many midwives have been undertaking the paramedical skill of peripheral intravenous cannulation (PIVC) for some time, even before socio-political influences resulted in a reduction in junior doctors' hours (Department of Health [DH] 2002). This chapter will examine the legal and professional issues associated with PIVC. The actual equipment, technique and procedure for PIVC will not be addressed as these aspects are well documented elsewhere (Ingram & Lavery 2007, Johnson & Taylor 2006, Scales 2005, Trim 2005). The chapter is primarily aimed at midwives who already perform PIVC or those seeking to gain competency in the skill, to pause and reflect on their practice. It will also be of relevance to other health care professionals with a specialist interest in the subject matter.

Peripheral intravenous cannulation: redefining the role of the midwife

The government's modernising agenda committed to strengthening education/training as well as inter-professional working and leadership in the health service, means that midwifery practice cannot be static (DH 2000, 2001a, 2004a). It has to be a dynamic process that keeps evolving and adapting to change. PIVC is already an integral part of many midwives' practice, at least for those practising within the United Kingdom (UK). Midwives' professional and medico-legal responsibility in relation to PIVC goes beyond the realms of their pre-registration education/training programme. Midwives work in different settings; most are employed within the National Health Service (NHS) and care for women at home or hospitals. A small percentage of midwives are self-employed, commonly referred to as independent practitioners. Whatever the setting, PIVC can be an invaluable skill especially when dealing with a maternity emergency such as major haemorrhage. At the University of Nottingham close collaboration with Nottingham University Hospitals NHS Trust has resulted in PIVC skill development workshops being incorporated within the pre-registration curricula. These sessions are usually open to midwives who want to develop their knowledge and proficiency on PIVC or those wanting to access the session as an update. Midwives and students embracing this topic within the professional issues/preparation for professional practice module, are encouraged to seek experience via direct supervision from an experienced colleague (or sign-off mentor(s) in the case of students) skilled in the practice of PIVC, link/liaison teachers who work on the labour suite or doctors such as anaesthetists. It is found that involving other disciplines fosters good working relationships. Through negotiation and inter-professional collaboration, some anaesthetists are willing for midwives and students to accompany them to day surgery, where the skill of PIVC can readily be practised with consent from clients.

Being skilled at PIVC assists midwives in their autonomous role, and helps to meet the diverse, changing and complex health care needs of childbearing women. Women do not have to wait for a doctor to be available to site the cannula, for

Box 6.1

Possible indications for peripheral intravenous cannulation in midwifery practice

- To administer intravenous bolus injections e.g. antibiotics.
- To commence intravenous fluids/blood transfusion as per medicine prescription chart.
- Commencement of syntocinon infusion.
- Prior to an epidural (usually whilst waiting for the anaesthetist).
- In an emergency such as major postpartum haemorrhage.

example for the administration of intravenous antibiotics, hydration prior to an epidural or the commencement of syntocinon infusion during induction of labour. Ultimately this reduces time delays and frustrations, culminating in women's satisfaction with their care. Moreover, pregnancy and childbirth are unpredictable events. The midwife is often the main professional carer with women during labour, and may find a number of situations necessitate PIVC as detailed in Box 6.1.

Legal and professional responsibilities of the midwife

The legal and professional implications of PIVC as highlighted by Hyde (2002) are manifold. Midwives wishing to undertake the procedure should not do so unless they are competent and working within the remit of their employer's guidelines, policies and procedures. The employer is not under any legal obligation to support the individual midwife unless she has completed an appropriate education/training programme and competency package to provide evidence of proficiency.

Developing competency in new skills

Competence can be defined as knowledge, skill or judgement that equips the midwife to perform her professional duties safely and effectively. Because PIVC is a relatively new skill being embraced by midwives, Rule 6 of the Nursing and Midwifery

Council (NMC 2004, p. 19) *Midwives Rules and Standards* delineates the midwife's responsibility and sphere of professional practice. Therefore, developments in midwifery practice that frequently become inextricably linked to the role of the midwife, may become incorporated into the initial preparation of midwives via the pre-registration curricula, e.g. perineal repair. Other developments that require midwives to learn new skills that are not necessarily an integral part of the midwife's role should be the responsibility of the employing authority. This can be realised through a locally agreed guideline, with input from supervisors of midwives to ensure the NMC standards are reflected and fulfilled.

Midwives are responsible for maintaining and developing the competence they have acquired during initial and subsequent midwifery education. Practice does not take place in a vacuum. It occurs in a context of continuing change and development that must be sensitive, relevant and responsive and have the capacity to adjust, where and when appropriate to service demands in order to be effective. Providing an integrated and holistic approach to care during pregnancy and childbirth takes effort and vision. The burgeoning growth in a midwife's role and professional responsibilities extends to many new skills. The NMC (2008a) *'The Code: Standards of conduct, performance and ethics for nurses and midwives'* guides the midwife to practise safely, autonomously and accountably within their sphere of professional practice. It outlines three key areas

that need to be considered when developing new skills, these are previously outlined in Chapter 2, and relates to maintenance of professional knowledge, competence and acknowledgement of personal limitations in order to exercise accountability and achieve safe practice. To achieve this Figure 6.1 reflects the statutory and expected standard of professional behaviour and practice highlighting that, because midwives are personally accountable for their practice, they must have a clear understanding of the dimensions of accountability before carrying out PIVC. It also provides a framework for the midwife to enhance and strengthen her practice providing that this is realised in accordance with professional knowledge, competence and employer's guidelines, policies and procedures. Before undertaking the task of peripheral intravenous cannulation, the midwife will fulfil her professional and legal obligations if she has a sound knowledge base and skills relating to venepuncture, intravenous bolus injections, administration and care of intravenous fluids.

Education/training

The midwife must complete a programme of education and training for PIVC similar to that detailed by the Royal College of Nursing [RCN] (2005) competency framework. Box 6.2 outlines a programme for PIVC. It is necessary that midwives are able to work within defined parameters to

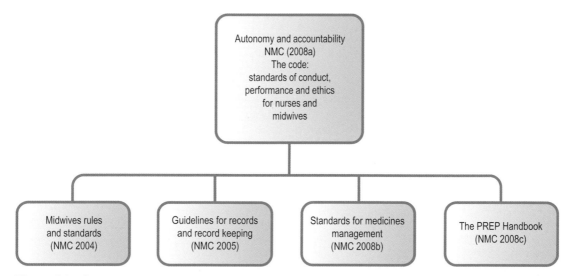

Figure 6.1 • Statutory and expected standard of professional behaviour/practice.

Box 6.2

Content of what an educational programme for peripheral intravenous cannulation may include

- Aims and learning outcomes.
- Knowledge of cannulation devices and rationale for their use.
- Knowledge of how to select the best site for cannulation.
- Knowledge of local NHS Trust policies/guidelines and Patient Group Directions.
- Medico-legal/professional responsibilities.
- Risk management issues (including prevention, recognition and management of complications).
- Infection control.
- Ethical considerations.
- Competencies and proficiencies to be achieved.
- Methods of assessment:
  - work-based learning packages.
  - e-learning.
  - problem-solving activities.
  - reflective activities.
  - demonstration or simulation with direct observation/supervision.
  - formal examination.
  - portfolio of evidence to account for the development of knowledge, experience, skills, proficiencies, details of when the skill was practised (e.g. time, date and name of the supervising practitioner) and practice-based assessments.

achieve proficiency in the skill. Some NHS Trusts, for example, will specify the number of PIVCs that midwives should undertake before they are deemed competent. Whilst others will recognise the heterogeneity of midwives in that each midwife has individual needs, and will become competent at their own pace. In such instances a minimum number for achievement may be specified, as some will achieve competency in the skill after a few attempts whilst others will need to practise the skill many times before they feel confident in their abilities to determine that they are proficient. Training mannequins for demonstration and simulation in skills and competency centres or the practice environment should be available, as well as other resources such as DVDs, CD-ROMs and web-based learning packages.

Accountability

There are numerous ways in which professional accountability may arise in midwifery practice. The concept of clinical governance has highlighted the need for midwives to adhere to quality standards whilst recognising their professional accountability in every sphere of their practice (Dimond 2006, Sale 2005, Swage 2000). Midwives are legally answerable for their professional conduct, omissions in care, their actions as well as any harm they may have caused to the woman during the course of their professional practice. This element of accountability remains whether or not the midwife acted on the advice or directions of a colleague or doctor. Midwives accounting for their actions, may take the form of being liable for litigation damages through the civil courts should the conditions relating to the law of negligence be met (Dimond 2006). They must, therefore, be familiar with the NMC (2004) *Midwives Rules and Standards* as well as *The Code* (NMC 2008a). In relation to the latter, midwives should consider the individuality of the client group for which they care. This means keeping in mind any aspect of women's culture, lifestyle, communication and religious needs that might impact on cannulation. Additionally, they must be conversant with risk management, the purpose of midwifery supervision and how to exercise their accountability in justifying the rationale for the intervention of PIVC. Their decision making should be based on best evidence, and ensure that women have been given every opportunity to give valid consent.

Legal responsibility

Midwives have a legal responsibility to women, their employer, their professional body and themselves, and should be conversant with local policies and guidelines in relation to cannulation. In the UK the law stipulates that all health care professionals must take *reasonable* care to avoid acts or omissions, which can be reasonably foreseen as being likely to cause injury to the recipient of their care. Pivotal to this is that all practising midwives must have an understanding of the law and how it relates to their actions. Midwives have a duty of care to mothers and babies, and if they should deviate from their duty of care, or cause actual harm, they become liable. In other words they are responsible for their actions. Minimising and preventing infection is a part of the midwife's responsibility that can be realised by following correct hand-washing procedures (Teare et al 2001). Good hand hygiene is often cited as the single most effective weapon in the arsenal of infection control (Chalmers & Straub 2006, DH 2003, 2004b, 2005, Hindley 2004, Ingram & Lavery 2005, 2006). The midwife is, therefore, charged with the responsibility of thinking through the actions that are taken in relation to cannulation. Not undertaking a practice in which she is neither proficient nor confident in performing should always be the guiding principle.

Consent: informed or valid

There is no concept of informed consent in law. A midwife seeking consent must determine to what a reasonable person is likely to attach significance. The DH (2000) *NHS Plan* provides assurance that consent must be sought from all NHS service users. This has resulted in the DH (2001b) *Reference guide to consent* establishing key principles that the midwife should be familiar with, known as the *12 key points on consent: the Law in England and Wales*. The law makes it clear that consent can be withheld or withdrawn at anytime providing that the individual has the mental capacity (Hotopf 2004). The midwife should consider issues of consent and how they relate to cannulation when seeking it from a woman for PIVC; establish that information framing will result in full comprehension of the issues, i.e. the reason(s) for the intervention and the associated risks.

The midwife must bear in mind that consent not based on understanding cannot be deemed to be valid. This is especially challenging during labour when the woman is usually in pain and might be anxious. Box 6.3 outlines a five-point plan *aide memoir* for the midwife when seeking consent for PIVC, which can be applied to other clinical situations.

Negligence

The concept of negligence law relates to conduct that falls below the standards of behaviour established by law to protect others from unreasonable risk of harm or damage. It comes under the law of Torts (Dimond 2006) and deals with acts or omissions that culminates in harm. The notion of the *'unreasonable person'* is crucial in this context as it provides the standard by which a midwife's professional conduct is judged. 'Tort' law is the term employed to describe

---

Box 6.3

Five-point plan when seeking consent for peripheral intravenous cannulation

- Information communicated is clear, accessible and comprehensible.
- An explanation of the purpose for the intervention/treatment is readily communicated to the woman.
- The existence of any alternatives is related to the woman to help her make an informed decision, and also respects, promotes and supports the woman's rights, preferences and cultural beliefs.
- Any substantial risks including side-effects of the intervention/treatment are outlined. It is crucial that the midwife establishes whether or not the woman has a known latex allergy.
- Women are provided with every opportunity to seek clarification and ask questions to ensure they fully understand the significance of PIVC.

Consent can only be valid if the woman receiving the information perceives it as having addressed all of the above key components.

---

a body of law that seeks to provide resolution for civil wrongs that do not arise out of contractual obligations. A woman injured as a result of PIVC as outlined in Box 6.4 may be able to mobilise the law of Torts to pursue damages, i.e. compensation from the midwife or employing organisation legally responsible or 'liable' for damages.

Proof of negligence

The midwife could be negligent if she does not follow local policy and guidelines and is not adequately educated/trained or assessed to be competent in performing cannulation. Negligence would be proven if it is clear that the practitioner carrying out the cannulation owed the woman a duty of care and if in

---

Box 6.4

Case study: negligence

A woman who had an intravenous cannula sited by a midwife during labour experienced complications due to damage caused during venous access, and has written a letter of complaint during the postnatal period, claiming that the midwife was negligent in her duty of care.

performing the skill the duty of care was not exercised and, as a result of this, harm was done to the woman. In making judgement on whether or not the midwife (defendant) had acted unreasonably in her duty of care, the woman (claimant) has the burden of proof to demonstrate in her evidence, beyond any reasonable doubt, the midwife's culpability. In law negligence has three necessary elements:

- A duty of care.
- Breach in that duty of care whether by omission or neglect.
- This act of omission/neglect resulted in harm/ damage.

This forms the basis of professional standard by which a midwife, doctor or nurse would be judged, taking into consideration knowledge, skills, experience and competence. Here the Bolam principle (Bolam v Friern Hospital Management Committee 1957) is usually applied, which is based on the standard of care and skill of a competent midwife that is commensurate with her field of practice, as judged by her peers. Judgement would be formulated as a rule that the midwife is not negligent if actions taken were reflective of practice at the time the incident occurred and is deemed as proper by a responsible body of opinion (the expert witnesses).

Reasonable care

The standard of care expected of midwives, nurses or doctors will depend on the nature of their employment, as well as their designation and experience. A registered midwife who performs PIVC is expected to exhibit skills mindful of the conditions of the Bolam principle, and the dimensions of her professional accountability.

Vicarious liability

In law vicarious liability occurs when one person is held responsible for the negligence of another. Usually, this applies in an employment context, where the employer is responsible or liable for the reasonable actions of employees whilst they are on duty. Compensation may have to be paid out due to the midwife's negligent actions or omissions. It is important that midwives understand they may find themselves involved in disciplinary, professional, criminal or civil proceedings. Midwives employed by the NHS may find that their employer will accept responsibility for their practice around PIVC providing they undertook the appropriate education/training programme approved by the organisation. Additionally, they must have adhered to clinical guidelines, policies, followed risk management procedures and demonstrated evidence based care (Hyde 2002). Service providers must protect their employees via indemnity cover for clinical negligence liabilities. Clinical Negligence Scheme for Trusts (CNST) is a statutory indemnity scheme managed by the NHS Litigation Authority. However, independent midwives are not protected by this scheme. They will need their own indemnity cover in case of any complaint of negligence and the pursuit of a compensation claim. It is hoped that independent midwives through social enterprise, an initiative welcomed by the UK government (DH 2007), will be able to have affordable insurance cover via the commissioning process.

Record keeping

The quality of record keeping reflects the standard of professional practice. Therefore, effective record keeping is one of the hallmarks of a skilled and safe practitioner. Conversely, careless or incomplete record keeping often highlights wider problems with an individual's practice. Midwives will be familiar with the mantra 'if it is not recorded, it has not been done'. Rule 9 of the *Midwives Rules and Standards* (NMC 2004) highlights the requirements for record keeping. The midwife should use this in conjunction with the NMC (2005) *Guidelines for records and record keeping* that requires an accurate, contemporaneous and comprehensive record of actions relating to all aspects of treatment, care planning and delivery. Any actions or omissions on the midwife's part must not compromise the safety of women. In terms of PIVC professional judgement must be used to decide what is relevant and what should be recorded. As concise information is required, Figure 6.2 is a good example of best practice, where an adhesive label covering essential components of PIVC can be completed and inserted in the woman's records. The principal aim of the label is to help and safeguard against infection. In essence this standardises the information health care professionals need to record about the intervention and their adherence to risk-management procedures, including infection control and health and safety issues. This allows for transparency when records are audited.

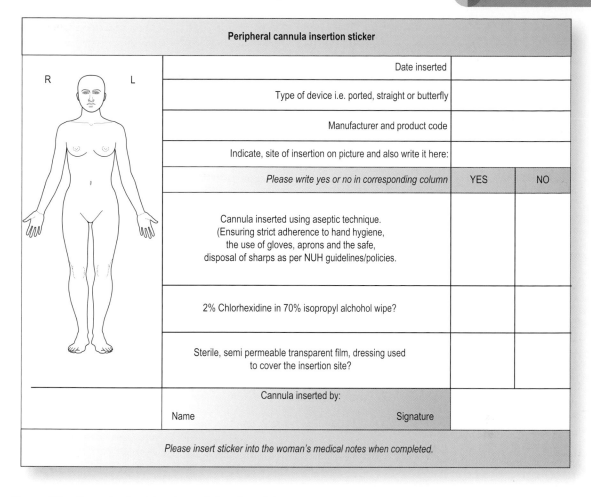

Peripheral cannula insertion sticker		
Date inserted		
Type of device i.e. ported, straight or butterfly		
Manufacturer and product code		
Indicate, site of insertion on picture and also write it here:		
Please write yes or no in corresponding column	YES	NO
Cannula inserted using aseptic technique. (Ensuring strict adherence to hand hygiene, the use of gloves, aprons and the safe, disposal of sharps as per NUH guidelines/policies.		
2% Chlorhexidine in 70% isopropyl alchohol wipe?		
Sterile, semi permeable transparent film, dressing used to cover the insertion site?		
Cannula inserted by: Name Signature		

Please insert sticker into the woman's medical notes when completed.

Figure 6.2 • Example of peripheral cannula insertion sticker. (Reproduced with kind permission from Nottingham University Hospitals NHS Trust.)

Health care records are any document which records any aspect of care that may be called in evidence before a court of law by the Care Quality Commission, new health and social care regulator in England or in order to investigate a complaint at local level. Midwives should be mindful that these records may also be used in evidence by the NMCs Fitness to Practise Committee. In order to fulfil professional and legal duties of care, record keeping relating to PIVC should be able to account for the assessment and the care that has been planned and provided. It should also include relevant information given to the woman for the care intervention, her care needs and condition as well as the measures taken to respond to these needs. Records should provide evidence that the midwife has understood and honoured her duty of care and all reasonable steps have been taken to care for the woman. Figure 6.3 reinforces the midwife's accountability in the context of record keeping.

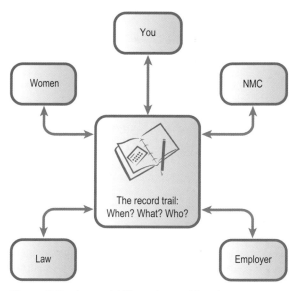

Figure 6.3 • Accountability and record keeping.

Table 6.1 Intravenous peripheral cannulation – skills checklist

	Date and sign	
	Achieved	Not achieved
Prepares woman taking in consideration comfort		
Explains procedure and communicates well with the woman in language she can understand in order to obtain consent		
Identifies the causes of needle stick injury		
Identifies strategies to avoid needle stick injury		
Explains the procedure to deal with needle stick injury		
Identifies the best sites for cannulation		
Explains the criteria for cannula choice and fixation dressings		
Has knowledge of the complications of cannulation		
Demonstrates preparedness in assembling equipment ahead of the procedure, i.e. considers use of latex-free equipment, tourniquet, chooses appropriate size cannula, gloves, sharps bin, 2% chlorhexidine in 70% isopropyl alcohol wipe, needles syringes, blood collecting bottles and IV fluids (if required) and appropriate allergy-free fixation dressings		
Takes precautions to prevent/minimise infection, e.g. maintains asepsis including thorough hand-washing and considers woman's HIV and hepatitis status		
Demonstrates empathy in minimising pain/discomfort, e.g. use of local anaesthetic, talking, attending and listening to the woman		
Employs good technique to stabilise the vein and immobilise the limb		
Secures the cannula by applying appropriate dressing		
Safely disposes of sharps and other relevant equipment following the procedure		
Record keeping: complete contemporaneous records, i.e. cannula size, date and time of insertion, dressing used and any special orders/follow-up.		

Table 6.1 provides a checklist for midwives to use when supervising others acquiring the skill of cannulation. This can form part of the midwife's ongoing professional portfolio, as well as a knowledge, skills and competency package.

Conclusion

Increasingly midwives have to enhance not only their practical skills but also their knowledge, clinical judgement and decision-making skills in order to respond to service demands. Working in new ways can result in a radical shift for midwives as they push the margins of their historically defined professional boundaries to develop new skills. Peripheral intravenous cannulation is now an integral part of contemporary midwifery practice. Therefore, as an autonomous and accountable practitioner it is the midwife's responsibility to ensure that her knowledge, skills and competence are kept up to date. In order to make informed decisions and exercise professional judgement this should include the associated risks of the procedure, infection control and legal and professional issues. There is no set guidance on the maintenance of competence that states when practice should be updated. It should be noted that each midwife is responsible for reviewing and updating her own practice. A hallmark of best practice is to update at least every 3 years (NMC 2008c). It is important that midwives are adequately prepared to meet the challenges of their professional role.

Key practice points

- Women must be fully informed of the rationale for PIVC as well as the risks.
- Women deemed to be mentally competent can exercise their autonomy and choose not to undergo PIVC.
- Practice must be current, reasonable and evidence-based.
- Records provide evidence of communication, care provided, decision making, adherence to infection control policy and the rationale for PIVC.

- Midwives must work in accordance with their statutory framework, NMC standard and ethical principles.
- Employers may be held liable for the actions of the midwives they employ, if they incur liabilities in the course of the employer's business, even though the employer may not be directly at fault.

References

Bolam v Friern Hospital Management Committee, 1957. WRL 582.

Chalmers, C., Straub, M., 2006. Standard principles for preventing and controlling infection. Nurs. Stand. 20 (23), 57–65.

Department of Health, 2000. NHS plan: a plan for investment, a plan for reform. Available online: www.dh.gov.uk Accessed 22 March 2008.

Department of Health, 2001a. Making a difference: the nursing, midwifery and health visiting contribution – the midwifery action plan. Available online: www.dh.gov.uk Accessed 22 March 2008.

Department of Health, 2001b. Reference guide to consent for examination or treatment. Available online: www.dh.gov.uk Accessed 22 March 2008.

Department of Health, 2002. Guidance on working patterns for junior doctors: a document produced jointly by the department of health. The National Assembly for Wales, The NHS Confederation and the British Medical Association. Available online: www.dh.gov.uk Accessed 22 March 2008.

Department of Health, 2003. Winning ways: working together to reduce healthcare associated infection in England. Available online: www.dh.gov.uk Accessed 22 March 2008.

Department of Health, 2004a. The NHS Knowledge and Skills Framework (NHS KSF) and the development review process. Available online: www.dh.gov.uk Accessed 22 March 2008.

Department of Health, 2004b. Towards cleaner hospitals and lower rates of infection. Available online: www.dh.gov.uk Accessed 22 March 2008.

Department of Health, 2005. Saving lives: a delivery programme to reduce healthcare associated infection (HCAI) including MRSA. Available online: www.dh.gov.uk Accessed 22 March 2008.

Department of Health, 2007. Welcoming social enterprise into health and social care: a resource pack for social enterprise providers and commissioners, Available online: www.dh.gov.uk Accessed 27 May 2008.

Dimond, B., 2006. Legal aspects of midwifery. Books for Midwives Press, Cheshire.

Hindley, G., 2004. Infection control in peripheral cannulae. Nurs. Stand. 18 (27), 37–40.

Hotopf, M., 2004. Mental capacity and valid consent. Psychiatry 3 (3), 8–10.

Hyde, L., 2002. Legal and professional aspects of intravenous therapy. Nurs. Stand. 16 (26), 39–42.

Ingram, P., Lavery, I., 2005. Peripheral intravenous therapy: key risks and implications for practice. Nurs. Stand. 19 (46), 55–64.

Ingram, P., Lavery, I., 2006. Prevention of infection in peripheral intravenous devices. Nurs. Stand. 20 (49), 49–56.

Ingram, P., Lavery, I., 2007. Peripheral intravenous cannulation: safe insertion and removal technique. Nurs. Stand. 22 (1), 44–48.

Johnson, R., Taylor, W., 2006. Skills for midwifery practice, second ed. Churchill Livingstone, Edinburgh.

Lewis, G. (Ed), 2007. The confidential enquiry into maternal and child health (CEMACH) saving mothers' lives: reviewing maternal deaths to make motherhood safer – 2003–2005 the seventh report of the confidential enquiries into maternal deaths in the United Kingdom. CEMACH, London.

Nursing and Midwifery Council, 2004. Midwives rules and standards. NMC, London.

Nursing and Midwifery Council, 2005. Guidelines for records and record keeping. NMC, London.

Nursing and Midwifery Council, 2008a. The code: standards of conduct, performance and ethics for nurses and midwives. NMC, London.

Nursing and Midwifery Council, 2008b. Standards of medicine management. NMC, London.

Nursing and Midwifery Council, 2008c. The PREP handbook. NMC, London.

Royal College of Nursing, 2005.
Competencies: an education and
training competency framework for
peripheral venous cannulation in
children and young people. Available
online: www.rcn.org.uk Accessed
21 March 2008.

Sale, D., 2005. Understanding clinical
governance and quality assurance:
making it happen. Palgrave
Macmillan, Houndmills.

Scales, K., 2005. Vascular access: a guide
to peripheral venous cannulation.
Nurs. Stand. 19 (49), 48–52.

Swage, T., 2000. Clinical governance in
health care practice. Butterworth
Heinemann, Oxford.

Teare, L., Cookson, B., Stone, S., 2001.
Hand hygiene. BMJ 323 (7310),
411–412.

Trim, J.C., 2005. Peripheral intravenous
catheters: considerations in theory
and practice. Br. J. Nurs. 14 (12),
654–658.

Further reading

National Patient Safety Agency, 2004.
Right patient – right care. www.npsa.
nhs.uk
*Emphasis placed on basic principles
of client identification to prevent
errors in practice.*

Raynor, M.D., Marshall, J.E., Sullivan, A.,
2005. Decision making in midwifery
practice. Churchill Livingstone,
Edinburgh.

*This text outlines decision making
frameworks that midwives can utilise
as their role shifts beyond the
traditionally defined professional
boundaries.*

Royal College of Nursing, 2003.
Standards for infusion therapy.
RCN, London.
*Gives useful information on infusion
devices and related complications.*

Tagalakis, V., Kahn, S.R., Libman, M.,
Blostein, M., 2002. The
epidemiology of peripheral
vein infusion thrombophlebitis:
a critical review. Am. J. Med.
113 (2), 146–151.
*Provides a critical perspective on one of
the common complications associated
with intravenous therapy/devices.*

Useful Website

www.socialenterprise.org.uk/
healthandcare for detailed
information on social enterprise
or
www.dh.gov.uk

Chapter Seven

7

Midwives undertaking ventouse births

Vicky Tinsley

CONTENTS

Introduction 67
Background: why some midwives
undertake ventouse births 68
The midwife ventouse practitioner:
barriers and opportunities 69
Ventouse extraction: the practicalities . . . 69
   Safety measures 69
   Guidelines 69
   Before vacuum extraction 69
   During vacuum extraction 70
Training and practice procedures 70
Recruitment of midwife ventouse
practitioners 70
The benefits of midwives undertaking
ventouse births 71
The procedure 71
Women's responses 71
Training 72
Accountability 72
   Record keeping 72
Personal reflections 72
Conclusion 74
Key practice points 74
References 74
Further reading 75

Before reading this chapter, you should be familiar with:
- Intravenous peripheral cannulation (see Chapter 6) and perineal suturing (see Chapter 10).
- Interpretation of cardiotocography (NICE 2007).
- Communication skills.
- Clinical governance/risk-management procedures.
- Clinical guidelines and local National Health Service (NHS) Trust policies.
- The importance of clinical competence when acquiring new skills and the maintenance of records such as professional portfolio.
- Guidelines for conducting a ventouse birth.
- The necessary equipment required to perform a ventouse birth.
- Legal and ethical considerations such as consent.

Introduction

The evidence base for one-to-one care in labour is strong and irrefutable (Hodnett et al 2007). Performing ventouse vacuum extraction is not about frustrating and disempowering midwives and women by introducing yet more medical intervention in the process of normal childbirth. Through working in a woman-centred way, midwives are well placed to ensure that medical interventions are only used when absolutely necessary to treat problems with the full involvement of the woman. Ventouse extraction should only be employed when midwives have exhausted all the skills in their repertoire in helping women to have a normal spontaneous birth. It is essential that midwives can articulate their effectiveness and justify the value in having them perform ventouse extraction, rather than being seen as cheaper providers of care. Ventouse extraction is a method used more commonly than forceps.

The ventouse uses a vacuum extraction – an instrument that applies traction. It can be used as an alternative to forceps. The cup clings to the baby's scalp by suction and is used to assist maternal effort. This chapter will identify why it is important to rethink the role of the midwife to develop competence in the skill of ventouse vacuum extraction. The aim of the chapter is twofold:

- To place emphasis on competence and fitness to practise by exploring the professional issues that must be fulfilled by any midwife who wishes to become a ventouse practitioner.
- To provide a clear account and a step-by-step guide for the procedure of ventouse extraction.

Background: why some midwives undertake ventouse births

Complete obstetric care (antenatal, intrapartum and postnatal) used to be a normal, essential part of British general practice (Smith & Jewell 1999). The norm now is for general practitioners (GPs) to provide only antenatal and postnatal care. The number of women giving birth under the care of their GP has steadily decreased from more than 85% to about 15% in 1975 (Royal College of Obstetrics and Gynaecologists 1981). Now in the 21st century this figure has further declined to well below 10%. Concomitantly there has been an increase in institutional birth (Marsh et al 1985). However, in a survey conducted by Hewison (2004) it was found that only 7% of GPs attended a birth within the last year of the study period.

Various factors have been proposed to explain the reluctance of GPs to be involved in intrapartum care. These include fear of litigation, the high cost of medical insurance, declining clinical competence, lack of training, interference with lifestyle, medico-political pressure, practice type, lack of role models, lack of time and training, inadequate remuneration and lack of role definition. Given the range and number of reasons it is not surprising that there has been a major reduction of intrapartum care by GPs (Smith 1992, Wiegers 2003, Young 1991). The current picture is that of a few enthusiasts to continue this work if at all possible. However, their numbers are dwindling.

A significant change in emphasis was signalled in 1992 with the publication of the House of Commons Health Committee report on maternity services (House of Commons Health Committee 1992). This publication ubiquitously known as the 'Winterton' report considered evidence which supported the view that home births in lower technology units were not detrimental to either the health of mother or baby in low-risk pregnancies. The report supported less medically orientated maternity care, more choice for women as to their intended place of birth and endorsed home birth as a valid option. This change in direction was supported by the Department of Health (DH 1993) report, *Changing childbirth*, which advocated greater choice for women on how and where they could give birth.

However, many GPs were reluctant to take up the challenge and gradually the community units previously known as 'GP units' have become known as 'midwife-led units'. The midwives had always provided most of the intrapartum care in a majority of GP units, but called in local GPs on the obstetric list to perform forceps births. In recent times the practice has been to transfer women needing more interventions, by ambulance to consultant units (Walker 2000). Over the last 20 years or so the ventouse vacuum method of facilitating birth has become widely used for certain problems in the second stage of labour. If GPs were no longer available to perform forceps births in community units, the logical next step was to train midwives to assist women to undergo ventouse extractions.

The latest policy document *Maternity matters* (DH 2007a) places great emphasis on choice, access and continuity of care in a safe service and builds upon the maternity services commitment outlined in *Our health, our care, our say* (DH 2007b). This is an important step towards meeting the maternity standards set out in the *National service framework for children, young people and maternity services* (DH 2004). Its aim was to ensure that all children and young people access services that are age related and recognize their needs are different.

Our health, our care, our say (DH 2007b) sets out the government's commitment to the importance of providing high-quality, safe and accessible maternity care through its commitment to offer all women and their partners a wide choice of type and place of maternity care and birth. The priority is to provide a choice of safe, high-quality maternity care for all women and their partners. This will enable pregnancy and birth to be as safe and satisfying as possible for both mother and baby, and provide support to new parents.

The main aim of these health reforms in England is to develop a patient-led NHS that uses the available resources as effectively and fairly as possible. Therefore, the principle should be that pregnancy and birth are normal life events supported by midwives. Thus one of the lynch pins to a quality maternity service is the decision making undertaken by individual midwives as well as those responsible for the organisation as to the best available evidence. To support this, midwives need to develop new skills as highlighted in the publication *Making a difference* (DH 1999), and are well placed to take on new initiatives.

The midwife ventouse practitioner: barriers and opportunities

Many midwives see the development of the midwife ventouse practitioner (MVP) as a step too far away from the principles of midwifery philosophy; a development which threatens the fundamental role of midwives. Some fear that this turns midwives into a hybrid doctor/midwife, or obstetric nurse/technician, and away from their role of a midwife as being 'with women'. Antagonists have feared that MVPs would be too quick to intervene when patience and other midwifery skills may be enough to result in a normal birth because 'they could do a ventouse'. Some midwives locally have also been concerned that, like perineal suturing and peripheral intravenous cannulation, this skill would eventually be required of all midwives.

However, many others have welcomed the initiative believing that it may restore pride in the profession and enhance client satisfaction (Charles 1999). The *Code* (Nursing and Midwifery Council [NMC] 2008) confirms that midwives may go outside traditional parameters to improve care, provided they are educated and trained appropriately and have the support of both managers and supervisors of midwives. Dimond (1999) suggests that it could be argued that there is no limit placed by legislation upon the activities which a midwife can perform provided that she has the skill, training and competence. Midwives should not be frightened to contemplate radical changes to the way in which they work. It could also be argued that there are dangers in the midwifery profession clinging emotionally to specific activities rather than providing a holistic service to women.

Ventouse extraction: the practicalities

Safety measures

Safety of ventouse extraction depends on careful consideration of a number of factors, several of which may be evaluated before the procedure, many during the procedure itself and a few after the procedure is completed.

Guidelines

Guidelines are an indispensable security net which ensures that all professional groups are confident that the roles undertaken by each group are appropriate. The nature and scope of the guidelines are locally determined and cover issues such as the criteria for referral to an obstetrician at booking; antepartum complications (e.g. when to refer in cases of hypertension or malpresentation); intrapartum problems (e.g. the criteria for changing care to the obstetrician); as well as issues that are common to all care groups (e.g. postpartum haemorrhage).

Before vacuum extraction

Fetal compromise as the primary or associated indication for vacuum extraction must be monitored carefully to ensure that additional stress from the procedure does not exceed recommended safety limits. Since outcome may be predetermined by the condition of the fetus *in utero*, caesarean section may be the safer option for birth if fetal compromise gives cause for concern. Indications for vacuum extraction should be separated into standard and special categories. In general, procedures in the standard group have a wider margin of safety than those in the special group. Special uses of the vacuum extractor will be contraindications for all but the most experienced operators. Because of the risks to the fetus and mother, vacuum extraction should not be attempted before the cervix is fully dilated. There may be a few exceptions to this rule in special circumstances, but only if strict criteria are followed.

Outcome with the vacuum extractor is closely related to the selection of suitable women which, in practice, may be made by considering the station of the presenting part, the degree of moulding and the position of the fetal head. When the head is visible at the outlet of the pelvis or is stationed on the pelvic floor, the procedure is easily performed and the risks to the fetus are minimal. On the other hand, mid-pelvic extractions demand a high level of technical skill as well as training in rotational vacuum extraction.

If labour is complicated by delay in the second stage, the possibility of a difficult extraction should be anticipated. Shoulder dystocia is also more common when this combination of factors is present; for these reasons, if the operator is not sufficiently experienced or has not been trained in the method of rotational vacuum extraction, caesarean section is the safer mode of birth for the fetus.

Vacuum extraction should not be attempted if cephalo pelvic disproportion is present, or when the station of the fetal head is high; the practice of applying a vacuum cup to the head in order to bring the presenting part down to a lower station so that birth may be completed with forceps should be discouraged.

During vacuum extraction

The importance of a correct application of the vacuum cup as a factor exercising a major influence on outcome cannot be overemphasized. Correct application of the cup depends on knowledge of the flexion point and the operator's ability to apply the cup over the ideal site on the fetal head. For malpositions the choice of cup should be one that includes the posterior design principle that allows correct application to the head when the flexion point is not readily accessible.

Training and practice procedures

Collins (1997) provides a useful insight into midwives extending their role within the Wiltshire Primary Care Trust. Locally, there were discussions through-out maternity at all levels which were as inclusive and consultative as possible and involved all key stake-holders. Trainees were to witness three ventouse extractions, after which they would undertake a min-imum of 10 ventouse extractions under supervision. After a final assessment, midwives were verified as competent to perform ventouse extraction following the agreed policy. The course is predominantly practice-based and is taught in conjunction with the consultant at the Central Delivery Suite (CDS) at

Princess Anne Wing (PAW) in Bath. The training programme also includes lectures, video guidance and simulated practice using models. All the trainees have also completed an ALSO® course. The length of time for training has varied from 4 months to 12 months with the average of 6–8 months. The training may take longer should the midwife work part time.

All the MVP births are part of an ongoing audit programme. They all complete a logbook of all the cases they are involved with and this also includes the ventouse extractions that are unsuccessful. More recently, the MVPs working in the community have also been keeping a record in a separate logbook of all cases that they are called to assess but in which they decide not to undertake a ventouse. These can then be shared with the group as a case discussion which encourages individual and collective learning.

Recruitment of midwife ventouse practitioners

Locally, an internal advertisement was placed for experienced midwives who wished to undertake this training using an employee specification for the required competencies. Each applicant was interviewed and asked to make a case presentation as part of the selection process. At the same time, obstetricians who would act as mentors and trainers for the midwives were identified and a local programme of theoretical and practical training was developed collaboratively. The midwives who were successful with their application came from both the consultant unit and from the birth centres. In the first group five midwives were trained. Training as it now exists then began in 1996.

Midwifery practice should remain sensitive, relevant and responsive to the needs of individual women and it was felt that this was achievable in this situation if midwives become competent in performing ventouse extractions. Until the introduction of the MVP if a woman had a prolonged second stage of labour or if fetal compromise occurred and there was no GP available or willing to perform an instrumental birth, she would need to undergo an ambulance journey to a consultant unit in the second stage of labour for an instrumental birth. This can be extremely traumatic for all concerned and midwives felt that they were failing to give quality care to women at a time when they were most vulnerable. It is also apparent that these women demonstrated a sense of loss when transferred to another unit; a loss not only of continuity and support from a familiar face but also of choice and control.

The benefits of midwives undertaking ventouse births

One of the unforeseen but important advantages has been the close links that have become established between the midwives and their medical colleagues, working together collaboratively in both the community birth centres and in the consultant units. This has led to a greater understanding of each other's roles, greater competence and enhanced clinical decision making. The MVPs have all reported increased levels of self-confidence in their practice. The short-term successes include the reduced rate of transfers in labour from the birth centres to the consultant unit (e.g. a 9% decrease as a result of a 24-hour MVP cover at Trowbridge) and an initial 10% increase in births. The response from women and their partners has also been overwhelming. The high degree of maternal and paternal satisfaction, demonstrated openly to the MVPs, has been extremely rewarding for all concerned.

The support that midwives required when undertaking new roles and responsibilities presents a significant challenge to all involved with the maternity services. *Maternity matters* (DH 2007a) recommended that the role of the midwife be reviewed and strengthened and argued that the midwife's role is a key one if midwives are to move away from the inappropriate imposition of a medical model of care. But midwives will only be able to balance the medical model of care with a midwifery model if they have the appropriate status within the policy-making and operational management of maternity services. In addition to this, the model of midwifery practice in birth centres can only emerge in practice if midwives are empowered to use their clinical judgement and to make clinical decisions for which they are responsible and held accountable (Hunter 2000). Any clinical decisions should continue to reflect the unique midwifery philosophy of care, which remains central to midwives' practice at the local level.

The procedure

This is detailed in Box 7.1.

Box 7.1

Procedure for midwife undertaking a ventouse extraction

- The procedure is explained and consent obtained.
- The woman is usually in the lithotomy position, but midwives should use their discretion. Locally, the MVPs have, on occasions, not placed the woman's legs in the lithotomy position.
- The bladder should be emptied.
- Local anaesthesia may be used with/combined with entonox analgesia.
- Locally midwife ventouse practitioners have not been trained to undertake pudendal nerve block.
- An episiotomy is not routinely carried out.
- The fetal heart needs to be recorded regularly in accordance with guidelines from the National Institute for Health and Clinical Excellence (NICE 2007).
- The cup of the ventouse is placed as near as possible to, or on the flexing point of the fetal head.
- The vacuum in the cup is increased gradually so to achieve a close application to the fetal head.
- It is essential to check that there is no maternal tissue within the vacuum cup.
- When the vacuum is achieved, traction is applied with the contraction and maternal effort.
- Traction is undertaken in a downward and backward direction.
- The vacuum is released and the cup then removed at the crowning of the fetal head as it will no longer regress.
- The woman can then use her own efforts and internal resources to push her baby out of the birth canal for the final part of the birth.
- Details of the birth are then documented in the woman's records.

Women's responses

The response from women and their partners has also been overwhelming. The degree of maternal and paternal satisfaction, demonstrated openly to the MVPs, has been extremely rewarding for all concerned. One woman commented:

I'm so glad Louise (midwife) was able to perform my ventouse. It meant I didn't have to be transferred to the consultant unit. I could stay in a unit I knew with staff that I knew. It also meant that my husband could spend more time with us.

Training

The length of training will depend on each individual midwife and is usually between 3 and 6 months. This comprises the following as identified in Box 7.2.

Accountability

Once a MVP is competent and performing ventouse extraction without supervision from the obstetric registrar, the MVP is held accountable for her own practice. Meticulous record keeping must take place at all times.

Record keeping

It is recommended that MVPs complete a logbook (see Figure 7.1) of all cases that they are involved in, including unsuccessful ventouse births and where they may decide against undertaking a ventouse birth. Furthermore, meeting regularly about every 8 weeks as a group to discuss cases enables midwives to reflect both individually and collectively to share learning opportunities.

Box 7.2

Theoretical component of ventouse birth training

- Reasons for ventouse extraction.
- Vaginal examinations.
- Checking for abnormalities.
- The equipment:
  - Description of machine and attachments.
  - Technical use of the machine.
  - Setting up of the machine.
- Video training and analysis.

Personal reflections

Box 7.3 details the comments reflective of some of the experiences of training and adaptation to the new role of the midwives in Wiltshire, including some perceived potential disadvantages. However, all the MVPs commented that the most difficult part of the role is making the actual decision to undertake the ventouse, ensuring that all the criteria

Box 7.3

Personal reflections by midwife ventouse practitioners on the advantages and disadvantages of this expanded role

'Practical training was dependent on chance, as obviously we couldn't just go to CDS (Central Delivery Suite) and ventouse a client on a whim.'

'It seemed to take ages (three months) to get going and then I had a good run of Ventouse deliveries. It's the luck of the draw. It would have been harder if there had been more of us doing it at the same time, chasing the same cases. The theory side was good, particularly looking at clinical decision-making processes and other surrounding issues.'

'I have personally benefited by increased knowledge, confidence and experience my clinical decision-making is more defined and I feel my practice has improved. It has given me more job satisfaction and self confidence in my clinical skills.'

'I was very impressed with (the Senior Midwife CDS) who helped those of us from the community units orientate ourselves with CDS rather than throwing us in at the deep end.'

'Continuity; to be able to see a case right through or even if called in I may have already met the women.'

'When a MVP is called in there is an expectation that she will be able to sort out the problem, i.e. deliver the baby. Because in these situations the stress and tension levels are quite high this can put a lot of pressure on the MVP. This does recede with time and gradually more experience and the support I received have been excellent.'

'The only possible disadvantage is to be called out when a MV delivery is not possible due to women not being within remit of the protocol, i.e. OT, OP position. But I always question the midwife on the phone to ascertain that the woman meets the ventouse criteria. I never mind if I find that I am called and not able to do a ventouse delivery. If I get a normal birth it's a bonus.'

Midwife ventouse practitioner logbook

Case no: ....   Date: ....   Time of birth: ....

Name: ....   Age: ....

Address: ....

Hospital No: ....   Consultant: ....

Gestation: ....   Gravida: ....   Parity: ....

History:

Induction: ....   Augmentation: 1st stage: ....

2nd stage: ....

Indication:

Abdominal palpation: ....   Contractions: ....

Exam PV: ....   Station: ....   Caput: ....   Moulding: ....

Comments on extraction:

Perineum:

Labour	Analgesia	Duty registrar
1st stage:	....	Others present
2nd stage:	....	
3rd stage:	....	
Total:	....	
Blood loss:	....	

Infant	Chignon	Resuscitation
Sex:	....	None: ....
Weight:	....	O_2 only: ....
APGAR:	....	IPPV mask: ....
Meconium:	....	IPPV intubated: ....

Figure 7.1 ● Example of midwife ventouse practitioner logbook.

for the policy matches the individual woman and her individual needs.

Conclusion

The vacuum extraction is a useful instrument in the selection available for operative modes of birth, provided the mother meets the criteria for such a procedure. Vacuum extraction reduces maternal injury and, hence, requires less analgesia, thus diminishing anaesthetic risk.

Expanding the midwife's role should not be undertaken lightly. To support those developments there must be extensive preparation and training. Supervised practice, clear protocols, on-going clinical audit and the appropriate equipment must all be available.

Managerial support, involvement from supervisors of midwives in the formulation of clinical guidelines, and both agreement and support from local obstetricians and GPs are all necessary to ensure that the midwives can undertake this extended role safely. The support that midwives require when undertaking new roles and responsibilities presents a significant challenge to all involved throughout the maternity services. *Changing childbirth* (DH 1993) and *Maternity matters* (DH 2007a) recommend that the role of the midwife be reviewed and strengthened. Page (1995) argues that the midwife's role is a key one if midwives are to move away from the inappropriate imposition of a medical model of care. But midwives will only be able to balance the medical model of care with a midwifery model if they have the appropriate status in the maternity

services within the policy making and operational management. In addition to this, the midwifery model can only emerge in practice if midwives are empowered to use their clinical judgement and to make clinical decisions on their own responsibility and accountability. However, any clinical decisions should continue to reflect the unique midwifery philosophy of care. It would appear that this remains central to the MVPs practice locally.

Key practice points

- If you are not trained to do it – do not do it!
- Midwives should personally choose to develop skills to undertake ventouse births. They are not mini doctors and there should be no managerial coercion.
- All clinical decisions and judgements should provide an enhanced outcome for women and their families.
- If performing a ventouse in a birthing centre, an ambulance should be called at the same time to prevent any delays in transferring should the ventouse not be successful.
- The promotion of normality in childbirth should be integral to the midwife's own philosophy of care.
- The importance of team work and multi-professional approaches to education, training and service developments cannot be underestimated.
- The development of good practice guidelines and clinical governance reporting structures embraces the general principals of risk management.

References

Charles, C., 1999. How it feels to be a midwife ventouse practitioner. British Journal of Midwifery 7 (6), 380–382.

Collins, A., 1997. Trust midwives extending their caring role in: everyday: an insight into the Wiltshire Health Care NHS Trust. Salisbury, Wiltshire.

Department of Health, 1993. Changing childbirth. The report of the Expert Maternity Group. Part 1. HMSO, London.

Department of Health, 1999. Making a difference. Strengthening the nursing midwifery and health visiting

contribution to health and health care. Department of Health, London.

Department of Health, 2004. National service framework for children, young people and maternity services. Department of Health, London.

Department of Health, 2007a. Maternity matters: access and continuity of care in a safe service. Department of Health, London.

Department of Health, 2007b. Our health, our care, our say. A new direction for community

services. Department of Health, London.

Dimond, B., 1999. The midwife consultant and the law. British Journal of Midwifery 7 (1), 38.

Hewison, J., 2004. Different models of maternity care: an evaluation of roles of primary health care workers. Department of Health, London.

Hodnett, E.D., Gates, S., Hofmeyr, G.J., Sakala, C., 2007. Continuous support for women during childbirth. The Cochrane Library of Systematic Reviews. Available online: http://

www.thecochranelibrary.com Accessed 6 July 2008.

House of Commons Health Committee, 1992. Second Report Session 1991–92: Maternity Services, Vol. 1. HMSO, London.

Hunter, M., 2000. Clinical freedom and responsibility. The paradoxes of providing intrapartum midwifery care in a small maternity unit as compared with a large obstetric hospital. Unpublished. Palmerston North, New Zealand.

Marsh, G.N., Cashman, H.A., Russell, I.T., 1985. General practitioner obstetrics in the northern region in 1983. Br. Med. J. 290, 901–903.

National Institute for Health and Clinical Excellence, 2007. Intrapartum care. NICE, London.

Nursing and Midwifery Council, 2008. The code: standards of conduct, performance and ethics for nurses and midwives. NMC, London.

Page, L., 1995. A vision for the future: to meet the challenge of changing childbirth. English National Board Midwifery Educational (ENB) Resource Pack; Number 6. ENB, London.

Royal College of Obstetrics and Gynaecology and Royal College of General Practitioners, 1981. Report on training for obstetrics and gynaecology for general practice: a joint working party. RCOG and RCGP, London.

Smith, L.F.P., 1992. Roles, risks and responsibilities in maternity care: trainees beliefs and the effects of practice obstetric training. Br. Med. J. 304, 1613–1615.

Smith, L., Jewell, D., 1999. General practitioners' contributions – What's really going on? In: Marsh, G., Renfrew, M. (Eds.), Community cased maternity care. Oxford University Press, Oxford.

Walker, J., 2000. Women's experiences of transfer from midwifery-led to a consultant-led maternity unit in the UK during late pregnancy and labour. J. Midwifery Womens Health 45 (2), 161–168.

Wiegers, T.A., 2003. General practitioners and their role in maternity care. Health Policy 66 (1), 51–59.

Young, G.L., 1991. General practice and the future of obstetric care. Br. J. Gen. Pract. 41, 266–267.

Further reading

Kirkham, M. (Ed.), 2003. Birth centres. A social model for maternity care. Books for midwives, Oxford.
This text provides the reader with an international perspective of birth within the low technological/high social support model of a birthing centre and highlights the roles, skills and relationships required by the midwife to ensure the maternity care they provide to women and their families in this environment is of the optimum standard.

Kirkham, M. 1999. The culture of midwifery in the NHS in England. J. Adv. Nurs. 30 (3): 732–739.
A useful resource in the context of professional autonomy. Highlighting that the challenges to professional autonomy are influenced by an array of factors not least a culture that reinforces blame and bullying.

Scottish Executive, 2002. Expert Group on Acute Maternity Services. Reference report. Scottish Executive, Edinburgh.
Explores the key issues facing midwives and other members of the multiprofessional/interdisciplinary team in relation to manpower training and the delivery of care using an integrated approach.

Chapter Eight

8

Forceps-assisted birth

Jean Wills, Jayne E. Marshall and Maureen D. Raynor

CONTENTS

Introduction 77
Rationale 78
Sharing best practice 79
Clinical practice rationale 79
Educational rationale 80
Implementation 81
Management rationale 81
Procedure for undertaking forceps birth . . 82
Instrument choice and basic procedure . . 83
Potential complications from
forceps-assisted births 83
Challenges 83
Establishing links 85
Reflections on a birth story 85
Record keeping 85
Conclusion 85
Key practice points 86
References 86
Further reading 87

Before reading this chapter, you should be familiar with:
- Professional accountability and liability.
- Statutory rules, standards and professional codes that govern the midwife's sphere of practice and responsibility for acquiring and developing competence in new skills.
- Legal and ethical decision-making frameworks in midwifery practice.

- Factors affecting the physiological process of spontaneous labour.
- Local Trust policies and national guidelines in relation to intrapartum care and management (including NICE 2007).
- Monitoring of fetal well being in labour.
- Risk-assessment and risk-management procedures including mode of birth.
- The value of inter-professional learning and working.
- Prevention, recognition and management of emergencies that may arise in midwifery practice such as postpartum haemorrhage, shoulder dystocia and neonatal resuscitation.
- Best-practice issues regarding perineal management during the intrapartum period and subsequent postpartum care of any perineal trauma.

Introduction

Studies such as those detailed in the Cochrane review (Hatem et al 2008) have shown that midwife-led births are associated with lower rates of intervention such as assisted vaginal births, leading to increased levels of maternal satisfaction. However, in order to provide women with continuity of care within a midwifery-led model, it could be argued that midwives skilled to perform assisted births such as the use of ventouse and forceps is one way of realising continuity of care and ensuring that such care is woman-centred. Thus, to promote the ethos of normal birth the role of the midwife in some National Health Service (NHS) Trusts in the United Kingdom (UK) has been extended to include the extra skills of fetal blood sampling, mid and low cavity forceps, and ventouse births. However, this position has not been designed to replace or compete with the medical staff but to improve and enhance the service and options provided to women. The aim is for the midwife, acting in the context of the assisted birth practitioner, to maintain continuity of care for women thus aiming to achieve a good birth experience for women with no medical intervention.

Aberdeen Maternity Hospital, and the two Leeds Hospitals, are regional referral units and have an instrumental delivery rate of approximately 16%. This figure is not dissimilar to those of other tertiary units in the UK. The Bulletin co-authored by Richardson and Mmata (2007) for the NHS Information Centre for England supports this. The authors reported that of the 593 400 NHS hospital births recorded by the Office of National Statistics via the birth registration system for England in 2005–2006, 11% resulted in instrumental births. Furthermore, the report highlights a major shift in the type of instrument used for assisted vaginal births. Whilst forceps were the instrument of choice during the 1980s (accounting for 83% of instrumental births) by 2002–2003, 68% of assisted births were via ventouse extraction.

In the context of using forceps for assisting a vaginal birth, this chapter aims to explore the role and professional responsibilities for those midwives interested in being trained to become assisted birth practitioners. It will, therefore, build on Chapter 7 that addresses the issue of births via ventouse or vacuum extraction. At the vanguard of change is the pioneering work and partnership forged between the University of Bradford and Aberdeen Maternity Hospital. This work will be highlighted as an example of best practice.

Rationale

In 2005 the first distance learning 'Assisted Birth Programme' enabling midwives to perform fetal blood sampling, ventouse and forceps births was launched as a joint venture between the University of Bradford and Aberdeen Maternity Hospital. This was in response to recent changes in local and national government policy brought about by both midwives and women challenging the medical model of control and interpretation of normality in childbirth, with more recent changes encouraging extended roles for both nurses and midwives developing around the Calman report (Department of Health [DH] 1993a) and Modernising medical careers (DH 2005). This programme, however, has sparked a debate between midwives, as many viewed this initiative as challenging the midwife's role as the guardian of normality for women (Anderson 2003).

The concept of 'normal' upon which recent midwifery practice has been built would appear to have been developed on an unstable foundation. Competing philosophies, cultural and social influences all shape an individual's understanding of words and any definition of 'normal' should be viewed as subjective, temporary and vulnerable to change. It is debatable as to how and who defines 'normal' for the midwife and women. An analysis of the history of midwifery reveals some insight into how and who has been responsible for the concept of normality in midwifery today and explains how social and political agendas have driven and shaped the working practices of the midwife. Some aspects of the art and science of midwifery and the concept of what is normal have changed over the years; however, some practices seem to have been relatively unaltered by the passage of time (Evenden 2000).

The 20th century witnessed an evolution in the provision and delivery of midwifery care, largely influenced by scientific, technological, sociological and political factors, which required maternity care to circumvent a wider field combining the art of midwifery and the science of obstetrics. This has enabled midwives to expand into a new era of care for women during childbirth. This evolution, as well as policy proposals (DH 2000), is advocating major changes in service provision and delivery, calling midwives to work in new ways and within new partnerships.

Many changes are documented and discussed within the midwifery profession and the NHS as a whole. These include changes in the way health care is allocated and provided (DH 1993b), extending the role of the midwife (DH 1999, Royal College of Midwives [RCM] 2002, Royal College of Obstetricians and Gynaecologists [RCOG] Scottish Committee 2005, Scottish Executive 2006) and the epistemology of the professions. Chapter 7 addresses midwives' acquisition of skills to undertake ventouse births, as it is acknowledged that whilst there have been several articles exploring midwives' personal experiences of becoming ventouse practitioners in stand-alone midwifery-led units (Charles 1999, Parslow 1997), there has been limited detail on how their role has been achieved and defined or on the standards and guidelines set and subsequent evaluation.

Concerns have been expressed by midwives and obstetricians that midwives may undertake a ventouse extraction to quicken the birth once they have been trained and so take the easy way out. Interestingly, a survey by Alexander et al (2002) evaluated the effect on practice of midwife ventouse practitioners and concluded that the number of ventouse births does not increase when midwives are able to use this skill themselves.

Studies exploring advanced practitioners and change management have highlighted problems with advanced practice, mainly that the roles and practice parameters are ill defined, whether the changes reflect 'medicalisation' or independence and if practitioners in advanced roles become too focused on their specialist area (Bryant-Lukosius et al 2004, Lewis 2003, Price et al 2000, Sookhoo & Butler 1999). Sociological, anthropological, gender studies and midwifery literature have also discussed the medicalisation or technological hegemony in midwifery and obstetric practice adversely affecting women's childbirth experiences (Crompton 1996, Jowitt 1993, Kirkham 2000, Menger 1993, Teijlingen et al 2000, Tew 1995). Further study is, therefore, essential to form a basis for extending research in this unexplored and innovative field of midwifery practice adding to existing literature on expanded midwife roles and midwifery/medical culture. Any conclusions and recommendations will also inform future workforce/workload planning at a strategic level.

Sharing best practice

Towards the end of January 1999, the consultant body from the Leeds Teaching Hospitals NHS Trust met to discuss a number of issues relating to the future of the obstetric services in Leeds. One of the major issues to be tackled was that of medical, nursing and midwifery staffing and service provision within the directorate. Faced with the implications of the Calman report (DH 1993a) enforcing the loss of junior medical staff at both senior house officer (SHO) and specialist registrar (SpR) grades, both the medical and midwifery team had to come up with different ways of working. It was acknowledged that to allow service provision to be altered both medical

and midwifery staff must be prepared to make fairly radical changes in their working practices. It was eventually jointly decided to train midwives with 2 years' labour ward experience to perform fetal blood sampling and assisted births using ventouse and low/mid cavity forceps. This initiative was actively supported by the Head of Midwifery and the Local Supervising Authority (LSA) responsible midwifery officer, who both negotiated vicarious liability for midwives in this expanded role. Following on from the successful evaluation of a pilot study (Wills & Deighton 2002) midwives were provided with the opportunity to undertake training on the midwife-assisted birth programme.

Leeds and later Aberdeen Maternity Hospital (AMH) senior medical and midwifery staff decided that midwives should be trained to perform fetal blood sampling and assisted births via use of both ventouse and low/mid cavity forceps, thereby enabling the best possible evidence-based care to be offered to women. A distance learning programme was written in a joint venture between Bradford University and AMH and, following interviews, initially 12 midwives were accepted for training which commenced in 2005. Women and supervision were the central drivers of the programme supported by the obstetricians and educationalists (Figure 8.1).

In Aberdeen the Head of Midwifery set up a working group composed of consultant obstetricians, Supervisor of Midwives and the Clinical Midwifery Manager for the labour ward to plan and monitor the way forward. The rationales for this programme were threefold, in that there was a clinical rationale, an educational rationale and a management rationale.

Clinical practice rationale

There was an identified need for this provision in clinical practice. The rationale for the introduction of the programme in Aberdeen was predominately a response to the reduction in junior doctors' hours and recognition that extending the role of experienced midwives to include assisted birth would enhance staff flexibility and improve the quality of care offered to labouring women. Additionally, in small obstetric units currently staffed by consultants with no middle-grade obstetricians, there is a need for skilled midwives to fill this gap. This resonates with current NHS policy that promotes a

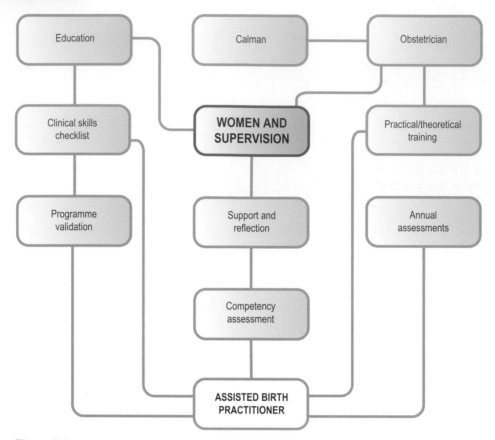

Figure 8.1 • Midwives performing assisted births: exploring new ways of working together.

lifelong learning approach as well as quality, efficiency and safe delivery of care (DH 2001, 2008). This encourages staff to break down barriers between different professional groups and promotes effective inter-professional team working. The key principles of the assisted birth midwife practitioner is outlined in Box 8.1.

Educational rationale

In planning this programme due account has been taken of the Quality Assurance Agency for Higher Education (QAAHE) Code of Practice for collaborative provision and flexible and distributed learning (QAAHE 2004).

The specific issues relating to the delivery, learner support and assessment of flexible and distributed learning are now outlined.

Box 8.1

Key principles of the assisted birth midwife practitioner programme

- It should be delivered in partnership with stakeholders who have identified a need for midwives to be skilled assisted birth practitioners.
- It should be responsive in order to meet the development needs of the labour ward team across the traditional boundaries of the obstetrician and midwife.
- It should be predominately work based and focused on 'competence in doing'.
- It should be woman centred in that the ultimate aim is to improve the quality and continuity of care offered to women.

Implementation

The responsibilities of the programme team at Aberdeen, the programme co-ordinator at Bradford and the participating practice areas were clearly documented in the programme specification (University of Bradford 2005). Students were provided with a clear schedule for the programme including assessment dates confirming their place on the course. This information was also available in the student handbook, prepared by the University of Bradford and given to students on the first day of the course. This handbook included tutor contact details and scheduled opportunities for tutor support.

Online resources were provided through the Blackboard Virtual Learning Environment (VLE); the programme co-ordinator has experience in this medium and provided structured student support. The VLE is reliable and capable of delivering resources of appropriate quality. Students have password protected access and appropriate internet access in their working environment or via their local library. Students were advised of the University computer purchase scheme but a personal home computer, although helpful, is not a course requirement.

This programme draws on the existing occupational standards, core knowledge and skills of experienced midwives and doctors to support a skills escalator approach to post-registration education (DH 2001). It utilises a full range of learning methods and there is clear demarcation of roles and responsibilities. The development of this programme has drawn on and developed staff skills in collaborative working, distance learning, work-based learning and online learning. All of these are likely to be an important part of future higher education provision and, therefore, this programme is a valuable learning experience for staff as well as students.

Management rationale

This programme is responding to a perceived need in Scotland and was supported by the lead clinician. Furthermore, the introduction of the assisted birth programme was, and continues to be, enthusiastically supported by the heads of midwifery, senior midwives on the labour ward and the consultant team. As Procter and Renfrew (2001) suggest, professional development and innovative practice

are important for all midwives to embrace if they are to offer the highest quality care to women. There has also been interest expressed in the rest of the UK. The demand for such a course is strong and long term. This is, therefore, a knowledge transfer project for the University of Bradford. However, as this provision is collaborative there are particular quality assurance issues to address (QAAHE 2004), for example having processes in place to audit, monitor and evaluate the quality of the programme in terms of theoretical and practical competence. An audit of each birth is completed by an independent professional the following day. This is to assess the woman's feelings on information giving, her understanding of the information, type and efficiency of analgesia, who performed the assisted birth and explore any concerns she may have.

The group set guidelines for midwife-assisted births, which were presented to the Obstetric and Gynaecology Committee and included in the labour ward guidelines. These defined the training required and the role of the trainers. Aims were set and the relevant method of recording and assessing progress agreed (Phillips & Bharj 1996).

Box 8.2 outlines the minimum requirements for midwives to be considered for the assisted birth programme. Midwives are required to keep a reflective diary of their experiences and a record of births undertaken (a minimum of 10 supervised births with each instrument are required before a midwife is ready to be assessed for competency). Once a midwife is deemed competent, her skills are assessed annually by a consultant obstetrician and a supervisor of midwives.

> ### Box 8.2
>
> **Midwife-assisted birth practitioner**
> **Requirements for training**
> - Effective registration on NMC Professional Register.
> - Have a minimum of 2 years' post-qualifying experience on a labour ward.
> - Be competent in cardiotocography (CTG) interpretation, perineal suturing and intravenous cannulation.
> - Evidence of studying at either degree or masters level.
> - Access to clinical experience on labour ward for the duration of the module.

Box 8.3

Guidelines for assisted births by midwives

Indications

- Maternal exhaustion.
- Failure to progress in 2ⁿᵈ stage of labour.
- Fetal compromise (when the midwife is competent).

Pre-requisites (Sullivan & Hayman 2008)

- Skilled, competent midwife able to acknowledge limitations and willingness to use ability to exercise skilled decision making, including inform obstetric registrar on duty/making referral as indicated.
- Term pregnancy (37 weeks and over).
- Maternal consent.
- Singleton pregnancy.
- Cephalic presentation 0 fifths palpable abdominally.
- Vertex at least 1 cm below the ischial spines: occipital anterior position.
- No asynclitism.
- Cervical os fully dilated.
- Membranes ruptured.
- Adequate analgesia.
- Bladder care, i.e. catheterisation.

Box 8.4

Role of the supervisor of midwives: midwife-assisted births

Role

- To facilitate safe, evidence-based practice and enhance continuity of care for women.
- Support midwives through the training and practice and continued support upon completion.

Supervisors input

- Multiprofessional working.
- Research knowledge of the subject.
- Communication and dissemination of information to all stakeholders.
- Defining safe parameters of practice.
- Development of evidence-based guidelines.
- Competency assessment following training.
- Validation of training programme.
- Clinical audit for clinical governance.
- Support for midwives.

Box 8.3 lists the criteria required before a midwife performs an assisted birth.

The proactive role and ongoing support of the supervisor of midwives in the development and implementation of the programme has played a crucial part in its success, see Box 8.4 above.

At the time of preparing this chapter there were three trained midwives in Aberdeen and Leeds, and five in Elgin. Elgin is a District General Hospital; the obstetric unit being staffed only by midwives and consultants with no middle-obstetric grades. Elgin hospital has approximately 1000 births per year, with an 11% instrumental birth rate. The role of the assisted birth practitioner in Elgin has been modified with regard to their unique needs and here it was decided to complete only the ventouse part of the programme.

The training programme includes a comprehensive list of clinical competencies, a competency assessment tool and performance indicators, as well as defining the level of training required and the role of the trainers, who should be at consultant level.

This programme enables midwives to gain a formally recognised standard of competence in their assisted birth role. The programme structure is specifically designed to support the development of the midwife's expanded role by encouraging collaborative clinical work-based training between midwife and consultant.

The framework of competencies being developed should clearly articulate a comprehensive and agreed framework of skills that each midwife needs to be capable of achieving in order to undertake the responsibilities of their role, in whichever environment they practice. The aim of the programme must be to guide and advance them from competent to expert. Therefore, while the competencies do not change as the midwife gains experience, performance within the competency should alter and improve.

Procedure for undertaking forceps birth

Although the procedure of assisted forceps births is considered to be outside the accepted definition of normality, the aim should be for this procedure to be perceived as unobtrusive as possible. Although Meakin (2004) suggests that the midwife's role is to summon appropriate personnel and stay by the woman's side when an assisted birth is undertaken, this would indicate clear demonstration of professional boundaries described by midwives for midwives. However, through partnership working the medical and midwifery professions can be enabled to practise within a more cohesive environment in order to deliver a service which can be shown to be of benefit both to the women and the joint professions as a whole. Ensuring the highest standard of care by midwives in this expanded role is of the utmost importance; therefore, all midwives have an annual competency assessment by an appropriate consultant and supervisor of midwives.

Instrument choice and basic procedure

Once the woman has adequate analgesia, there is little to choose between the vacuum extractor and the forceps for an instrumental birth. With more complex cases, operator experience and the specific details of each individual clinical situation are the key principles in determining whether to use a vacuum extractor or forceps. If birth should be expedited for fetal distress, then forceps may be more appropriate because the time taken to assist the birth is significantly less when compared to a ventouse.

Forceps consist of two blades with shanks that are joined together at a lock with handles to provide a point for traction. There are three main types of forceps that are suitable for different situations, each requiring a different level of proficiency of the operator:

- Outlet Forceps, e.g. Wrigleys Forceps.
- Mid-cavity Forceps, e.g. Neville-Barnes Forceps.
- Rotational Forceps, e.g. Keillands.

For the purposes of this chapter only the procedure for assisting birth using Wrigleys outlet forceps will be presented as midwives would not be expected to perform complex mid-cavity/rotational forceps births, i.e. Keillands forceps. It is usual for the forceps to be held discreetly in front of the labouring woman in order to visualise how they will be positioned per vaginam, and then placed around the fetal head. The left blade is inserted before the right blade with the midwife's hand protecting the vaginal wall from direct trauma. The forceps blades will then lie parallel to the axis of the fetal head

and between the fetal head and the pelvic wall. The blades are then locked and before applying traction their application must be checked. If the application is incorrect, then the midwife must reposition the blades or abandon the procedure. Traction should only be applied in conjunction with uterine contractions and expulsive efforts from the woman. The axis of traction changes during the assisted birth and is guided along the pelvic curve of Carus, with the forceps blades being directed to the vertical as the head eventually crowns (see Figure 8.2).

Potential complications from forceps-assisted births

The use of routine episiotomy when undertaking forceps births to reduce anal-sphincter trauma and subsequent faecal incontinence remains controversial. Whilst some studies have found that a restricted use of episiotomy was associated with a reduced risk of posterior perineal trauma than with a more liberal approach, randomised trials have shown there to be no prophylactic protective effect on the incidence of damage to the anal sphincter. On the other hand, when episiotomy was restricted, an increase in the incidence of damage to the anterior vaginal wall and labia has been observed.

Following a successful birth of the fetal head using forceps, midwives must also be prepared for the possibility of shoulder dystocia and subsequent postpartum haemorrhage. It is, therefore, important that there is always accurate application of the forceps and close adherence to standard techniques and guidelines which are essential for midwives developing safe and competent practice to minimise risk to mother and baby. Sullivan and Hayman (2008) assert that such procedures can only be learnt in clinical practice.

Challenges

Concerns over this expanded role have surrounded the training of SHOs in these procedures, the worry being that the midwife will become skilled to the detriment of the junior doctors' training programme. This has not been found to be the case in the units involved; the midwifery and medical staff now finding they work more closely together. It is envisaged that once the midwives are competent and confident they will then take on the role

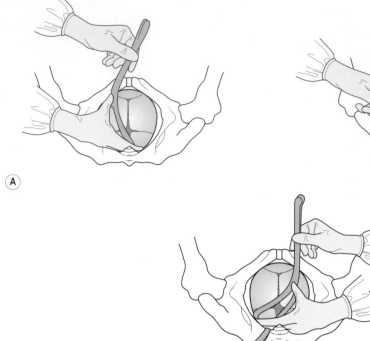

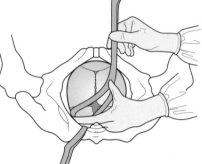

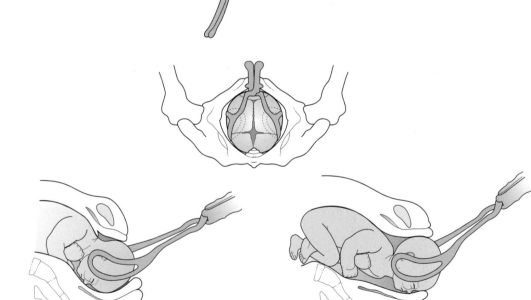

Figure 8.2 ● Procedure for forceps-assisted birth. (A) Applying the left forceps blade. (B) Applying the right forceps blade. (C) Locking and applying traction. (From WHO 2003, with permission.)

of teaching the SHOs. Other concerns have been around the additional time and workload of the midwives in this expanded role. A business plan has been written at Aberdeen as there is an awareness of the possibility of compromising the midwives' primary role. This will allow for the future service needs to be adequately resourced thus allowing for women, their partners and the midwife to share in a positive and fulfilling birth experience.

Once the Aberdeen/Leeds link is established this will allow for a later comparative study involving both units. If the programme becomes widely accepted and implemented it would be of value to undertake a further study to investigate the concept of post-traumatic stress syndrome in women following instrumental births. This would allow for the evaluation of differences, if any, in outcomes between assisted births performed by midwives and those performed by doctors.

Establishing links

Both Aberdeen, Elgin and Leeds practitioners hope to continue to train and support the expanded midwives' roles whilst at the same time forging links across both professional and national boundaries. This is to benefit both practitioners and women alike from this partnership working, informing best practice by:

• establishing communication pathways to allow for support and information sharing.
• exploring clinical work patterns influencing care at the point of delivery.
• developing new ways of working together.
• building an ongoing structure to support continued link working.

Reflections on a birth story

This expanded role will not be for every Health Board, NHS Trust, or every midwife, but practitioners in Aberdeen feel not only that is this the right direction to follow to enhance care for women, but also privileged to be part of such a new and challenging time for the midwifery profession as a whole. It could be argued that normality in midwifery is a moving concept sometimes viewed differently by the women experiencing maternity care. This begs the question whether the women

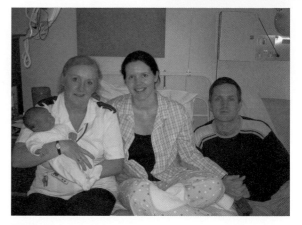

Figure 8.3 ● The day after an assisted birth with forceps. Craig and Bronwyn with baby Anakin.

in midwives' care ever get a chance to express their views of where normality for their birth should begin or end.

The following quote from a father highlights one family's experience of the effects midwives are having on labour and birth by performing assisted forceps births.

A forceps delivery was daunting, but having the midwife with previous care in my wife's labour to then follow on and perform the assisted forceps delivery offered a very reassuring sense of security and continuity. Allowing midwives to multitask such as this must be so rewarding and satisfying for them as much as us too.
(See Figure 8.3).

Record keeping

Rule 6 and 9 of the NMC (2004) Midwives Rules and Standards outline the parameters of the midwife's sphere of practice and requirements for records and record keeping. Box 8.5 identifies the salient points midwives acting as assisted birth practitioners must take into consideration to reduce the risk of litigation.

Conclusion

There is an identified clinical need for this programme. Staff develop knowledge and skills, which will enhance both quality and efficiency of

Box 8.5

Record keeping must reflect the following:

- Time and date.
- Initial assessment.
- Consent.
- Indication for the assisted birth.
- Analgesia – type, amount and time administered.
- Bladder care.
- Type of instrument used.
- Any difficulties encountered and management plan to remedy the problem(s).
- Monitoring of maternal/fetal well being throughout the procedure.
- Episiotomy (indication for/reason for not performing surgical procedure).
- Maternal/fetal/neonatal complications or injuries.
- Perineal repair:
  ○ diagrammatic representation to depict extent, type and degree of trauma,
  ○ time of repair,
  ○ additional analgesia needed to perform the repair,
  ○ method and material used,
  ○ thorough examination of the genital tract and anal sphincter prior to and following the repair,
  ○ post-partum analgesia,
  ○ health education information regarding perineal hygiene/care and healing.
- Tone of uterus, estimated blood loss and achievement of haemostasis.
- Maternal/neonatal outcome, including neonatal APGAR score and result of paired cord blood sampling.
- Name of midwife-assisted birth practitioner and other health care professionals present for the birth.
- Any aftercare/postpartum follow-up.

intrapartum care. The programme is educationally innovative while adhering to sound educational and quality principles. It is a good example of knowledge transfer and partnership working. When undertaking this new role it must be accepted that sufficient time is allocated to allow for the midwives training, support and study. This will involve the multiprofessional team of consultants, supervisors of midwives, midwifery managers and lecturers as well as the midwives themselves.

Prior to undertaking the course NHS Trusts need to ensure that they have secured vicarious liability for the extended role and that the obstetric consultants are willing to teach, observe and monitor midwives performing forceps-assisted births within their particular unit.

Key practice points

- An assisted vaginal birth is not without risks.
- The midwife as an accountable practitioner must recognise that adherence to standard technique, skilled application of the forceps and recognition of personal limitations are key to safe practice.
- Any midwife who uses forceps to aid birth must have the knowledge, understanding and be proficient in the skill (NMC 2004). This means attending to her educational needs and ensuring regular updates.
- The woman must be adequately briefed to achieve valid consent. This information must include benefits, risks and complications of the intervention.

References

Anderson, G., 2003. A concept analysis of 'normal birth'. Evidence Based Midwifery 1 (2), 48–54.

Alexander, J., Anderson, T., Cunningham, J., 2002. An evaluation by focus group and survey of a course for midwifery ventouse practitioners. Midwifery 18, 65–72.

Bryant Lukosius, D., DiCenso, A., Browne, G., Pinelli, J., 2004. Advanced practice nursing roles: development, implementation and evaluation. J. Adv. Nurs. 48 (5), 519–529.

Charles, C., 1999. How it feels to be a midwife ventouse practitioner.

British Journal of Midwifery 7, 380–382.

Crompton, J., 1996. Post-traumatic stress disorder and childbirth: 2. British Journal of Midwifery 4, 354–373.

Department of Health, 1993a. Hospital doctors: training for the future. (Calman report). HMSO, London.

Department of Health, 1993b. Changing childbirth, Part 1: report of the Expert Maternity Group. HMSO, London.

Department of Health, 1999. Making a difference. HMSO, London.

Department of Health, 2000. NHS Plan: a plan for investment, a plan for reform. www.dh.gov.uk

Department of Health, 2001. Working together, learning together: a framework for lifelong learning for the NHS. HMSO, London.

Department of Health, 2005. Modernising medical careers. HMSO, London.

Department of Health, 2008. High quality care for all: NHS next stage review final report (Darzi report). HMSO, London.

Evenden, D., 2000. The midwives of seventeenth-century London. Cambridge University Press, Cambridge.

Hatem, M., Sandall, J., Devane, D., Soltani, H., Gates, S., 2008 Midwife-led versus other models of care for childbearing women. Cochrane Database Syst. Rev. (4). Art No: CD004667. doi:10.1002/14651858.

Jowitt, M., 1993. Childbirth unmasked. Peter Wooller, Shropshire.

Kirkham, M., 2000. The midwife–mother relationship. Palgrave MacMillan, Hampshire.

Lewis, P., 2003. A framework for advancing practice. British Journal of Midwifery 11, 260–262.

Meakin, S., 2004. Procedures in Obstetrics. In: Henderson, C., Macdonald, S. (Eds.), Mayes' midwifery. A textbook for midwives. Bailliere Tindall, Edinburgh, pp. 970–986.

Menger, J., 1993. Post-traumatic stress disorder in women who have undergone obstetric procedures. Journal of Reproductive and Infant Psychology 11, 221–228.

Nursing and Midwifery Council, 2004. Midwives rules and standards. NMC, London.

Parslow, L., 1997. A midwife ventouse practitioner. Midwives 110, 165–166.

Phillips, M., Bharj, K., 1996. Developing a tool for the assessment of clinical learning. British Journal of Midwifery 4, 471–474.

Price, C., Han, S., Rutherford, I., 2000. Advancing nursing practice: an introduction to physical assessment. Br. J. Nurs. 9 (22), 2292–2296.

Proctor, S., Renfrew, M., 2001. Linking research and practice in midwifery. Balliere Tindall, London.

Quality Assurance Agency for Higher Education, 2004. Education training for advanced practice. QAAHE, London.

Richardson, A., Mmata, C., 2007. NHS maternity statistics, England: 2005–2006. Available online: http://www.ic.nhs.uk Accessed 7 December 2008.

Royal College of Midwives, 2002. Position paper No 26. Refocusing the role of the midwife. RCM, London.

Royal College of Obstetricians and Gynaecologists, 2005. The future of obstetrics and gynaecology in Scotland. Service Provision and workforce Planning Scottish Committee of the RCOG. RCOG, London.

Scottish Executive, 2006. Delivering care, enabling health. Scottish Executive, Edinburgh.

Sookhoo, M., Butler, M., 1999. An analysis of the concept of advanced midwifery practice. British Journal of Midwifery 7, 690–693.

Sullivan, C., Hayman, R., 2008. Instrumental vaginal birth. Obstetrics, Gynaecology and Reproductive Medicine 18 (4), 99–104.

Teijlingen, E., Lowis, G., McCaffery, P., Porter, M., 2000. Midwifery and the medicalization of childbirth; comparative perspectives. Nova Science Publishers, Huntingdon, New York.

Tew, M., 1995. Safer childbirth? A critical history of maternity care, second ed. Chapman Hall, London.

University of Bradford, 2005. Assisted Birth for Midwives HM-3200T: Programme Specification University of Bradford, School of Health Studies.

Wills, J., Deighton, S., 2002. Midwives performing instrumental deliveries: programme development and personal reflection. Pract. Midwife 5, 22–25.

World Health Organisation, 2003. Managing complications in pregnancy and childbirth. A guide for midwives and doctors. Available online: http://www.who.int/reproductive–health/impac/Procedures/Forceps_delivery_P33_P35.html

Further reading

Johanson, R.B., Menson, V., 2007. Vacuum extraction versus forceps for assisted vaginal delivery. Cochrane Database Syst. Rev. (4). Art No: CD000224. doi:10.1002/14651858.
This paper provides a good comparison of the evidence around the use of instruments to effect a vaginal birth with consideration for maternal and fetal well being.

Royal College of Obstetricians and Gynaecologists, 2005. Operative vaginal delivery; Guideline No. 26. RCOG, London.
Outlines the key principles to adhere to for safe outcomes when carrying out an assisted vaginal birth by either forceps or ventouse.

Chapter Nine

9

Facilitating vaginal breech birth at term

Jayne E. Marshall

CONTENTS

Introduction 90
Incidence of breech presentation 90
The evidence 90
Indications and contraindications
of vaginal breech birth 91
Potential complications of breech birth . . 92
Place of birth 92
Position for birth 93
Facilitating a breech labour and birth 93
Manoeuvres to assist the birth
of the breech 94
    For extended legs 94
    For extended arms: *Løvsets*
    manoeuvre 94
    For the after-coming head:
    Burns Marshall 96
    Mauriceau-Smellie-Veit 96
Professional responsibilities
of the midwife 97
    Responsibility to develop
    competence in breech birth 97
    Accountability 97
    Consent and trespass to the person . . . 99
    Negligence and a reasonable
    standard of care 99
    Vicarious liability 99
    Documentation and autonomous
    practice 99
Conclusion 100
Key practice points 100
References 101
Further reading 102
Useful websites 102

Before reading this chapter, you should be familiar with:

- Types of breech presentation.
- Diagnosis of breech presentation by abdominal examination, fetal heart auscultation and vaginal examination.
- Factors affecting the physiological process of spontaneous labour.
- Local Trust policies and national guidelines in relation to intrapartum care and management (including NICE 2007).
- The physiology and mechanism of breech birth.
- Monitoring of fetal well being in labour.
- Risk-assessment and risk-management procedures including mode and place of birth.
- Legal and ethical frameworks.
- Statutory rules, standards and professional codes that govern the midwife's sphere of practice and responsibility for developing competence in new skills.
- The value of inter-professional learning and working.

The term *midwife* is used throughout this chapter, but it is appreciated this may also apply to other health professionals, such as the obstetrician wishing to develop skills in this area of clinical practice.

Introduction

It is worth considering at the beginning of this chapter that a breech presentation at term is NOT an abnormality, it is just UNUSUAL and so a normal labour and spontaneous vaginal birth should not be excluded. Although in Western childbirth culture, a breech birth has the status of an 'emergency', in many parts of the world such a vaginal birth is part of normal practice (Burvill 2005). As Allison (1996) purports, this was also the case in the United Kingdom (UK) for most community midwives during the last century. However, following the Peel Report (Maternity Advisory Committee 1970), that gave rise to the move of childbirth from the home to the hospital environment, such skills of the midwife have been eroded as midwifery became subsumed into a medico-technocratic model where obstetric intervention prevailed: including the management of breech births.

However, since the early 1990s there has been much socio-political influence in the UK, aimed at improving childbirth choices and quality of maternity services for women, whilst also providing the opportunity for midwives to re-examine their role in providing a more holistic model of care to the pregnant woman (Department of Health [DH] 1993, 1998, 1999, 2003, 2004, 2007). Furthermore, the reduction in junior doctors' hours (DH 2002) has provided further opportunities for Trusts to embrace collaborative working between health professionals (DH 2001), that in some instances have led to a redefining of roles and responsibilities for the midwife and her medical colleagues.

In respect of facilitating a vaginal breech birth, Cronk (1998a, 1998b) and Reed (1999a, 2003) have clearly documented their experiences of supporting women to give birth naturally other than by caesarean section and are an inspiration to other midwives seeking to develop or re-establish skills in this area. However, not all breeches can, or should be, born vaginally. It is not the intent of this chapter to address the various type of breech presentation, the diagnosis and physiology and mechanism of a breech birth as these are well documented in other text (Burvill 2005, Chadwick 2002, Coates 2009, Lewis 2004), but to re-examine the knowledge and skills required to effectively facilitate **planned** vaginal breech births at term in both home and hospital settings. Consequently, the over-riding aim is to empower midwives with the confidence to develop/advance their skills in this area, recognising those situations where a vaginal breech can be contemplated and successfully achieved, and thus improve the choices available to childbearing women.

Incidence of breech presentation

Breech presentation is a longitudinal lie of the fetus with the buttocks in the lower pole of the maternal uterus. The incidence of breech presentation reduces as pregnancy progresses: being around 15% at 28 weeks to around 3–4% by term as a result of spontaneous version (Chadwick 2002). However, it is more common for the fetus to present by the breech where there is a multiple pregnancy, preterm labour, fetal abnormality such as hydrocephaly, Müllerian fusion of the uterus, placenta praevia, pelvic masses (fibroids and large ovarian cysts) and polyhydramnios.

Whilst the use of acupuncture techniques using moxibustion (see Chapter 3) and external cephalic versions for uncomplicated breech presentations at term (see Chapter 5) have had some effect on reducing the incidence of breech presentation, Hofmeyer and Kulier (2000) found that postural management of adopting the knee-chest position for varying time periods in late pregnancy showed no significant benefit for spontaneous breech version.

The evidence

The evidence regarding the safest mode for breech babies to be born has been somewhat controversial and misleading. Hannah et al (2000) had found in their randomised multi-centred Term Breech Trial that the safest way to give birth to a baby presenting by the breech was by planned caesarean section, as the outcomes were much better in this group than those from the planned vaginal birth group. This has had an effect on the choices offered to women who may be presenting with a breech towards the end of their pregnancy regarding the mode of birth and a consequential increase in planned caesarean sections.

By 2004 doubts had been cast on the results of Hannah et al's (2000) study. Although Kotaska (2004) had questioned the validity and ethical basis of using a randomised controlled trial for such a study, there had been other retrospective studies undertaken by Háheim et al (2004) and Ulander et al (2004) that also distrusted the results and recommendations. Work undertaken by Alarab et al

(2004) further claimed that vaginal birth was still a safe option for breech presentations. Interestingly, in the follow-up study to the Term Breech Trial, Whyte et al (2004) and Hannah et al (2004) discovered that the outcomes between the planned caesarean section group and the planned vaginal birth group after 2 years were comparable in both maternal health and child development; although more babies in the vaginal birth group initially required some form of resuscitation. In comparison, a small-scale trial in the Netherlands reported by Molkenboer et al (2006) showed that the outcomes for breech babies weighing over 3.5 kg who were born vaginally, were possibly worse at 2 years than babies of similar weight born by planned caesarean section.

A more recent study (PREMODA study) conducted in France and Belgium clearly concluded that, where planned vaginal breech birth is common practice and when strict criteria are met before and during labour, vaginal breech birth at term can still be a safe option (Goffinet et al 2006). In this study the maternity units taking part, maintained their usual policies and practice for advising women with a breech presentation at term and thus continued exercising their clinical judgment to make appropriate decisions in the best interest of woman and baby regarding mode of birth. This was in direct contrast with Hannah et al's (2000) study where any clinical judgment was ultimately removed from the health professional as women were randomly selected to each group which consequently affected the overall results.

For a successful outcome of a vaginal breech birth, the evidence also points to the most important factor being that of an experienced health professional to assist the woman. However, details as to whether this is a midwife or obstetrician is not specified. Where there were comparable birth outcomes between vaginal breech and planned caesarean section, the attending health professional had 10–20 years experience of vaginal breech births. Consequently, the Confidential Enquiry into Stillbirths and Deaths in Infancy [CESDI] (2000) recommended that the most experienced available practitioner should be present at a vaginal breech birth and that all maternity units have guidelines in place, including structured simulated training for all staff who may encounter vaginal breech births.

Indications and contraindications of vaginal breech birth

When assessing the feasibility to support a woman's decision to give birth vaginally, the midwife should be aware of the indications and contraindications of vaginal breech births as detailed in Table 9.1. A risk assessment should be made and discussed with each individual woman based on these details, including place of birth. The decisions that are subsequently made should be clearly articulated in the woman's records so that other health professionals who may be involved in the woman's care are also fully aware of the situation (Nursing and Midwifery Council [NMC] 2004, 2005, 2008).

Table 9.1 Indications and contraindications of vaginal breech birth

	Indications	Contraindications
Presentation	Flexed/extended	Incomplete
Fetal size	< 4000 g	> 4000 g
Maternal pelvis	Clinically adequate	Evidence of fetopelvic disproportion
Attitude of fetal head	Flexed/deflexed	Hyperextension
Fetal status	No fetal abnormality	Gross fetal abnormality: hydrocephaly Fetal growth restriction (*relative contraindication*)
Maternal status	No underlying medical condition/surgical indication	Surgical indications: placenta praevia, previous caesarean section x 2 / uterine surgery (*relative contraindication*) Medical conditions (*relative contraindication*)

Potential complications of breech birth

Whilst the significance of midwives being able to detect and minimise risk in all childbirth scenarios is clearly recognised, it is especially important that they are fully aware of the potential complications associated specifically with vaginal breech births at term. These are listed in Table 9.2. Awareness of these potential complications serves in providing the basis of the midwife's intrapartum care and facilitation of a safe vaginal birth. In the latest Confidential Enquiry into Maternal and Child Health [CEMACH] report on Perinatal Mortality in 2005 there were eight reported neonatal deaths at term of breech presentations due to intrapartum asphyxia (CEMACH 2007); however, the mode of birth or place of birth were not articulated.

Place of birth

If there are no contraindications identified and a vaginal breech birth is planned for the home environment it is important that the midwife is competent to facilitate the birth and has clear lines of communication and support from her colleagues, including the supervisor of midwives, with a second midwife being present for the birth itself. However,

Table 9.2 Potential complications of breech birth

Potential fetal/neonatal complication	Associated cause
Congenital abnormality: e.g. hydrocephaly	A cause for the presentation Mechanism of the birth itself poses risks
Congenital dislocation of the hip (↑ frank/extended breech)	Usually a complication of the presentation and **not** the birth process
Fetal asphyxia	Umbilical cord prolapse (↑ preterm labour) Cord compression Premature placental separation once the body has been born
Intracranial haemorrhage	Rapid decompression of the fetal skull causing tearing of the dura mater lining the brain and other major blood vessels
Fractures of the femur, humerus, clavicle and spine/spinal cord damage Dislocation of the hip, shoulder, neck Brachial nerve paralysis (Erb's Palsy) Soft-tissue damage to fetal liver, kidneys, spleen and adrenal glands Dislocation of fetal jaw/soft tissue damage to mouth and gums/feeding difficulties	Incorrect or excessive handling during the birth Abdominal area is roughly squeezed Baby's mouth incorrectly being used to create traction rather than the malar bones (cheekbones) in the Mauriceau–Smellie–Veit manoeuvre
Cold injury/thermal shock and hypoglycaemia	Ambient temperature too cool and baby loses heat during completion of the birth process
Potential maternal complication	
Urethral, vaginal and perineal trauma	Rapid birth of the baby's head
Effects of anaesthesia (local, regional, general), infection, haemorrhage, thromboembolic disorders, etc.	Risks of operative procedures
Psychological distress, affecting attachment to baby, feeding difficulties and traumatic stress disorder	Unexpected vaginal breech birth with lack of time to discuss options

according to NICE (2007) a breech is considered to be a malpresentation indicative of risk, and recommends the labour and birth should be planned to take place in an obstetric unit. Outside of the hospital environment, any decision to transfer the woman from the home should be made promptly, taking into consideration the time it would take to complete. An action plan for the labour and birth should be made with the woman including identifying those situations where midwives would make the decision to transfer to hospital: namely where there is a lack of progress or fetal compromise.

If the midwife encounters a woman in labour at home with a breech presentation where a hospital birth had initially been planned, she should remain calm whilst making a careful assessment of the risk to the woman and baby, taking into consideration the parent's wishes before a decision to transfer to hospital is made. This will depend on the stage of labour, fetal position and maternal medical and obstetric history. If the woman was nearing the second stage of labour, assistance should be promptly summoned while supporting her to give birth at home rather than in a cramped and cool ambulance. On the other hand, if a decision is made to transfer to hospital, the midwife should alert the hospital of the transfer and ensure that the paramedics are equipped for neonatal resuscitation. The fetal heart and maternal condition should be monitored and recorded throughout the journey to hospital. The midwife must always be prepared for the birth in transit as it may progress more rapidly than initially anticipated. In such a situation, the driver should be asked to stop the ambulance in order for the midwife to assist the birth and undertake any necessary manoeuvres safely. It is worth considering taking a number of towels/blankets to wrap the baby should it be born in transit, skin-to-skin contact and early breast feeding to maintain thermoregulation, i.e. warmth and reducing the likelihood of hypoglycaemia and hypothermia.

Position for birth

The woman's position can significantly affect the physiological labour and birth process and the one that is adopted should ideally be her choice. Unlike with cephalic presentations, there has been no research undertaken to ascertain the optimal position for women to give birth vaginally to a breech presentation at term. Much of the text describing vaginal breech births tends to assume the woman should give birth in the hospital environment on the bed in a semi-recumbent, adapted lithotomy position. This position, however, affects the normal physiological process of labour where the fetus struggles to be born against gravity, consequently increasing the need for the midwife to undertake manoeuvres and assist the birth. In contrast, Burvill (2005, p. 114) defines a physiological breech birth as:

> one in which the mother births her baby in the position in which she feels most comfortable, under her own power, her uterine contractions and gravity working in harmony.

While gravity helps to expel the fetus, it is the expulsive contractions and angle of the pelvis that assists in facilitating a physiological breech birth, requiring little assistance from the midwife, except in the birthing of the after-coming head. The experiences of midwives competent in facilitating vaginal breech birth have clearly demonstrated this with their 'hands off the breech' approach, when the woman either adopts a standing or an 'all fours position'/'English pray' position (Burvill 2005, Cronk 1998, Reed 2003, Royal College of Midwives [RCM] 2005). Where the mother is on 'all fours' or leans up on the bed/settee or on her birth partner (see Figure 9.1), the baby's trunk descends through the pelvis at 45° and is able to move more freely around the curve of Carus of the maternal pelvis. Not only does this position provide an excellent view of the birth process and access to the baby's face as it is born over the perineum, there is also ample space for the midwife to undertake any manoeuvres should they be necessary to assist the birth of the baby.

Facilitating a breech labour and birth

When undertaking intrapartum care of a woman presenting with a breech at term, there are some important issues for the midwife to consider that are pertinent to the breech scenario. These have been summarised in the *Intrapartum checklist* as detailed in Box 9.1.

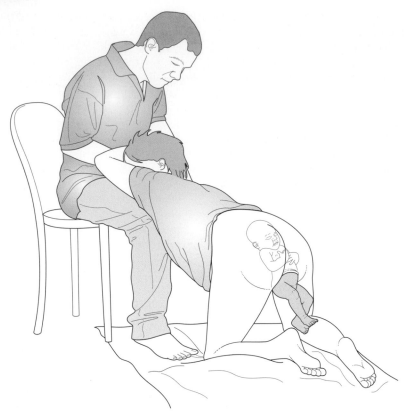

Figure 9.1 • The baby descending in the 'English pray' position.

Manoeuvres to assist the birth of the breech

The following manoeuvres were originally developed to facilitate a breech birth with the woman positioned on the bed, but may be utilised when the woman is on 'all fours' or standing. However, with the benefits of gravity encouraging descent of the fetus in the latter positions, the likelihood of the midwife needing to adopt such measures is reduced. Nevertheless, it is important that the midwife is both aware of, and skilled in such manoeuvres and maintains such competence.

For extended legs

If the fetal legs are not born spontaneously, it is likely they are extended. Gentle pressure, as shown in Figure 9.2, can be applied in the popliteal fossa (back of the knee) of one of the legs to encourage flexion that will assist in the birth of the leg. This can be repeated for the other leg if necessary.

For extended arms: *Løvsets manoeuvre*

This manoeuvre is used when the arms fail to appear during the birth of the baby's trunk and chest as a result of them being extended above the head. If the arms are not released then labour will be obstructed.

The baby is held at the iliac crests with thumbs over the sacrum and downward traction is applied whilst the baby is rotated 180° (see Figure 9.3). Care must be taken to always keep the baby's back towards the woman's front, i.e. the baby's ***back*** must be ***uppermost*** in a semi-recumbent position or the baby's ***abdomen*** is ***uppermost*** in an all fours position. It is important that the baby is not grasped by the flanks or abdomen as this may cause intra-abdominal trauma resulting in kidney, liver or spleen injury.

Box 9.1

Intrapartum check list for vaginal breech labour and birth at term

- **Monitoring of progress**:

  If the physiological process of labour does not progress, this should be clearly documented and assistance sought. The use of oxytocics to augment a breech labour should be avoided (due to the additional effects this can have on fetal well being) and caesarean section be undertaken.

- **Analgesia:**

  Opiates are discouraged as they can affect fetal well being. However, in the hospital setting epidural analgesia reduces the woman's mobility that consequentially affects the physiological process of birth.

- **Regular fetal heart monitoring undertaken and documented**:

  Continuous electronic fetal heart monitoring *in hospital.* Pinard or sonicaid auscultation every 15 minutes during and following a contraction in the first stage and following each contraction in the second stage *at home* (NICE 2007 recommendations).

- **Check for cord prolapse if membranes rupture and buttocks are not engaged.**

- **Meconium stained liquor:**

  Distinction should be made between meconium that is passed by the fetus as a consequence of the abdomen and buttocks being compressed during descent through the birth canal and liquor that is truly meconium stained as a result of fetal compromise.

- **Check for full dilatation before encouraging the woman to push:**

  The woman may experience a premature urge to push as the fetal body can pass through the cervix prior to full dilatation: the fetal head could become entrapped causing asphyxia increasing perinatal morbidity and mortality.

- **The umbilical cord may be loosened gently (RARELY required):**

  This may be undertaken to prevent constriction of blood vessels as the baby's body is born. In the 'all fours' position, the condition of the baby can be easily monitored by observing the chest movements.

- **Encourage a physiological birth with minimum handling (*hands off the breech*):**

  To allow the baby to be born by gravity and propulsion and reduce trauma to the baby.

- **Vault of the fetal skull should be born slowly**:

  To avoid rapid decompression resulting in intracranial haemorrhage.

- **Be aware and skilled in manoeuvres:**

  To assist the birth of the breech if problems arise with fetal descent and to control the birth of the baby's head.

- **DO NOT PERFORM BREECH EXTRACTION (routine use of manoeuvres/interventions to expedite birth):**

  This can cause delay and obstruction, e.g. fetal arms pulled upwards, head extended backwards.

- **Care of the baby following birth should include:**

  Appropriate resuscitation including suction of the oropharynx and inspection of the vocal cords (if thick meconium), maintaining the baby's body temperature, early feeding and paediatric assessment for signs of birth trauma.

- **Postnatal examination of the mother:**

  To assess the physical condition including any birth trauma and discuss the birth and its outcome whilst assessing psychological well being.

- **Documentation**:

  Is vitally important throughout the labour and birth, to include specific details of all discussions and referrals, and the time they were initiated. As the breech is born, the time that each stage is reached and any manoeuvres undertaken should also be recorded. Additionally documentation should account for immediate condition of the baby, including any resuscitation measures taken, and the condition of the mother following the birth.

Løvsets manoeuvre enables the baby's posterior arm lying in the sacral curve, to rotate and lie anteriorly under the pubic arch. The anterior arm is then born and the baby can be rotated back in the opposite direction in order for the second arm to be born. If the arm is not born spontaneously, it is usual to splint the humerus with two fingers, flex the elbow and sweep the arm across the face and downwards across the baby's chest ('cat-lick' manoeuvre).

Should the woman have adopted the all fours position, it is important that the baby's **abdomen** remains uppermost. Therefore, if the baby's left arm is extended, the baby should be rotated to the

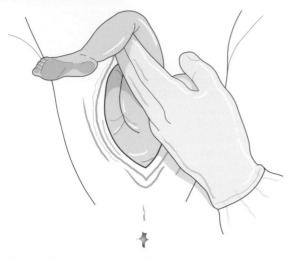

Figure 9.2 ● Assisting the birth of extended leg by applying pressure on the popliteal fossa. (From Fraser and Cooper 2009, with kind permission of Elsevier.)

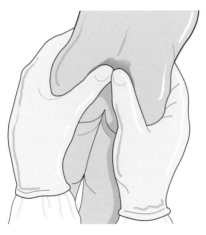

Figure 9.3 ● Correct grasp for Løvsets manoeuvre for extended arms. (From Fraser and Cooper 2009, with kind permission of Elsevier.)

left by applying downward traction on the pelvic girdle in order to release the arm. This process is then repeated for the right arm if necessary.

For the after-coming head

Burns Marshall

This particular manoeuvre facilitates movement of the baby's head through the maternal pelvic outlet, but is only possible when the woman is in a semi-recumbent, adapted lithotomy position. The baby is allowed to 'hang' until the head descends onto

the perineum when after about 1 to 2 minutes, the nape of the neck becomes visible and the sub-occipital region is born. The baby's ankles are grasped and, while maintaining traction to prevent the neck from extending and resulting in possible cervical spine fracture, the sub-occipital region is pivoted through an 180° arc under the pubic arch, until the mouth and nose are free of the vulva (see Figure 9.4A). This should be undertaken slowly to prevent sudden changes in pressure to the baby's head and undue stretching of the perineum. The perineum can be guarded to prevent sudden escape of the head (Figure 9.4B). It is essential that the midwife observes that the baby has descended sufficiently to ensure that it is the sub-occipital region that pivots under the pubic arch and not the neck to avoid fracture of the cervical vertebra and crushing of the spinal cord.

Mauriceau-Smellie-Veit

Although the baby's head is facilitated through the same 180° arc as in the Burns Marshall manoeuvre, the Mauriceau-Smellie-Veit manoeuvre provides more control with the birth of the head and places less strain on the baby's back. This particular manoeuvre can be undertaken in a variety of positions that the woman may adopt for the birth:

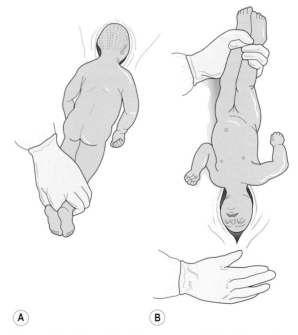

(A)   (B)

Figure 9.4 ● Burns Marshall manoeuvre for the after-coming head. (A) Correct grasp around the fetal ankles. (B) The sub-occipital region pivots 180° under the pubic arch: the mouth and nose are free of the vulva. (From Fraser and Cooper 2009, with kind permission of Elsevier.)

semi-recumbent, sitting, the adopted lithotomy position or in the 'all fours' position. As this manoeuvre facilitates maximum flexion of the baby's head, it can be used to advantage when the head is extended and descent is delayed. Furthermore, it allows for slow birthing of the baby's head and thus reduces the risk of intracranial haemorrhage.

In the semi-recumbent position, the midwife should first support the baby on one of her arms, with her first and ring fingers placed on the baby's malar bones (cheekbones), pulling the jaw down and increasing flexion. It is important that the midwife avoids placing her finger in the baby's mouth to prevent fracture to the jaw or trauma to the mouth and gums that can result in the baby having difficulties with feeding. The other hand is placed across the baby's shoulders with the midwife's middle finger on the occiput to increase flexion. The outer fingers can apply gentle traction on the baby's shoulders. Maintaining flexion, the head is delivered until the sub-occipital region appears and then the baby's head is slowly pivoted gently and slowly **upwards** around the symphysis pubis following the curve of Carus, delivering the chin and face first (see Figure 9.5A).

In an all fours position, the baby's head is flexed by tipping the occiput **forwards** with the middle finger of the right hand and by gentle pressure on the baby's malar bones with the fingers of the left hand (see Figure 9.5B and C). The vault of baby's head should be born slowly and gently to facilitate gradual adaptation of the head to the changing pressures imposed by the birth process. This should be in a **downwards** direction following the pelvic curve of Carus.

Professional responsibilities of the midwife

Responsibility to develop competence in breech birth

The European Union (EU) and Article 42 of Directive 2005/36/EC that determine the basis of the midwifery education and training programmes of member states, clearly state that midwives are at least entitled to take up and pursue a breech birth, but only in URGENT cases (NMC 2009). However, as it is normal for 3–4% of all pregnancies to present with a breech at term, midwives should have the knowledge and skills to support women who choose to birth their baby vaginally as stated in the Standard requirements and Guidance of Rule 6 (NMC 2004). As obstetricians are expected to have such skills according to the guidance by the Royal College of Obstetricians and Gynaecologists [RCOG] (2006), it is argued that so should midwives, who are not only the main intrapartum carer, but are usually the first health professional the woman has contact with in labour.

In order to avoid a total loss of these skills in the midwifery profession, midwives with experience in facilitating vaginal breech birth have a professional responsibility not only to maintain their own knowledge and skills, but also to pass these on to other midwives, including student midwives. This can be achieved by 'normalising' breech births at term in the midwifery curricula, as well as in the clinical area and in skills and competency centres through simulation in skills drills, Interprofessional Team Objective Structured Clinical Examination [ITOSCE] with paramedics or obstetricians and through supervision of midwifery. The regular use of life-size mannequins or a doll and pelvis to go through the mechanism of vaginal breech birth and possible manoeuvres, can effect development and maintenance of the skills involved and also inspire midwives with confidence in their abilities to then transfer into their clinical practice.

Accountability

Midwives are accountable for their actions and omissions in care. This also applies to the information and advice they give to women, which must be based on the best available evidence so that the woman has every opportunity to make an informed decision. All the options available to the woman must be presented, including risks and benefits, should their baby be presenting by the breech. Failure to do so may constitute a breach in the duty of care on the part of the midwife should any harm to the woman and baby result from the act/omission (Dimond 2006). The continued endorsement of caesarean sections as the only safe option for breech presentation because of the lack of experienced health professionals skilled in vaginal breech birth, Evans (2007) proclaims to be bordering on the criminal and a failure to address the ethical principle of non-maleficence (do no harm). All decisions made and actions taken should be undertaken safely

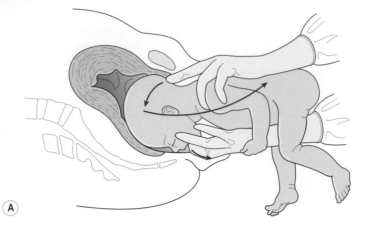

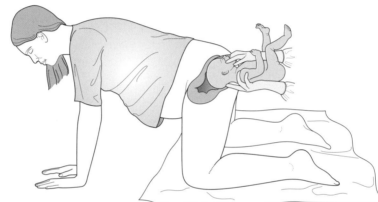

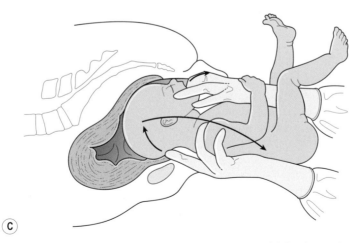

Figure 9.5 • Mauriceau-Smellie-Veit manoeuvre for the after-coming head. (A) Semi-recumbent/sitting/adapted lithotomy position showing position of hands and *downward* direction of flexion whilst pivoting *upwards* through an 180° arc under the pubic arch. (B and C) 'All fours' position demonstrating how the occiput is tipped *forwards* to achieve flexion, pivoting *downwards* under the symphysis pubis to facilitate birth of the head. (A and C adapted from Sweet & Tiran 1997, with permission of Elsevier).

and appropriately, and in accordance with the ethical principle of beneficence: in the best interests of the woman and baby.

Consent and trespass to the person

Should the midwife use her professional judgment and decide to undertake a manoeuvre to assist the breech birth, as this will involve her making some contact with the person of the woman, it is important she obtains the woman's consent in order to avoid a claim of legal tort of trespass to the person. It is recommended that the midwife discusses the reasons for manoeuvres, including their benefits and risks, with the woman, obtains her consent to undertake any necessary manoeuvres and records this in advance of labour, to enable her to fully understand their significance.

Negligence and a reasonable standard of care

The Clinical Negligence Scheme for Trusts (CNST) that encourages and supports the effective management of claims and risk, requires that all Trusts contributing to the scheme, have referenced, evidenced-based multidisciplinary policies for key conditions/situations on labour wards. One of these policies relates to breech presentation that includes external cephalic version and selection for vaginal birth. Part of the midwife's legal accountability is being conversant with local policies and guidelines, risk management and midwifery supervision in respect of vaginal breech births. A case of negligence may be proven if the midwife does not follow local policy and guidelines or if she is not competent or adequately trained to facilitate vaginal breech births. For negligence to be proven in law, it has to be shown that the midwife facilitating the birth owed the woman a duty of care which was not exercised (breached) and, as a result, harm occurred.

Should there be an alleged case of negligence, the basis for the professional standards by which a midwife would be judged, in respect of her knowledge, skills and competence is founded on the Bolam principle (Bolam v Friern Hospital Management Committee 1957). This relates to the standard of care expected of the ordinary skilled midwife that is commensurate with others in her area of practice and as judged by her peers: such standards being

reasonably expected at the time the alleged negligent act took place. A midwife who facilitates vaginal breech births, therefore, is expected to demonstrate skills conscious of the Bolam principle and her professional accountability.

Vicarious liability

It is usual that where a midwife has been found negligent while acting in the course of her employment, her employer (the National Health Service [NHS] Trust) will accept liability and thus compensation would be paid out for the negligent action or omission. Independent midwives, however, will need to ensure they have adequate personal indemnity insurance should there be any claim for compensation as a result of alleged negligence on their part. Furthermore, midwives may find themselves involved in disciplinary, professional and civil hearings as a result of their actions. It is, therefore, important that midwives who facilitate planned vaginal breech birth ensure that their employer will accept responsibility for their practice, providing they have the required knowledge and skills and have followed risk-management procedures.

For some midwives to facilitate vaginal breech births this may mean they have to be instrumental in changing attitudes among colleagues in clinical practice, be it in the community or the hospital setting. This may also necessitate a change in Trust policy that embraces midwives being granted the authority to use their clinical judgment and skill to appropriately advise and assist women to birth their breech babies vaginally. As a result, the midwife would be working within her contractual obligations to her employer, who in turn would accept any liability.

Documentation and autonomous practice

The quality of record keeping is reflective of the standard of the midwife's professional practice and the extent of her autonomy in making clinical decisions (Marshall 2005). The midwife should be conversant with Rule 9 (NMC 2004) and the contents of the *Guidelines for records and record keeping* (NMC 2005) as her records may be scrutinised by her supervisor of midwives at the annual supervisory meeting, or used to investigate a complaint at local level. Furthermore, the records may also be accessed by the Care Quality Commission: the new health and social care regulator in England, a court of law or used as evidence by the NMC's Fitness to Practise Committee. Throughout this chapter, the importance of the midwife's record keeping has been highlighted in relation to the discussions with the woman about the mode and place of birth for the breech birth, including the benefits and risks. Specific details relating to the intrapartum documentation is also evident in the *Intrapartum check list*.

It is particularly important that where the woman is reluctant to consider anything other than a vaginal breech birth, regardless of the midwife's professional advice of the contraindications and consequential risks, the midwife seeks the advice of her supervisor of midwives and other experienced colleagues to offer support in managing the situation to the best of her abilities. Respecting the autonomy of the woman in this situation would be unethically sound. It is essential that the midwife clearly documents *all* the details of such advice as she can be held accountable for any omissions in this respect should an adverse outcome result (NMC 2004, 2005). It is recommended that entries are made in the records by the supervisor of midwives and other colleagues in support of the midwife's clinical judgment. However, the midwife has a legal duty of care to provide midwifery care to the woman in whatever environment the woman chooses to give birth: including a vaginal breech birth.

Conclusion

As an autonomous, accountable practitioner, the midwife has responsibility to offer women true choice regarding mode of birth and promote normal physiological birth in relation to breech presentations at term. This includes being familiar with the current evidence and re-developing the skills midwives once had to facilitate vaginal breech births at term where there are no contraindications. However, it is imperative that such skills are seen as part of the normal physiological birth process rather than viewed as a rare maternity 'emergency'

by education providers, medical colleagues and employers. This is the challenge that midwives must meet in order to fully address their professional and legal duties to the childbearing woman, who presents with a breech at term.

Key practice points

- A physiological labour and spontaneous vaginal birth is a viable option for women with an uncomplicated pregnancy and breech presentation at term.
- Midwives should be aware of the indications for and potential complications of a vaginal breech birth in order to minimise risk and encourage a successful outcome.
- Midwives must ensure their advice to women regarding mode of birth for breech presentations at term is evidence-based and founded on ethical principles.
- Trust policy should embrace midwives developing/advancing their skills in the facilitation of vaginal breech births at term in uncomplicated pregnancies.
- A physiological birth should be encouraged where the breech is born with the aid of gravity and propulsion and *NOT* traction: adopting the principle of *'hands off the breech'*.
- Midwives should be skilled in manoeuvres to assist the birth of the breech, being aware of the situations in which to use them.
- There should be a comprehensive action plan made with the woman and clear lines of communication with colleagues and the supervisor of midwives, especially when the vaginal breech birth is planned in the home environment.
- Midwives should be fully conversant with their statutory responsibilities and professional and legal accountability in respect of vaginal breech births at term.
- Collaborative learning and working practices are vital to ensure the skill of facilitating vaginal breech births is re-established in normal midwifery practice so that women are provided with *all* available options.
- Skilled and experienced practitioners are the key to physiological vaginal breech births.

References

Alarab, M., Regan, C., O'Connell, M.P., Keane, D.P., O'Herlihy, C., Foley, M.E., 2004. Singleton breech delivery at term: still a safe option. Obstet. Gynecol. 103 (3), 407–412.

Allison, J., 1996. Delivered at home. Chapman and Hall, London.

Bolam v Friern Hospital Management Committee, 1957. WRL 582.

Burvill, S., 2005. Managing breech presentation in the absence of obstetric assistance. In: Woodward, V., Bates, K., Young, N. (Eds.), Managing childbirth emergencies in community settings. Palgrave Macmillan, Basingstoke, Hampshire, pp. 111–139.

Chadwick, J., 2002. Malpresentations and Malpositions. In: Boyle, M. (Ed.), Emergencies around childbirth. Radcliffe Medical Press, Oxon, pp. 63–81.

Coates, T., 2009. Malpositions of the occiput and malpresentations. In: Fraser, D.M., Cooper, M.A. (Eds.), Myles textbook for midwives. Fourteenth ed. Churchill Livingstone, Edinburgh, pp. 573–605.

Confidential Enquiry into Maternal and Child Health [CEMACH], 2007. Perinatal Mortality 2005: England Wales and Northern Ireland. CEMACH, London.

Confidential Enquiry into Stillbirths and Deaths in Infancy [CESDI], 2000. Seventh Annual Report. Maternal and Child Health Research Consortium, London.

Cronk, M., 1998a. Midwives and breech births. Pract. Midwife 1 (7/8), 44–45.

Cronk, M., 1998b. Hands off the breech. Pract. Midwife 1 (6), 13–15.

Department of Health, 1993. Changing childbirth, Part 1: report of the Expert Maternity Group. HMSO, London.

Department of Health, 1998. A First class service: quality in the new NHS. HMSO, London.

Department of Health, 1999. Making a difference: strengthening the nursing, midwifery and health visiting contribution to health and healthcare. HMSO, London.

Department of Health, 2001. Working together, learning together. A framework for lifelong learning in the NHS. HMSO, London.

Department of Health, 2003. Building on the best: choice, responsiveness and equity in the NHS. The Stationary Office, London.

Department of Health, 2004. The NHS Knowledge and Skills Framework (NHS KSF) and the development review process. HMSO, London.

Department of Health, 2007. Maternity matters: choice, access and continuity of care in a safe service. HMSO, London.

Department of Health The National Assembly for Wales, the NHS Confederation and the British Medical Association, 2002. Guidance on working patterns for junior doctors. HMSO, London.

Dimond, B., 2006. Legal aspects of midwifery. Books for midwives, Cheshire.

Evans, J., 2007. First do no harm. Pract. Midwife 10 (8), 22–23.

Fraser, D.M., Cooper, M.A., 2009. Myles textbook for midwives. fourteenth ed. Elsevier, Edinburgh.

Goffinet, F., Carayol, M., Foidart, J.M., Alexander, S., Uzan, S., Subtil, D., Bréart, G., PREMODA Study Group, 2006. Is planned vaginal delivery of breech presentation at term still an option? Results of an observational prospective survey in France and Belguim. Am. J. Obstet. Gynecol. 194 (4), 1002–1011.

Háheim, L.L., Albrechtsen, S., Nordbø Berge, W., Bórdahl, P.E., Egeland, T., Henriksen, T., Øian, P., 2004. Breech birth at term: vaginal delivery or elective caesarean section? A systematic review of the literature by a Norwegian review team. Acta Obstet. Gynecol. Scand. 83 (2), 126–130.

Hannah, M.E., Hannah, W.J., Hewson, S.A., Hodnett, E.D., Saigal, S., Willan, A.R. Term Breech Trial Collaborative Group, 2000. Planned caesarean section versus planned vaginal birth for breech presentation at term: a randomized multi-centre trial. Lancet 356, 1375–1383.

Hannah, M.E., Whyte, H.D., Hannah, W.J., Hewson, S., Amankwah, K., Cheng, M., et al., 2004. Term Breech Trial Collaborative Group. Maternal outcomes at two years after planned caesarean section versus planned vaginal birth for breech presentation at term: the international randomized multi-centre trial. Am. J. Obstet. Gynecol. 191 (3), 917–927.

Hofmeyer, G.J., Kulier, R., 2000. Cephalic version by postural management for breech presentation. In: The Cochrane Library, Issue 3. Update Software, Oxford. CD000051.

Kotaska, A., 2004. Inappropriate use of randomized trials to evaluate complex phenomena: case study of vaginal breech delivery. BMJ 329, 1039–1042.

Lewis, P., 2004. Malpositions and malpresentations. In: Henderson, C., Macdonald, S. (Eds.), Mayes midwifery: a textbook for midwives. thirteenth ed. Balliere Tindall, London, pp. 884–917.

Marshall, J.E., 2005. Autonomy and the midwife. In Raynor, M.D., Marshall, J.E., Sullivan, A. (Eds.), Decision making in midwifery practice. Elsevier, Edinburgh, pp. 9–21.

Maternity Advisory Committee, 1970. Domiciliary and maternity bed needs. Chairman Peel Sir John. HMSO, London.

Molkenboer, J.F., Roumen, F.J., Smits, L.J., NiJhuis, J.G., 2006. Birth weight and neurodevelopmental outcomes of children at two years of age after planned vaginal delivery for breech presentation at term. Am. J. Obstet. Gynecol. 194 (3), 624–629.

National Institute for Health and Clinical Excellence, 2007. Intrapartum care: care of healthy women and their babies during childbirth (NICE Clinical Guideline 55). Developed by the National Collaborating Centre for Women's and Children's Health. NICE, London.

Nursing and Midwifery Council, 2004. Midwives rules and standards. NMC, London.

Nursing and Midwifery Council, 2009. Standards for pre-registration midwifery education. NMC, London.

Nursing and Midwifery Council, 2005. Guidelines for records and record keeping. NMC, London.

Nursing and Midwifery Council, 2008. The Code: Standards of conduct, performance and ethics for nurses and midwives. NMC, London.

Reed, B., 1999a. Knee deep at a home birth. Pract. Midwife 2 (8), 46.

Reed, B., 2003. A disappearing art: vaginal breech birth. Pract. Midwife 69, 16–18.

Royal College of Midwives, 2005. Normal breech birth. Available online: www.rcmnormalbirth.org.uk/ default.asp?sID=1099658440484 Accessed 24 February 2008.

Royal College of Obstetricians and Gynaecologists, 2006. Clinical green top guidelines for management of breech presentation No 20b. RCOG, London.

Sweet, B.R., Tiran, D. (Eds.), 1997. Mayes' Midwifery, 12th edn Elsevier, Edinburgh.

Ulander, V.M., Gissler, M., Nuutila, M., Ylikorkala, O., 2004. Are health expectations of term breech infants unrealistically high? Acta Obstet. Gynecol. Scand. 83 (2), 180–186.

Whyte, H.D., Hannah, M.E., Saigal, S., Hannah, W.J., Hewson, S., Amankwah, K., et al., 2004. Outcomes of children at two years after planned caesarean section birth versus planned vaginal birth for breech presentation at term: the international randomized term breech trial. Am. J. Obstet. Gynecol. 191 (3), 864–871.

Further reading

Breech birth: the mechanism of delivery displayed, 2000. Pract. Midwife 3 (2), 20–22.
Clearly demonstrates the mechanism of the birth of a breech presentation at home in the 'all-fours' position through text and photographs.

Evans, J. 2005. Breech birth: What are my options? AIMS, Taunton.
An informative and empowering text that discusses the major issues surrounding breech birth and explains the options for women and midwives to consider that are reinforced by the inclusion of poignant personal birth stories.

Reed, B., 1999b. Knee-deep: the photo story. Pract. Midwife 2 (10), 16–17.
The photographic account of a breech birth presenting with a knee, attended by Becky Reed [see Reed B 1999a] with narrative from the mother's perspective.

Useful websites

www.radmid.demon.co.uk
www.rcmnormalbirth.org,uk

Chapter Ten

10

Perineal management and repair

Christine Kettle and Maureen D. Raynor

CONTENTS

Introduction 104
Background 104
Education/training 104
Classification of spontaneous perineal
tears 105
Assessment of perineal trauma 105
Current evidence 106
  Management of perineal tears
  (first and second) and episiotomy:
  non-suturing issues 106
  Implications for practice of
  non-suturing perineal muscles 107
  Implications for practice of non-suturing
  of the perineal skin 108
Suture techniques 108
Suture materials 108
  Suture materials and technique:
  recommendations for practice 108
Management of complex perineal trauma 110
  Third-degree tears 110
Risk factors 110
Repair of sphincter trauma 110
Principles and technique of repair 110
Who should carry out primary repair
of obstetric anal injuries? 111
Management of other types of complex
trauma 112
  Tear in rectal mucosa (buttonhole) . . . 112
  Bilateral vaginal tears 112
  Management of tears to the labia
  minora 112
  Periurethral lacerations 113
  Management of perineal haematoma . 114

Female genital mutilation 114
  Classification and prevalence
  of female genital mutilation 114
  Female genital mutilation:
  legal context 114
  Female genital mutilation:
  the evidence base 116
Assessment and care planning for
labour 116
  Procedure for de-infibulation 117
  Female genital mutilation
  and perineal suturing 117
Immediate postnatal care 117
Perineal care postpartum: practice
implications 117
Perineal care clinic 117
Medico-legal implications 118
Key practice points 118
References 119
Further reading 120

Before reading this chapter, you should be familiar with:
- Maternal physical and psychological morbidity after birth.
- Impact of morbidity on women's lives and relationships.
- Recommendations of (NICE 2008) antenatal care guidelines and postnatal care guideline (NICE 2006).
- Recommendations of CEMACH (Lewis 2007).
- Skills for health competencies for postnatal care.

- Anatomy and physiology of the external female genitalia and pelvic floor musculature.
- Strategies to prevent perineal trauma during childbirth.
- Current classification of pelvic floor trauma.
- Procedure for undertaking a medio-lateral episiotomy.
- Basic surgical skills including knot tying and correct handling of instruments.
- Procedure for undertaking routine repair of episiotomy or second-degree tears.
- Cultural diversity education/training.

Introduction

The main focus of this chapter will be on the advanced skills required by midwives to assess, classify and repair more complex perineal trauma. It will review the current evidence underpinning the methods and materials used for repair of episiotomy, second, third and fourth-degree tears. In addition, it will address the challenges and professional issues presented to midwives who want to advance their practice and develop proficiency in repairing complex trauma. It will also cover aspects of female genital mutilation relevant to the chapter, the importance of postnatal follow-up and describe multi- and interdisciplinary working in order to reduce associated maternal morbidity.

Background

The impact of perineal trauma can be extremely distressing for a new mother during the early postnatal period when she is trying to cope with hormonal changes, the demands of her baby and pressures imposed as a result of her changing role. Most women are unprepared for the associated discomfort, which is a concern given that more than 300 000 women (Kettle et al 2002) will experience some type of perineal damage following childbirth in the United Kingdom (UK) and millions more worldwide. Perineal trauma is not a new phenomenon, in fact it has occurred throughout the ages and is documented as far back as 2050 BC (Derry 1935). Today midwives utilise current evidence and advanced skills in an endeavour to reduce both the rate and extent of perineal trauma experienced by women. For those women who are unfortunate to sustain perineal

injury it is important that skilled midwives and doctors repair the trauma, using the best suturing techniques and materials, in order to minimise any associated short-term and long-term morbidity. Most maternity hospitals do not provide dedicated 'perineal care clinics' for women with problems and, therefore, have no means of monitoring the long-term physical and psychological effects of perineal trauma following childbirth.

Education/training

The midwife's role has evolved dramatically over the past decade with new challenges presenting as a result of the reduction in junior doctors' hours, new ways of working, women's expectations and cultural diversity. Midwives are keen to develop new skills and advance their practice in order to address the demands of the fast-changing maternity services. However, it is important before any new skills or responsibilities are embraced that knowledge gaps are identified, adequate training programmes are available and competency is reached.

Given that midwives in the UK usually repair most of the episiotomies and tears (first or second degree) that occur following spontaneous vaginal birth, it is concerning that there are no national guidelines relating to the way that the procedure is taught, supervised and assessed. Indeed, a large proportion of midwives do not learn to undertake the procedure of perineal repair until after they are qualified. This can result in wide variations in techniques and materials used due to the fact that the individual midwife/doctor usually adopts the method first taught by their peers, which is quite often not based on robust evidence. A large proportion of midwives also lack basic surgical skills and have poor knowledge of tissue handling, knot tying and the correct use of instruments.

When undertaking perineal repair, midwives must recognise their limitations and be prepared to seek assistance from an experienced colleague as and when necessary to ensure that the procedure is carried out correctly. However, in today's economic climate many hospitals have reduced staffing levels, which result in a reduction in the capacity to supervise or teach colleagues new skills. This may result in a workforce lacking in perineal repair skills and may lead to midwives making the decision to leave tears unsutured. This can be prevented by ensuring that experienced colleagues are available in the workplace to provide ongoing supervision and support for those midwives requiring assistance in developing their perineal repair skills. Midwives who are appropriately trained are more likely to provide a consistent, high standard of repair, which may also reduce the extent of short-term and long-term morbidity associated with perineal trauma. The implications for midwives wishing to engage with repairing complex trauma are detailed at the beginning of the chapter.

Classification of spontaneous perineal tears

When reviewing the literature regarding the classification of spontaneous perineal trauma there is disparity in its definition. This can be confusing to midwives and doctors and may lead to incorrect or inappropriate categorisation. In order to elucidate what structures are involved Sultan (1999) proposed the classification identified in Table 10.1, which has now been adopted by the National Institute for Health and Clinical Excellence (NICE 2007) and the Royal College of Obstetricians and Gynaecologists (2007) as well as the International Consultation on Incontinence (Norton et al 2002).

Table 10.1 Definition/classification of perineal tear (NICE 2007)

Degree	Tear
First degree	Involving injury to the skin only
Second degree	Involving injury to the perineal muscles, but not the anal sphincter
Third degree	Involving injury to the perineum and the anal sphincter complex: 3a: < 50% of external anal sphincter thickness torn 3b: > 50% of external anal sphincter thickness torn 3c: internal anal sphincter torn
Fourth degree	Injury to perineum involving the anal sphincter complex (external anal sphincter and internal anal sphincter) and anal epithelium

It is important for midwives to understand the anatomy and physiology of the pelvic floor and to be able to differentiate between perineal tears involving the external anal sphincter (EAS) and internal anal sphincter (IAS), as depicted in Figure 10.1.

Assessment of perineal trauma

Following completion of the third stage of labour, the midwife responsible for the woman's care must carry out a thorough and systematic examination of the perineum even if it initially looks intact. It is important to explain to the woman why the examination is necessary and to place her in a comfortable position (unsupported lithotomy) so that the trauma is easily visualised, using good lighting. There is no need to use lithotomy poles to support the woman's legs during examination or repair of perineal trauma as this may bring back locked in memories of previous sexual abuse or flashback relating to female genital mutilation (FGM). The external genitalia must be inspected for lacerations and the labia parted to facilitate examination of the anterior, posterior and lateral vaginal walls. It is important to visualise the apex of the vaginal trauma and to identify anatomical landmarks, including the hymenal remnants. A rectal examination must be carried out as part of the initial assessment to ensure that any trauma to the IAS or EAS is not missed (NICE 2007). The woman should be reassured and given an explanation as to why the procedure is necessary and her consent obtained.

The midwife inserts her index finger into the woman's anus and she is then asked to try to contract her anal sphincter (Figure 10.2). The EAS looks similar to striated red meat, such as beef, as compared to the IAS, which is lighter in colour and has been described as being similar to the colour of chicken. If the EAS is torn, the separated ends of the torn muscles will be observed to retract backwards into either side of the ischiorectal fossa. If the woman has an effective epidural she will not be able to contract her EAS muscle. The IAS can be quite difficult to identify as it is a thickened continuation of the circular smooth muscle of the bowel and it is only 2–3 mm in thickness. If there is any doubt about the extent of trauma or structures involved the midwife must seek assistance from a more experienced colleague.

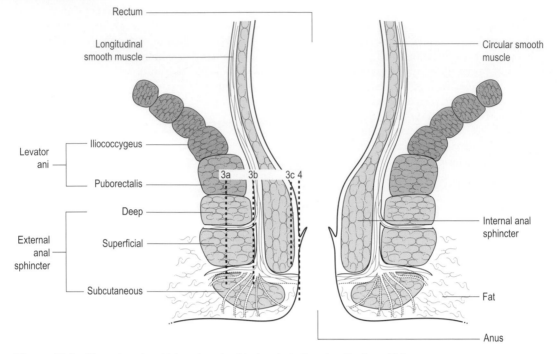

Figure 10.1 • The external and internal anal sphincters including classification of injury.

Current evidence

Management of perineal tears (first and second) and episiotomy: non-suturing issues

Non-suturing perineal muscles and skin

There have been several small studies that have attempted to evaluate the effects of leaving perineal tears unsutured following childbirth. The research to date includes two small retrospective cohort studies carried out in England and two small randomised controlled trials (RCTs) carried out in Sweden and Scotland (Clement & Reed 1999, Fleming et al 2003, Head 1993, Lundquist et al 2000).

The two small studies carried out by Head (1993) and Clement and Reed (1999) involving 55 and 107 women respectively, found no difference in short-term morbidity or wound-healing rates in perineal trauma left to heal without suturing. The validity of these findings are questionable due to the small sample sizes and recall bias as data were collected from women over a period of 6 months to 15 years retrospectively. It is also difficult to establish if the outcomes were better or worse for women with sutured or unsutured trauma due to the fact that there were no matched comparison groups.

Results from the small RCT carried out by Lundquist et al (2000) involving 78 primiparous women in Sweden, which compared non-suturing versus suturing of first-degree and second-degree tears, found a non-significant increase in short-term discomfort (burning sensation and soreness) associated with non-suturing, but no difference in wound healing between the groups. The second RCT undertaken by Fleming (2003) involving 74 primiparous women in Scotland found no significant difference in pain at 10 days and 6 weeks between the non-sutured and sutured groups. However, the study found that wound healing was significantly poorer with non-suturing up to 6 weeks postpartum. Fleming described the method used to measure wound healing, although it was unclear how healing was defined and assessed in the study conducted by Lundquist et al (2000).

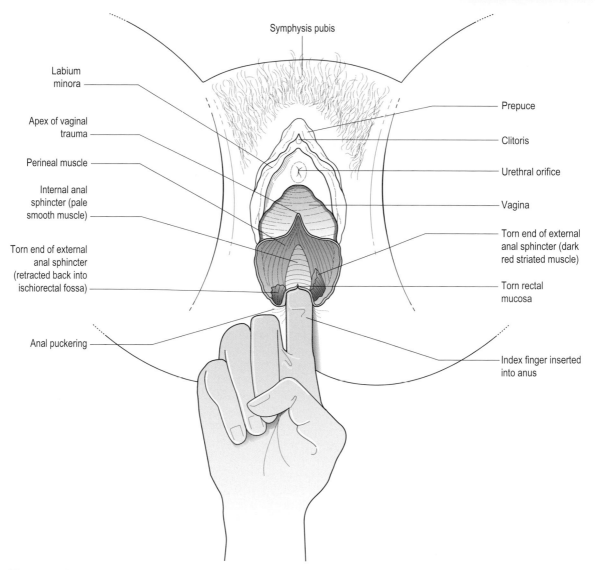

Symphysis pubis

Labium minora

Apex of vaginal trauma

Perineal muscle

Internal anal sphincter (pale smooth muscle)

Torn end of external anal sphincter (retracted back into ischiorectal fossa)

Anal puckering

Prepuce

Clitoris

Urethral orifice

Vagina

Torn end of external anal sphincter (dark red striated muscle)

Torn rectal mucosa

Index finger inserted into anus

Figure 10.2 • Examination of the external anal sphincter and internal anal sphincter (examiner should ask the woman to contract her anal sphincter).

Implications for practice of non-suturing perineal muscles

The evidence from these small studies must be carefully interpreted due to their limitations and insufficient sample size required to detect clinically important outcomes.

- There is no long-term evidence available to evaluate the consequences of leaving perineal muscle unsutured.

- Midwives must be cautious about leaving perineal trauma unsutured unless it is the woman's explicit wish.

Non-suturing of perineal skin

There have been two RCTs carried out that compared a two-stage method of repair (vagina and perineal muscle are sutured but the perineal skin is left unsutured) to the more traditional three-stage method (vagina, perineal muscle and skin are sutured) (Gordon et al 1998, Oboro 2003). The study undertaken by Gordon et al (1998) in England, which involved 1780 women who sustained a first or second-degree tear, or episiotomy, following spontaneous vaginal birth, found no significant difference in perineal pain at 10 days postpartum between groups. In contrast, the multicentre RCT conducted in Nigeria by Oboro et al (2003) involving 823 women who sustained a second-degree tear or episiotomy found that leaving the perineal skin unsutured reduced perineal pain at 48 hours, 14 days, 6 weeks and 3 months following birth. Both RCTs found that leaving the perineal skin unsutured but apposed increased rates of wound gaping at 48 hours compared with suturing. At 10 days Gordon et al (1998) reported that non-suturing of the skin increased wound gaping at 10 days. However, Oboro et al (2003) found no significant differences in wound gaping at 14 days postpartum. At 3 months postpartum the two RCTs reported reduced rates of superficial dyspareunia in the groups that had the perineal skin left unsutured compared to the sutured groups.

Implications for practice of non-suturing of the perineal skin

- There is evidence of some benefit associated with leaving perineal skin unsutured compared with sutured skin in terms of reducing pain and superficial dyspareunia.
- Midwives must be aware that there is an increased risk of wound gaping in the non-sutured skin groups.

Suture techniques

Current evidence from a Cochrane systematic review of seven RCTs ($n = 3822$ primiparous and multiparous women) found that continuous suture techniques compared with interrupted sutures for perineal closure (all layers or perineal skin only) was associated with less pain and reduction in analgesia use up to 10 days postpartum. It is interesting to note that subgroup analysis showed that there is an even greater reduction in pain when continuous suturing techniques were used for all layers compared to skin only. Subgroup analysis also showed some evidence of reduction in dyspareunia

experienced by participants in the groups that had continuous suturing for all layers. Meta-analysis showed a reduction in suture removal in the continuous suturing groups versus interrupted, but no significant differences were seen in the need for re-suturing of wounds or long-term pain (Kettle et al 2007). In addition, it has economical advantages in that the continuous technique requires one packet of suture material per perineal repair compared to two or more packets for the interrupted method (Kettle et al 2002).

Suture materials

Three randomised controlled trials (Gemynthe et al 1996, Kettle et al 2002, McElhinney et al 2000) comparing rapidly absorbed polyglactin 910 (Vicryl Rapide) to standard polyglactin 910 (Vicryl) found no overall difference in short-term perineal pain between groups. However, two of the trials (Gemynthe et al 1996, Kettle et al 2002) found a significant reduction in pain when walking at 10–14 days postpartum. Only one of the trials (McElhinney et al 2000) reported a reduction in superficial dyspareunia at 3 months postpartum. All three RCTs found that Vicryl Rapide compared to standard Vicryl was associated with a significant reduction in the need for suture removal up to 3 months following childbirth.

Suture materials and technique: recommendations for practice

In light of the current evidence the recommended suture technique and material for the repair of second-degree tears and episiotomy are:
- The continuous non-locking suturing technique for all layers (level 1a evidence). For every 5 women sutured using the continuous suturing technique (for all layers) there will be one less complaining of pain up to day 10 postpartum compared to the interrupted method.
- Vicryl Rapide suture material 2–0 on 36 mm tapercut needle (level 1b evidence).

  If the trauma is very deep the perineal muscles can be closed using a two layer continuous non-locking technique as illustrated in Figure 10.3.

  Note: these recommendations are based on evidence presented within the NICE Intrapartum Care Guidelines (NICE 2007).

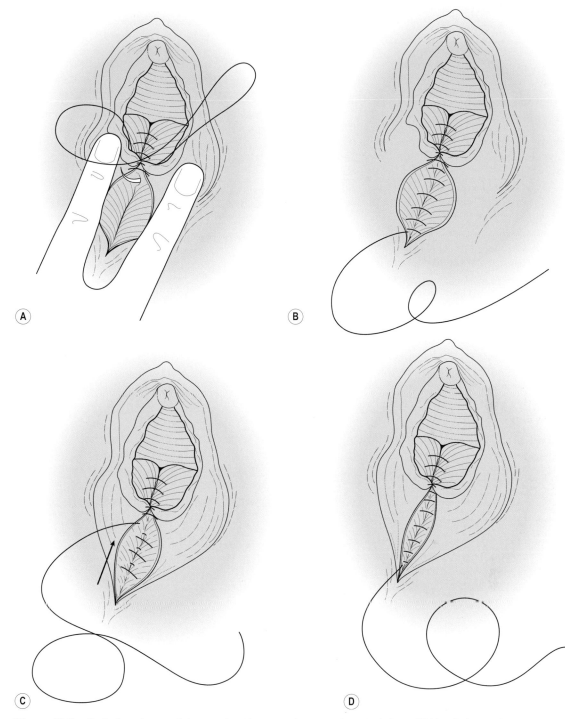

Figure 10.3 • Illustrating closure of deep perineal trauma using a two layer technique. (A) Needle inserted to commence closure of perineal muscles. (B) First layer of sutures inserted to close the deeper trauma. (C) 2–3 continuous sutures inserted, working from lower end of perineal muscle trauma to introitus (this facilitates closure of 2nd layer (i.e. working from introitus to lower end of the trauma). (D) Second layer inserted to close superficial trauma. Now ready to insert continuous subcutaneous sutures to close perineal skin.

Management of complex perineal trauma

Third-degree tears

Suture techniques for repair of the external anal sphincter muscle

Current evidence from a Cochrane systematic review of three RCTs ($n = 279$ primiparous and multiparous women) that compared the overlap versus end-to-end techniques for EAS repair found there was no statistically significant difference in perineal pain, dyspareunia, flatus incontinence and faecal incontinence up to 12 months postpartum (Fernando et al 2006). However, on trial ($n = 52$ women) carried out by Fernando et al (2004) found a lower incidence in faecal urgency and anal incontinence score in the overlap group compared to the end-to-end group. The trial also reported a lower risk of deterioration of anal incontinence symptoms at 12 months in the overlap group but no difference in quality of life. All three trials were of good methodological quality; however, there were considerable heterogeneity in the outcome measures, time points and reported results.

Suture material for repair of the internal and external anal sphincter muscles

Currently there has been very little research undertaken to assess the best suture material to use for repair of the EAS or IAS. It is usual practice to use absorbable monofilament sutures such as 3–0 polydiaxanone (PDS) as it is thought to lessen the risk of infection compared to braided material such as 2–0 polyglactin (coated Vicryl®). PDS takes 180 to 210 days to be absorbed as compared to coated Vicryl, which takes 56 to 70 days (Ethicon INC 2004).

One RCT ($n = 112$ women) carried out by Williams et al (2006) compared PDS 3–0 to coated Vicryl 2–0 and found no significant difference between groups in rates of anal incontinence, perineal pain or suture migration up to 12 months postpartum. However, the study was not powered to look at changes in infection rates (Williams 2006). Based on this evidence the RCOG (2007) Green-top Guideline No 29 recommends either monofilament sutures such as polydiaxanone (PDS) or coated braided sutures such as standard Vicryl 2–0 for repair

of the EAS muscle. The guideline also recommends either 3–0 PDS or 2–0 standard Vicryl for repair of the IAS muscle.

Risk factors

The main factors that are associated with an increased risk of third and fourth-degree tears have been identified in a number of retrospective studies (Fenner 2003, Fitzpatrick 2001, Sultan 1994a, 1994b).

Repair of sphincter trauma

It is important that the midwife/doctor has a sound understanding of the anatomy and physiology of the IAS and EAS prior to undertaking the repair (Figure 10.1).

The entire anal sphincter complex extends for approximately 3 cm along the anal canal and the IAS overlaps the EAS by approximately 1.7 cm (DeLancey et al 1997). The EAS lies in close proximity to the puborectalis and is attached posteriorly to the coccyx by some of its fibres. It surrounds two-thirds of the anal canal and is comprised of dark striated muscle, which is under voluntary control. The EAS is responsible for the squeeze tone of the rectal canal and 10% to 20% of the resting tone, thus preventing uncontrolled passage of flatus and faeces.

The IAS is a thickened continuation of the circular smooth muscle of the rectum that overlaps and lies superior to the EAS. This pale involuntary muscle provides the majority of the resting tone of the anus (80% to 90%) and forms an important component of the faecal continence mechanism. It assists the EAS to maintain closure to prevent involuntary passage of flatus or faeces, which is of great importance when sleeping.

Principles and technique of repair

The midwife/doctor should evaluate the full extent of the injury by carrying out a systematic examination of the external genitalia, vagina and rectum prior to commencing the repair. The findings should be carefully documented according to the recommended classification (Table 10.1). The repair should be carried out as detailed in Box 10.1:

Box 10.1

Principles and technique of repair

1. An experienced practitioner (midwife/doctor) should undertake or supervise the less experienced operator.

2. The repair should be carried out under spinal or general anaesthesia in an operating theatre, with good lighting and aseptic conditions.

3. If a fourth-degree tear has occurred, the torn anal epithelium should be repaired with either interrupted or continuous standard Vicryl 3-0 or Vicryl Rapide 2-0 sutures attached to a 31 mm round bodied needle (the knots must be placed in the lumen of the anal canal).

4. If disrupted, the internal anal sphincter should be repaired with interrupted mattress sutures using either standard Vicryl 2-0 or PDS 3-0.

5. The external anal sphincter is repaired using either the overlap technique or end-to-end (Figure 10.4) with PDS 3-0 or standard Vicryl 2–0 suture material. The choice of technique will depend on the degree of trauma and operators preference (if the sphincter is less than 50% (3a tear) it will not be possible to perform an overlap repair).

6. Following repair of the anal sphincter complex the vagina, perineal muscles and skin should be repaired using Vicryl Rapide 2-0 suture material and the continuous suture technique.

7. It is important to carry out a rectal examination following completion of the procedure to ensure that sutures from the vaginal and perineal muscle repair have **not** perforated through the rectal mucosa.

8. Count swabs, instruments and needles to ensure that they are all accounted for and complete documentation. A diagram is useful to illustrate the full extent of the trauma.

9. Inform the woman regarding the full extent of the injury and give advice regarding diet, pain relief, hygiene, pelvic floor exercises and the importance of attending for follow-up.

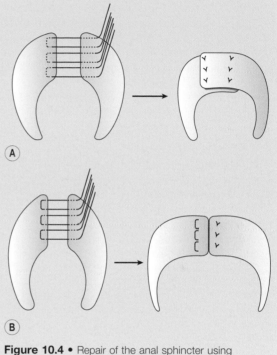

Figure 10.4 • Repair of the anal sphincter using (A) overlap or (B) end-to-end techniques.

Who should carry out primary repair of obstetric anal injuries?

Injury to the anal sphincter complex during vaginal birth may have significant consequences if it is not identified and appropriately repaired by a skilled midwife/doctor. There is some debate between colorectal surgeons and obstetricians as to who is the most appropriate person to carry out repair of primary obstetric anal sphincter injuries in terms of better outcomes. However, in a survey of colorectal practice undertaken in the UK by Fernando et al (2002), 7% of colorectal surgeons performed more than 10 primary sphincter repairs per year, 30% performed less than 5 per year and 60% had never performed the procedure. According to the RCOG (2007) Green-top Guideline No.29 (The management of third and fourth degree perineal tears) 'appropriately trained practitioners' should deal with this type of complex trauma and that attempts to repair anal sphincter injuries by inexperienced practitioners may result in increased morbidity. Therefore, one could argue that the most appropriate person to undertake the repair is one that has received formal training, has undergone

Box 10.2

Recommendations for repair of sphincter trauma

- It is important that the midwife/doctor has a sound understanding of the anatomy of the perineum and anal sphincter complex.
- Prevention of complex trauma is the best treatment.
- It is advisable that complex perineal trauma is repaired in theatre under regional or general anaesthetic by an experienced practitioner.
- There is weak evidence of benefit associated with the overlap technique for primary repair of the external anal sphincter compared with the end-to-end method.
- There is very little evidence regarding the best suture material to use for repair of the external anal sphincter or internal anal sphincter. However, findings from one small randomised controlled trial carried out by Williams et al (2006) suggest that either PDS 3-0 or coated braided Vicryl 2-0 can be used for repair of the EAS and IAS.
- Women should be warned that there is a possibility of PDS suture material perforating through the perineal skin, which may cause discomfort.
- Midwives who would like to advance their skills to repair more complex trauma such as third/fourth-degree tears must seek approval from their employing organisation, undergo a recognised structured training programme, practice under supervision until competency is reached and maintain their proficiency.

a period of supervised repairs and has reached competency. It is also important that the midwife/doctor maintains knowledge, skill and competence by regular practice and updating. Box 10.2 provides recommendations for repair of sphincter trauma.

Management of other types of complex trauma

Tear in rectal mucosa (buttonhole)

Occasionally a tear in the rectal mucosa may occur without involving the anal sphincter complex. This type of injury is not classified as a third or fourth-degree tear; however, similar principles must be adhered to when repairing this type of trauma to minimise the risk of recto-vaginal fistula. The disrupted rectal mucosa must be repaired by an experienced operator using interrupted or continuous sutures with the knots placed in the lumen of the rectum. A second layer of tissue should be approximated and sutured over the repaired rectal mucosa prior to closing the vagina, perineal muscles and skin using a continuous suture technique.

Bilateral vaginal tears

If bilateral or multiple vaginal tears occur, these can be repaired using a non-locking continuous suture technique and Vicryl Rapide 2–0 suture material (see Figure 10.5A). The midwife should identify each apex of the vaginal tears and suture each laceration separately, taking care to restore anatomical alignment without narrowing the vagina. Once the hymenal remnants are reached the suturing material can be secured using an Aberdeen or loop knot. The midwife should then continue suturing the other vaginal tears using the same technique before continuing to close the perineal muscles and skin using the same non-locking continuous suturing method. It is important that the hymenal remnants are reconstructed as illustrated (Figure 10.5B).

It may be necessary to insert a vaginal pack for 24 hours if there are multiple superficial vaginal lacerations that persist in bleeding and are difficult to suture. If the perineal muscle trauma is very deep it may be necessary to close the trauma in two layers using the continuous non-locking suture technique as illustrated (Figure 10.3).

Management of tears to the labia minora

If this type of trauma occurs, it is important that it is carefully repaired by an experienced midwife/doctor otherwise the woman may experience perineal discomfort and also she may develop psychological problems due to concerns over altered body-image. Tears to the labia minora should be repaired with Vicryl Rapide 3–0 suture material and a continuous non-locking technique with sub-cutaneous skin closure as illustrated in Figure 10.5A. Prior to undertaking the repair the operator must ensure that the area is adequately anaesthetised using lignocaine 1% and a fine needle (25 mm gauge).

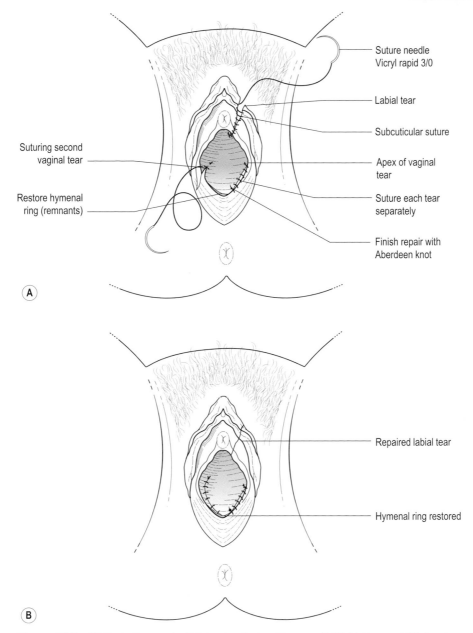

Figure 10.5 • (A) Illustrating repair of bilateral vaginal wall tears and left labial tear and (B) showing complete repair of the left labial and vaginal trauma including reconstruction of the hymenal ring.

Periurethral lacerations

Tears near to the urethra are called periurethral lacerations and they are sometimes bilateral and quite often very superficial (first degree). If these are not bleeding excessively they could be left unsutured; however, the woman must be instructed to part the labia daily during bathing to ensure labial fusion does not occur. This type of injury, although appearing very minor, can be very painful and cause voiding difficulties. Therefore, sometimes it is advisable to repair the trauma with continuous non-locking stitches and Vicryl Rapide 3-0 suture material. An experienced midwife/doctor must carry this out and care must be taken to ensure that the area is adequately anaesthetised prior to commencing the procedure.

113

If the laceration(s) are close to the urethra an indwelling catheter should be inserted prior to carrying out the repair and it should be left in situ for 24 hours.

Management of perineal haematoma

A haematoma may occur in the vulva, vagina or perineum following birth due a concealed ruptured vessel, which continues to bleed. The incidence is approximately 1 in 500 vaginal births and it is usually associated with an episiotomy or perineal tear; however, it can occur in situations where the perineum appears to be intact. The haematoma presents as a swelling, which becomes very painful and can lead to hypovolaemic shock and collapse if it is not promptly recognised and treated. The treatment of a perineal haematoma by an experienced practitioner is outlined in Box 10.3. Please note if the haematoma is small and not expanding it can be treated conservatively with ice packs to control the bleeding, analgesics for pain relief and antibiotics to prevent infection. The haematoma should resolve and be absorbed within approximately 2–3 weeks postpartum.

Female genital mutilation

Midwives as lead professional for the majority of women during pregnancy have a responsibility to make sensitive enquiries during the antenatal period in order to identify women who have had female

---

Box 10.3

Treatment of a perineal haematoma

1. Treatment of shock and stabilising the woman's condition.
2. Exploration of the trauma in theatre under a spinal or general anaesthetic, with good light and aseptic conditions.
3. Evacuation of the haematoma.
4. Identification and ligature of the bleeding vessel.
5. Closure of the perineal wound ensuring that the dead space is closed.
6. Occasionally a drain or pack is inserted for approximately 24 hours post operatively.
7. Postoperative administration of antibiotics and strong analgesics.
8. Postnatal follow-up at 6 weeks.

---

genital mutilation (FGM). Key recommendations from the NICE (2008:23) states:

Pregnant women who have had female genital mutilation should be identified early in antenatal care through sensitive enquiry. Antenatal examination will then allow planning of intrapartum care.

FGM also known as female cutting or female circumcision graphically depicts the range of procedures involving partial or complete removal of the female genital organs. It has serious implications for the physical, reproductive and psychosexual health and well being of girls and women.

Classification and prevalence of female genital mutilation

The classification of FGM is well documented (WHO 2001, 2006, 2008) and is summarised in Figure 10.6. FGM is a global problem; a common practice in many countries, predominantly Africa. It is estimated that in excess of 100 million women and girls have had FGM (WHO 2008). Although FGM is becoming a widespread phenomenon in the UK, the true scale of the problem is unclear. A statistical study based on population census and survey, funded by the Department of Health (DH) reveals that about 66 000 of women with FGM reside in England and Wales in 2001. It is reported that 16 000 of girls under 15 years old are at high risk of FGM III in England and Wales, with a further 5000 at high risk of FGM I and FGM II (Dorkenoo et al 2007). However, these figures will have increased with the rise in immigration and influx of refugees and those seeking asylum status.

Female genital mutilation: legal context

FGM has been illegal in the UK since 1985. The Female Genital Mutilation Act 2003 strengthens and amends the loop holes in the *1985 prohibition of female circumcision* legislation (Home Office 2004). It is now an offence for UK residents to perform FGM abroad, even in countries where the practice is legal. Anyone involved in the practice of FGM could be incarcerated for 14 years. To date,

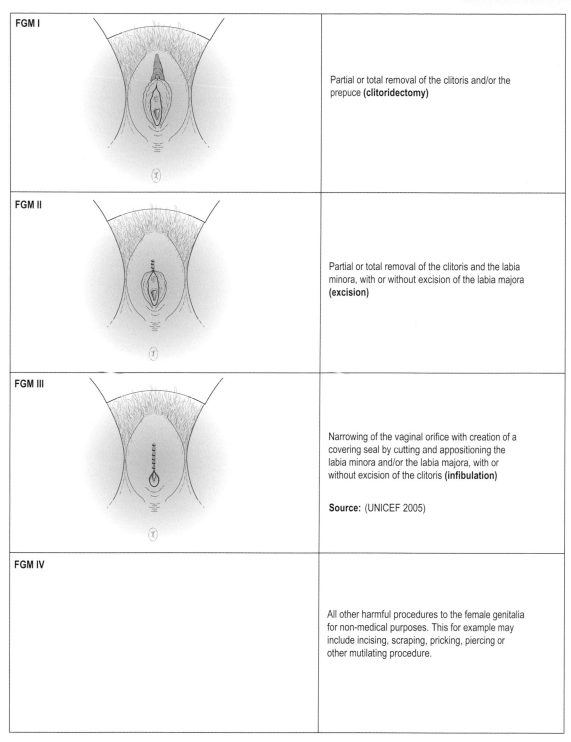

FGM I		Partial or total removal of the clitoris and/or the prepuce **(clitoridectomy)**
FGM II		Partial or total removal of the clitoris and the labia minora, with or without excision of the labia majora **(excision)**
FGM III		Narrowing of the vaginal orifice with creation of a covering seal by cutting and appositioning the labia minora and/or the labia majora, with or without excision of the clitoris **(infibulation)** **Source:** (UNICEF 2005)
FGM IV		All other harmful procedures to the female genitalia for non-medical purposes. This for example may include incising, scraping, pricking, piercing or other mutilating procedure.

Figure 10.6 • World Health Organisation's classification of female genital mutilation.

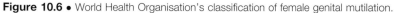

there have been no successful prosecutions in the UK. Lockhat (2004) surmised that the Law tends to take a 'Eurocentric' view on decision-making processes in families, including parental responsibility. Direct action is, therefore, needed to engage and work with affected communities (Dorkenoo 2006). It is illegal to suture the vagina so that the structures are apposed, i.e. the vagina cannot be closed as in FGM III. Clear explanations must be provided to the woman and her partner regarding the requirements of the law, including child protection.

Female genital mutilation: the evidence base

Despite the WHO (2001, 2007, 2008) stating that FGM III is present in 90% of women from northern Sudan and 98% of women from Somalia, there is a dearth of reliable research evidence regarding the effect of FGM on outcomes for mothers and babies. However, the findings by the WHO (2006) study group on FGM have provided a useful turning point. It clarifies the significant health risks at childbirth, including the increased likelihood that the woman and baby could perish. The current triennial report on the Confidential Enquiries into Maternal Deaths in the UK (Lewis 2007) provides sobering information relating to a woman with FGM III who died as a consequence of haemorrhage following caesarean section. This operation might not have been necessary had the woman been allowed to birth vaginally with the aid of a medio-lateral episiotomy or anterior episiotomy/de-infibulation procedure.

Assessment and care planning for labour

The worst-case scenario would be for an unbooked woman with FGM III to present in established labour with second stage imminent and the midwife or doctor being ill-prepared to make the appropriate response. A significant proportion of these women may be asylum seekers or refugees. Many of whom may also be from black African countries and may have difficulty communicating their needs and accessing care (Lewis 2007). They are likely to present late in pregnancy with no antenatal care including screening. The DH (2006) states that care planning should be predicated on some key principles as outlined in Box 10.4:

Box 10.4

Main principles of vaginal assessment antenatally to plan intrapartum care in the presence of FGM III (DH 2006)

- Women might not disclose information regarding female genital mutilation (FGM) voluntarily during initial antenatal consultation when mutual respect and trust is not yet established between them and their midwife. Moreover women may not understand the full implications for childbearing.

- Although the WHO (2008) outlines why the term FGM should be used, many women do not identify with the term 'mutilation' and might find it offensive. The midwife must be culturally sensitive and avoid terminology that could be perceived as pejorative and damaging to women's self-esteem. *Have you had the cut?* or *have you been closed?* are innocuous questions and less likely to be perceived as a threat (Momoh 2005).

- In order to help eradicate FGM the midwife should be critical of the practice without being critical of the women.

- On antenatal assessment by a specialist midwife or doctor skilled in caring for women with FGM, it should be determined whether the physical barrier will impede a normal birth. If this is the case de-infibulation procedure is recommended.

- Women should be asked whether they wish to be fully opened or opened until the urethral opening is fully exposed.

- Careful and sensitive discussion with the woman and her partner should take place on the degree of opening and its implications.

- Antenatal care provides an opportune time for health education/health promotion on psychosexual health and to explore child-protection issues especially if the gender of the baby is known to be a girl.

- Due attention should be given to ethical considerations such as dignity, respect and consent.

- Women should be helped to reach an informed decision. This may mean having to use advocacy/interpreting service.

- Women should be in control at all times, as the interpreter is not permitted to make decisions on behalf of women.

The midwife must ensure that the interpreter is not supportive of the practice of female genital mutilation, has the appropriate language skills and will respect the woman's decision and ensure confidentiality.

Procedure for de-infibulation

De-infibulation is reversal or opening of FGM III to facilitate a spontaneous vaginal birth. Momoh (2005) recommends antenatal reversal during the second trimester around 20 weeks' gestation, but many women elect not to have the procedure, choosing instead to have a medio-lateral episiotomy. Women who opt to be opened may choose to have the procedure performed during labour via local anaesthesia.

Skill and sensitivity is important, but no special training is required to divide the scar tissue in an emergency situation. The DH (2006) DVD demonstrates the procedure clearly, i.e. the ease of inserting a sterile Spencer Wells forceps under the scar tissue that has been previously anaesthetised. Local anaesthetic is required for the procedure before dividing the scar tissue in the midline using a sterile scissors or surgical blade. It must be remembered that although de-infibulation is popularly referred to as 'reversal' this is somewhat of a misnomer. The procedure aims to ensure full restoration of the vaginal opening but cannot replace the tissue removed via the initial FGM. For those women who choose to undergo deinfibulation, they must be involved in the decision making on whether they want to be fully opened or opened until the urethra is exposed. The DVD available via the DH (2006) provides clear guidance on how to perform the procedure. Relevant professional bodies such as the Royal College of Midwives (www.rcm.org.uk), Royal College of Obstetricians and Gynaecologists (www.rcog.org.uk) and Royal College of Nursing (www.rcn.org.uk) provide information on their website for practitioners on FGM.

Female genital mutilation and perineal suturing

If the deinfibulation is carried out in the antenatal period the edges of the wound will need to be sutured preferably using 3.0 Vicryl rapide and the continuous suturing technique. Suturing (antenatal or intrapartum) is important to decrease the likelihood of the raw edges of the wound adhering in the midline as reinfibulation in the UK is illegal.

Immediate postnatal care

Perineal trauma that has been correctly approximated anatomically and sutured using the continuous technique and Vicryl Rapide© suture material will heal within 2 weeks of childbirth by primary intention. This is probably due to the fact that the perineal area immediately after parturition provides optimal conditions, which are necessary for the promotion of quality healing, providing that there are no adverse factors such as haematoma formation or infection.

Postnatally, it is important to obtain a baseline observation of the trauma site, as information from this initial assessment will assist with the planning and provision of the woman's care. It will also provide an opportunity for the midwife to give advice regarding pain relief, hygiene, pelvic-floor-muscle exercise, diet and rest (see Chapters 3 and 14). During the early postnatal period if there are any concerns about healing, infection or severe pain, referral should be made to the appropriate practitioner or to a dedicated 'perineal care clinic' in those units that have this facility. In the case of FGM it is even more important to reinforce health education/promotion, especially in relation to prevention of morbidity, the flow of urine, lochia/menstruation and the changes to sensation that will be experience on the resumption of sexual intercourse.

Perineal care postpartum: practice implications

As stated in the pre-requisites at the start of the chapter, midwives and other health-care professionals should ensure that they are familiar with relevant postnatal guidelines, such as NICE (2006) guideline on postnatal care, which give advice on all aspects of postnatal care, including perineal management. The relevant sections of NICE (2007) intrapartum care guideline that focuses on the initial assessment of the mother following birth and perineal care should also be used to inform knowledge base and practice.

Perineal care clinic

Women who sustain complex perineal trauma following childbirth should be offered routine referral to a dedicated 'perineal clinic'. Currently there are a number of clinics throughout the UK; however, most have different models of care, which vary according to local expertise and financial resources.

The University Hospital of North Staffordshire has a 'perineal care clinic' that is led by a specialist midwife and backed by two lead obstetricians. All women who sustain a third or fourth-degree tear following birth are given a routine appointment to attend the clinic for review at 6 weeks postpartum. In addition, midwives, GPs, specialist community public health nurses, practice nurses and consultants refer women with other problems such as dehisced perineal wounds, urinary and faecal incontinence, superficial dyspareunia, and concerns about subsequent births. The women attending the clinic receive sensitive, appropriate and effective treatment in a friendly environment; and for those women that require further investigations, such as endo-anal scan or anorectal physiology tests, appropriate referral is made. The specialist midwife works closely with other disciplines including the obstetric physiotherapists, colorectal surgeon, urogynaecologist and continence advisors who attend a monthly multidisciplinary meeting to discuss and plan appropriate care for women with complex problems. Both the physical and psychological aspects of their care are addressed, which if left untreated can impact negatively on the dynamics of mother–baby interaction, domestic relationships and lifestyle.

Medico-legal implications

Currently there is a steady increase in litigation related to obstetric anal sphincter injury. The majority of cases are related to failure to identify the extent of injury following birth, which may result in complications such as rectovaginal fistulae and anal incontinence. Other sources of litigation include inappropriate placement of episiotomy incisions, incorrect anatomical approximation of perineal wounds and psychological trauma.

If the woman sustains trauma to the anorectal complex this is not considered to be negligent (see Chapter 2) unless inappropriate or substandard care was given at the time of birth. However, failure to recognise the degree of injury and carry out a satisfactory repair according to recommended guidelines may result in litigation. It is important to inform the woman regarding the full extent of the perineal injury sustained and also to reassure her that it has been repaired to a high standard using the best suture technique and materials. In the case of FGM, the midwife must not on any account succumb to pressure from the woman, her husband or other family members to contravene the Law by reclosing the vagina.

Key practice points

- Midwives must be aware of the employing authority's policies and guidelines relating to perineal assessment, repair and postnatal management.
- A robust plan of care should be devised during the antenatal period for women with female genital mutilation.
- Perineal tears must be thoroughly inspected, using good lighting and the extent of injury carefully documented in the hospital case notes.
- It is important to carry out a rectal examination, as part of the initial assessment to ensure that injury to the anorectal complex is not missed.
- Midwives must be aware of the legal implications associated with inadequate or incorrect repaired perineal trauma.
- Midwives must be appropriately trained to carry out the procedure of perineal repair, recognise their own limitations and seek assistance when required.
- If the woman refuses to be examined it is essential to inform her of the potential risks, which may occur if trauma to the anal sphincter complex is missed.
- Women who explicitly request not to have sutures inserted must be given the opportunity to discuss their concerns with the person providing care. It is important to document in the medical records the full extent of the trauma being left unsutured and also that the risks have been discussed. This should be witnessed and countersigned by a second health professional.
- Following completion of the repair it is vital to document a comprehensive account of the procedure in the medical notes (it is useful to include a diagram to illustrate the extent of the trauma). Black ink should be used and the midwife/doctor should sign and print his/her name.
- Following completion of the repair all instrument, sharps and swabs must be accounted for and documented in the records.
- Women should be given information regarding the extent of perineal trauma sustained, and how and when to seek advice if problems occur.
- Being at the vanguard of change, midwives must build capacity through partnership working within the multidisciplinary team as well as multi-agency collaboration to eradicate female genital mutilation. This includes child protection agencies and women's advocacy and empowerment services. Above all the midwife must be suitably informed to care for women with female genital mutilation appropriately and work within the legal framework when repairing the perineum.

References

Clement, S., Reed, B., 1999. To stitch or not to stitch? A long term follow up study of women with unsutured perineal tears. Pract. Midwife 2 (4), 20–28.

DeLancey, J.O.L., Toglia, M.R., Perucchini, D., 1997. Internal and external anal sphincter anatomy as it relates to midline obstetric lacerations. Obstet. Gynecol. 90, 924–927.

Department of Health, 2006. Female genital mutilation DVD. DH, London.

Derry, D.E., 1935. Note on five pelves of women of the Eleventh Dynasty in Egypt. Journal of Obstetrics and Gynaecology of the British Empire xiii, 490–495.

Dorkenoo, E., 2006. Female genital mutilation: politics and prevention. Hurst, London.

Dorkenoo, E., Morrison, L., MacFarlane, A., 2007. A statistical study to estimate the prevalence of female genital mutilation in England and Wales: summary report. FORWARD, London. Available online: www.forwarduk.org.uk Accessed April 2008.

Ethicon, I.N.C., 2004. Product Catalogue. Ethicon, Oxford.

Fenner, D.E., Genberg, B., Brahma, P., Marek, L., DeLancey, J.O.L., 2003. Fecal and urinary incontinence after vaginal delivery with anal sphincter disruption in an obstetric unit in the United States. Am. J. Obstet. Gynecol. 189, 1543–1550.

Fernando, R.J., Sultan, A.H., Radley, S., Jones, P.W., Johanson, R.B., 2002. Management of obstetric anal sphincter injury – A systematic review and national practice survey. Biomedical Central (BMC) Health Services Research 2–9.

Fernando, R.J., Sultan, A.H., Kettle, C., Radley, S., O'Brien, P.M.S., 2004. Obstetric anal sphincter injury – does repair technique affect the outcome? BJOG 111, 115.

Fernando, R., Sultan, A.H., Kettle, C., Thakar, R., Radley, S., 2006. Methods of repair for obstetric anal sphincter injury. Cochrane Database Syst. Rev. Issue 3. Wiley, Chichester.

Fitzpatrick, M., McQuillan, K., O'Herlihy, C., 2001. Influence of persistent occipito-posterior position on delivery outcome. Obstet. Gynecol. 98 (6), 1027–1031.

Fleming, E.M., Hagen, S., Niven, C., 2003. Does perineal suturing make a difference? The SUNS trial. BJOG 110, 684–689.

Gemynthe, A., Langhoff-Roos, J., Sahl, S., Knudsen, J., 1996. New VICRYL formulation: an improved method of perineal repair? British Journal of Midwifery 4 (5), 230–234.

Gordon, B., Mackrodt, C., Fern, E., Truesdale, A., Ayers, S., Grant, A., 1998. The Ipswich Childbirth Study: 1. A randomised evaluation of two stage postpartum perineal repair leaving the skin unsutured. BJOG 105 (4), 435–440.

Head, M., 1993. Dropping stitches. Nurs. Times 89 (33), 64–65.

Home Office, 2004. Circular 10/2004 The female genital mutilation Act 2003. Home Office, London. Available online: www.circulars. homeoffice.gov.uk Accessed 3 January 2008.

Kettle, C., Hills, R.K., Jones, P., Darby, L., Gray, R., Johanson, R., 2002. Continuous versus interrupted perineal repair with standard or rapidly absorbed sutures after spontaneous vaginal birth: a randomised controlled trial. Lancet 359 (9325), 2217–2223.

Kettle, C., Hills, R.K., Ismail, K.M.K., 2007. Continuous versus interrupted sutures for repair of episiotomy or second degree tears. Cochrane Database Syst. Rev. Issue 4. Wiley, Chichester.

Lewis, G. (Ed.), 2007. The Confidential Enquiry into Maternal and Child Health (CEMACH). Saving mothers' lives: reviewing maternal deaths to make motherhood safer 2003–2005. The seventh report on Confidential Enquiries into Maternal Deaths in the United Kingdom. CEMACH, London. Available online: www. cemach.org.uk Accessed 3 January 2008.

Lockhat, H., 2004. Female genital mutilation: treating the tears. University Press Middlesex, London.

Lundquist, M., Olsson, A., Nissen, E., Norman, M., 2000. Is it necessary to suture all lacerations after a vaginal delivery? Birth 27 (2), 79–85.

McElhinney, B.R., Glenn, D.R.J., Harper, M.A., 2000. Episiotomy repair: vicryl versus vicryl rapide. Ulster Med. J. 69 (1), 27–29.

Momoh, C., 2005. Female genital mutilation. Radcliffe, Oxford.

National Institute for Health and Clinical Excellence, 2006. Routine postnatal care of women and their babies – Clinical Guideline No 36. NICE, London.

National Institute for Health and Clinical Excellence, 2007. Intrapartum care: Care of healthy women and their babies during childbirth Clinical Guideline No 55. NICE, London.

National Institute for Health and Clinical Excellence, 2008. Antenatal care. Routine care for the healthy pregnant women Clinical Guideline No 62. NICE, London.

Norton, C., Christiansen, J., Butler, U., Harari, D., Nelson, R.L., Pemberton, J., 2002. Anal incontinence. In: Abrams, P., Cardozo, L., Khoury, Wein, A. (Eds.), Incontinence. 2nd ed. Health Publication Ltd, Plymouth, pp. 985–1044.

Oboro, V.O., Tabowei, T.O., Loto, O., Bosah, J.O., 2003. A multicenter evaluation of the two-layer repair of perineal trauma after birth. BJOG 1, 5–8.

Royal College of Obstetricians and Gynaecologists, 2007. Management of third and fourth degree perineal tears following vaginal delivery. Green-top Guideline No 29 (revised version). RCOG, London.

Sultan, A.H., 1999. Obstetric perineal injury and anal incontinence. Clinical Risk 5, 193–196.

Sultan, A.H., Kamm, M.A., Bartram, C.I., Hudson, C.N., 1994a. Perineal damage at delivery. Contemporary

Reviews in Obstetrics and Gynaecology 6, 18–24.

Sultan, A.H., Kamm, M.A., Hudson, C.N., Bartram, C.I., 1994b. Third degree obstetric anal sphincter tears: risk factors and outcome of primary repair. Br. Med. J. 308, 887–891.

UNICEF, 2005. Female genital mutilation/cutting: a statistical exploration. Available online: http://www.who.int.

Williams, A., 2006. Author's reply: How to repair an anal sphincter injury after vaginal delivery: results of a randomised controlled trial. BJOG 113 (8), 977–978.

Williams, A., Adams, E.J., Tincello, D.G., Alfirevic, Z., Walkinshaw, S. A., Richmond, D.H., 2006. How to repair an anal sphincter injury after vaginal delivery: results of a randomised controlled trial. BJOG 113, 201–207.

World Health Organisation Study Group on Female Genital Mutilation and Obstetric Outcome, 2006. Female genital mutilation and obstetric outcome: WHO collaboration prospective study in six African countries. Lancet 367 (9525), 1835–1841.

World Health Organisation, 2001. Management of pregnancy, childbirth and the postpartum period in the presence of female genital mutilation: Report of a WHO Technical Consultation. WHO, Geneva.

World Health Organisation, 2008. Eliminating female genital mutilation: an interagency statement (OHCHR, UNAIDS, UNDP, UNECA, UNESCO, UNFPA, UNHR, UNICEF, UNIFEM and WHO). WHO, Geneva. Available online: www.who.int Accessed 7 July 2008.

Further reading

Henderson, C., Bick, D. (Eds.), 2005. Perineal care: an international issue. Quay Books, Wiltshire. A useful text that provides a good overview of perineal care from a global perspective.

HMSO, 2004. The Children's Act. HMSO, London. Available online: www.opsi.gov.uk/acts2004 *Provides guidance on the Law and child protection.*

Royal College of Nursing, 2006. Female genital mutilation. RCN, London. Available online: www.rcn.org.uk *A useful educational resource for health-care professionals.*

11

Haemodynamic assessment and monitoring in maternity care

Louise C. Stayt

CONTENTS

Skill outline 121
Rationale and background 121
Procedure 122
   Haemodynamic physiology 122
   Haemodynamic changes during
   pregnancy 123
   Non-invasive haemodynamic
   assessment 123
   Invasive haemodynamic assessment . 127
Professional responsibilities 131
Key practice points 131
References 132
Further reading 133

Before reading this chapter, you should be familiar with:
- The physiological adaptation of the woman's body to pregnancy.
- Pregnancy associated cardiovascular changes.
- The principles and procedures of assessing vital signs including respiratory rate, pulse rate, blood pressure and temperature.
- The physiology of pulse and blood pressure, including an understanding of Korotkoff sounds.
- The significance of assessing blood pressure during pregnancy.
- Risk-management procedures.
- Principles of maternal cardio-pulmonary resuscitation.
- Key recommendations of Confidential Enquiry into Maternal and Child Health (CEMACH) report: Saving mothers' lives (Lewis 2007).

Skill outline

Haemodynamic assessment incorporates all the necessary observations assessments and measurements required to comprehensively evaluate cardiovascular function and sufficiency. Haemodynamic assessment and monitoring includes non-invasive techniques such as skin-perfusion assessment, temperature measurement, pulse measurement, non-invasive blood-pressure measurement, and invasive techniques such as arterial blood pressure (BP) monitoring and central venous pressure monitoring.

Rationale and background

Although rare, many complications can occur during pregnancy which may lead to haemodynamic instability (Carlin & Alfirevic 2006). Pregnancy-related complications are detailed in Box 11.1.

Box 11.1

Complications of pregnancy
- Severe pre-eclampsia and eclampsia.
- Disseminated intravascular coagulation (DIC).
- Haemolysis, elevated liver enzyme, low platelet count (HELLP) syndrome.
- Haemorrhage.
- Pulmonary oedema.
- Pulmonary emboli.
- Ruptured uterus.

(Edwards 1998, Luppi 1997, Oliveira et al 2002)

Box 11.2

Pre-existing medical conditions

- Myocardial infarction.
- Congenital heart disease.
- Dysrhythmia.
- Cerebral pathology – aneurysm, subarachnoid haemorrhage.
- Sepsis.
- Traumatic injury.
- Drug abuse.

(Edwards 1998, Luppi 1997, Oliveira et al 2002)

Other pre-existing medical conditions may also give rise to haemodynamic instability during pregnancy. These are detailed in Box 11.2.

Childbearing women may become acutely ill at any time during pregnancy, labour and puerperium. Early recognition of complications, correct diagnosis and prompt treatment interventions are critical to the health and well being of the pregnant woman and unborn child (Dhond & Dob 2000). The midwife is the most senior practitioner at 70% of UK births (Wilson & Symon 2002) and, therefore, has a professional responsibility to recognise the warning signs (Dimond 2006).

The Confidential Enquiry into Maternal and Child Health (CEMACH) (Lewis 2007) acknowledges that delays in recognition of life-threatening illness contribute to avoidable maternal deaths. In addition, the National Confidential Enquiry for Patient Outcome and Death (NCEPOD) found that 66% of patients admitted to intensive care units exhibited physiological instability for more than 12 hours prior to their admission (NCEPOD 2005). National Institute for Health and Clinical Excellence (NICE 2007) also acknowledge that the recognition of acute illness is often delayed and its subsequent management may be inappropriate. This may result in late referral and avoidable admissions to critical care, and may lead to unnecessary deaths, particularly when the initial standard of care is suboptimal. Accurate and effective haemodynamic assessment may assist in the early recognition of life-threatening illnesses in the pregnant woman. The purpose of this chapter is to help to equip midwives with the necessary knowledge and skills to effectively assess and monitor women in their care.

Procedure

Haemodynamic physiology

Cardiac output

Cardiac output (CO) is the amount of blood the heart pumps in 1 minute and is a function of heart rate (HR) and stroke volume (SV). Stroke volume is the amount of blood ejected from the heart in each ventricular contraction and heart rate is the number of heart beats per minute (Seeley et al 2007).

$$CO = SV \times HR$$

The heart transports blood to deliver oxygen and nutrients to the cells and to remove waste products. CO is an indicator of how well the heart is carrying out this function. CO is principally regulated by the demand for oxygen by the cells of the body. CO is raised in response to high metabolic oxygen demand to maintain oxygen supply to the cells, whereas during rest when cellular demand for oxygen is low CO is at baseline (Seeley et al 2007). Cardiac output is regulated by alteration in the SV or the HR. Stroke volume is dependent on several factors: preload, afterload and contractility.

Preload

Preload is the degree to which the muscle fibres in the ventricles are stretched prior to contracting. Muscle fibres within the ventricles are stretched by the blood volume in the ventricles at end-diastole. According to Frank–Starling's law of the heart the more the ventricle is filled with blood during diastole then the greater the volume ejected during the systolic contraction. In other words the greater the venous return the greater the stroke volume (Guyton & Hall 2005). Therefore, an increase in venous return will increase preload and, in turn, increase stroke volume. A decrease in venous return will reduce preload and, in turn, decrease stroke volume. Decreased pre-load is usually caused by hypovolaemia. Causes of hypovolaemia include haemorrhage, dehydration, vomiting and diarrhoea, and burns (Guyton & Hall 2005).

Afterload

Afterload reflects the pressure that the ventricles in the heart have to generate in order to eject the blood out of the heart chambers and through the arterial vascular system. Afterload is a reflection of the resistance to blood ejected from the left ventricle (Seeley et al 2007). The resistance offered by the peripheral circulation is known as the systemic vascular resistance (SVR), whereas the resistance offered by the vasculature of the lungs is known as the pulmonary vascular resistance (PVR). An increase in afterload reduces cardiac output whereas a decrease in afterload increases cardiac output. Increased afterload may be caused by vasoconstriction. Decreased afterload may be caused by sepsis, anaphylaxis, drug overdoses, high spinal cord damage, and local anaesthetic epidurals.

Contractility

Contractility refers to the heart's ability to pump blood and reflects the sufficiency and function of the myocardium (Guyton & Hall 2005). Reduction in contractility may be caused by myocardial infarction, arrthymias, valve dysfunction, cardiac tamponade and pulmonary embolism.

Blood pressure and mean arterial pressures

BP is a product of cardiac output and vascular resistance:

BP = CO × SVR

Consequently, alterations in BP are due to changes in cardiac output, systemic vascular resistance or both. Mean arterial pressure (MAP) is the average pressure required to push blood through the circulatory system (Dougherty & Lister 2005). Mean arterial pressure may be derived mathematically with the following equation:

$$\text{MAP} = \frac{\text{diastolic BP} + (\text{systolic BP} - \text{diastolic BP})}{3}$$

Organ perfusion relies on an adequate mean arterial pressure. Most organs need a MAP of 70 mmHg for normal perfusion and functioning.

Haemodynamic changes during pregnancy

There are many physiological changes in the cardiovascular system during pregnancy. Maternal blood volume increases to 40% above normal by 30 weeks' gestation.

Therefore, cardiac output increases by 40% due to an increased stroke volume and heart rate (Dhond & Dob 2000). In addition, there is a decrease in systemic vascular resistance due to increased levels of prostacyclin and arteriovenous shunting to the placental bed (Dhond & Dob 2000). Since CO increases and SVR decreases there should not be a discernable change in a pregnant woman's BP; however, a slight decrease of 10–15 mmHg in MAP is considered to be normal.

Non-invasive haemodynamic assessment

General observations

Alterations in BP are a late sign of a compromised circulation; therefore, midwives are required to recognise earlier, often very subtle, signs of compromised cardiovascular function. General appearance can give a good indication of a woman's overall haemodynamic status (Moreau 2005). First impressions count and if the woman looks unwell she probably is.

Level of consciousness

Level of consciousness and mood state can be a very sensitive indicator of cardiovascular function (Reynolds 1999). Cerebral blood flow is maintained between a MAP of 60 and 140 mmHg. An alteration of cardiac output will, therefore, influence cerebral perfusion. A reduction in cerebral perfusion leads to drowsiness, confusion, agitation and a reduced level of consciousness through to unconsciousness (Smith 2003). A rapid assessment of a woman's conscious level may be facilitated with the acronym AVPU detailed in Box 11.3. A reduction in the AVPU to responding to voice or below requires immediate medical attention with priority given to protecting and maintaining the patient's airway.

Box 11.3

AVPU level of consciousness scale

Alert = Alert and orientated, opens eyes spontaneously.
Voice = Only responds or opens eyes to voice.
Pain = Only responds or open eyes to pain.
Unconscious = No response to voice or pain stimuli.

Colour

A woman's overall colour gives an indication of skin perfusion. Pale, cool skin may signify reduced peripheral perfusion. Inspection of the oral mucous membranes for pallor is recommended, particularly in people with dark skin, as facial pallor may be difficult to detect (Moreau 2005). Peripheral cyanosis is a blue tinge to the fingers or extremities and is caused by inadequate circulation. Peripheral cyanosis is commonly caused by exposure to cold, vasoconstriction, mild and moderate hypotension, and cardiac failure. Central cyanosis is indicated by a blue tinge to the tongue, mucous membranes, gums and lips, which can radiate across the jaw line to the patients earlobes (Sheppard & Wright 2003). Central cyanosis signifies a severe compromise of the circulatory or ventilatory systems and reflects poor perfusion and oxygenation. Central cyanosis indicates a more catastrophic and life-threatening event such as severe anaemia, congenital heart disease, heart failure, hypothermia, respiratory failure, myocardial infarction or pulmonary embolism. Central cyanosis is an ominous sign and requires immediate medical attention.

Skin temperature

Skin temperature is a useful guide to establishing haemodynamic status and may be used to determine severity of hypovolaemia or shock. During hypovolaemia, blood will be diverted away from the skin and the peripheries in order maintain central temperature and conserve circulation to the major organs. Typically peripheries will, therefore, feel cool to touch during hypovolaemia or shock. However, the pregnant woman with hypovolaemia or shock may present with warm peripheries. This is due to the circulating progesterone during pregnancy which causes peripheral vasodilation and reduction in systemic vascular resistance (Edwards 1998).

Skin condition

Inspect the woman for signs of oedema. Peripheral oedema is an indicator of impaired venous return or movement of blood through the heart (Reynolds 1999). Inspect the skin's turgor, as a reduced skin turgor may represent dehydration. Assessment of skin turgor is carried out by gently squeezing a small area of skin on the forearm. The skin is then released. If the skin quickly returns to its original shape the individual has a normal skin turgor. If, however, the skin only returns to its original shape over 30 or more seconds, the skin has poor turgor and may signify dehydration (Moreau 2005).

Capillary refill

Capillary refill is the rate at which blood refills empty capillaries. Capillary refill is measured by gently pressing a fingernail until it turns white, and then timing how many seconds are needed for colour to return once the nail is released. Normal refill time is 2 seconds or less. Capillary refill time may be used to indicate adequacy of peripheral perfusion. A refill time of greater than 2 seconds may signify an impaired perfusion to the peripheries. Capillary refill time does vary greatly amongst individuals and, therefore, it is a measurement that is best considered in conjunction with other clinical indicators of poor perfusion.

Temperature

Although core temperature is not directly reflective of cardiovascular function it has been included, as temperature is an important aspect of the overall assessment. An increased temperature is often the first indicator of infection and sepsis, both of which may impact cardiovascular function. Normal temperature ranges between 35.9°C and 37.5°C (Moreau 2005). In order to distinguish the reading from the pulse rate, it is good practice to document temperature recording on an observations chart utilising a cross (see Figure 11.1).

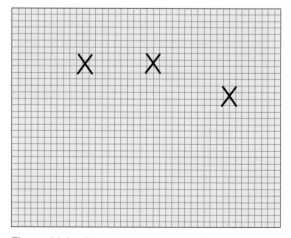

Figure 11.1 ● Temperature documentation.

Pulse check

A person's pulse is a wave of pressure or distention that is transmitted along the pliable arterial walls in response to the systolic contraction of the heart. A pulse may be palpated and measured to determine an individual's heart rate. When assessing a pulse the rate, rhythm and amplitude of the pulse should be noted. A normal heart rate varies greatly amongst individuals; however, tachycardia is usually defined as a rate of over 100 beats/minute and bradycardia is defined as a rate slower than 60 beats/minute (Dougherty & Lister 2005). Due to an increase in blood volume during pregnancy the maternal heart rate increases by 15–20 beats/minute. Therefore, during pregnancy a mild tachycardia is normal (Edwards 1998). The pulse should have a regular sequence which reflects the coordinated action of the heart's conduction system and myocardium. Disruption to either of these systems may lead to an irregular pulse rhythm reflecting the uncoordinated contraction of the heart (Dougherty & Lister 2005). Measuring the amplitude of the pulse is a reflection of the pulse strength and elasticity of the arterial wall (Guyton & Hall 2005).

An arterial pulse may be palpated in any artery that lies close to the surface to the body. The most easily accessed and most often used site for pulse measurement is the radial artery; other sites include carotid, femoral and brachial plexus. During times of circulatory insufficiency or reduced peripheral perfusion, peripheral pulse may be increasingly difficult to palpate. The extent of perfusion insufficiency may be assessed by firstly palpating the peripheral radial site and progressing to the central pulses (brachial and then carotid). Differences in the strength of pulse between the peripheral and central pulses can then be ascertained. Similarly, lower-limb perfusion may be assessed by firstly palpating the pulse in the dorsalis pedis, then the posterior tibial, then the popliteal and, finally, the femoral pulse.

The pulse should be measured by placing the first, second or third finger along the appropriate artery and pressing gently. Utilising the thumb to palpate the pulse should be avoided as the thumb has a strong pulse itself. The pulse should be counted for 60 seconds and documented. It is good practice to document pulse with a clear dot on the correct number connected to the previous reading with a straight line (see Figure 11.2). Curved connecting lines or unclear dots may easily lead to a misinterpretation of heart rate.

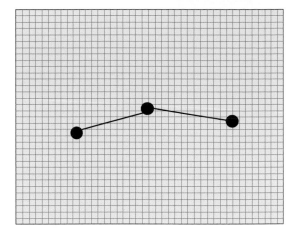

Figure 11.2 • Pulse rate documentation.

Non-invasive arterial blood pressure

BP is a critical component of a person's vital signs and allows evaluation of their cardiovascular status (Thomas et al 2002). BP measurement is the most frequently performed clinical procedure and many important clinical and therapeutic decisions rely on its accuracy (Eşer et al 2007). However, BP measurement is frequently performed inaccurately by health-care providers (Armstrong 2002, Oliveira et al 2002). Correct evaluation of BP is indispensable in the early diagnosis of pre-eclampsia, as an increase in BP is the first clinical sign of the disease (Oliveira et al 2002).

Normal BP values vary greatly amongst individuals; however, generally a range of 100/60 to 140/90 mmHg is considered normal. Hypotension is generally defined as a systolic BP of less than 100 mmHg. Hypertension is generally defined as systolic pressure of greater than 150 mmHg and/or a diastolic pressure of greater than 100 mmHg (Seeley et al 2007). However, there is a physiological decrease in BP during the second trimester of pregnancy (Oliveira et al 2002) and mean arterial pressure may decrease by 10–15 mmHg (Edwards 1998). Therefore, an elevated BP is never normal during pregnancy and may be an early indicator of pre-eclampsia.

There are two main non-invasive methods of measuring BP: the auscultatory method and the oscillatory method.

Auscultatory blood pressure measurement

The auscultatory method is an indirect method of measuring arterial BP in the brachial artery of the arm (Sheppard & Wright 2003). The auscultatory method utilises a sphygmomanometer which consists of a cuff with a rubber bladder within, an inflating bulb and a manometer and control valve. Sphygmomanometers may be mercury or anaeroid. BP is measured by utilising a stethoscope to identify Korotkoff sounds. The cuff is inflated until the radial pulse is no longer palpable. The systolic BP measurement is the point at which a clear tapping sound is audible. The diastolic pressure is measured at the point when the sound can no longer be heard (Dougherty & Lister 2005).

There are a number of limitations and sources of error associated with the manual auscultatory method: poor hearing, user error, and failure to interpret Korotkoff sounds correctly. In addition it has been found that users display a terminal digit preference and tend to record pressures ending in 0 or 5 (Broad et al 2007). Users have also been found to record the expected pressure of the particular person rather than the actual reading (Dougherty & Lister 2005).

Cuff size may greatly influence the accuracy of BP measurement (Oliveira et al 2002). If the cuff is too small it may lead to an overestimation of BP and if the cuff is too large BP may be underestimated. The cuff width should be 40% of the arm circumference and cuff length should be 80% of the arm circumference (Sheppard & Wright 2003). Several cuff sizes should, therefore, be available in clinical practice in order to obtain more precise and accurate BP measurements. The cuff should be applied 2–3 cm above the antecubital fossa allowing easier access to the brachial artery. The cuff bladder should be placed directly over the brachial artery. Ideally, the arm should be placed at the level of the fourth intercostal space, 45° from the axial line with the patient in the sitting position (Eşer et al 2007, Mort & Kruse 2008). There is a significant difference in BP measurement of patients in the recumbent and supine position; therefore, it is important that when comparing BP measurements that they are carried out in the same position each time (Eşer et al 2007).

Automated oscillatory blood pressure measurement

Automated intermittent oscillometric devices are frequently utilised in arterial BP measurement (Thomas et al 2002). An oscillometric cuff is inflated around a proximal limb and inflated until all oscillations in cuff pressure caused by arterial pulsations are extinguished. The occluding pressure is then lowered in a stepwise fashion so that oscillations re-appear over a discrete interval. The alteration in oscillatory amplitude during deflation is transduced into mean, systolic and diastolic pressures, which are displayed on a monitor screen (Oh et al 2003).

Since the BP is measured by sensing the variations of pressure in the cuff by the pulsing of the artery underneath it, the correct placement of the cuff is essential for accurate BP readings (Oh et al 2003). Measurement error is found to be less frequent with calibrated oscillatory devices than manual auscultation; however, there are a number of limitations. Automated devices have 95% confidence intervals within the normatensive range, however, the confidence intervals are very much reduced outside of the normal BP range (Amoore et al 2008, Oh et al 2003). In addition any arrythmias may increase the likelihood of erroneous measurements. Cuff misplacement may also contribute to inaccuracies.

BP should be recorded utilising the format depicted in Figure 11.3.

Respiratory rate

Respiratory rate is a key predictor of cardiac arrest and admission to intensive care (Kennedy 2007). Jevon and Ewans (2007) suggest that a deterioration or change in respiratory rate may be the first indication of critical illness. The rate and pattern of a pre or postpartum women's breathing is, therefore, extremely significant. Despite this, respiratory rate is the most frequently omitted or incorrectly documented vital sign (Moore 2007).

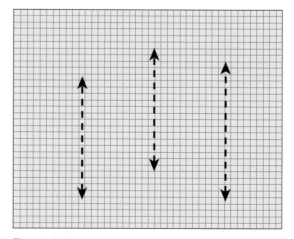

Figure 11.3 ● Blood pressure documentation.

The respiratory rate should be measured by counting the number of breaths over a full minute, as the critically ill women may develop irregular or laboured breathing. For accuracy, a woman should be resting for at least 5 minutes before the respiratory rate is measured (Kennedy 2007). During the interpretation of the recording the midwife should consider recent physical activity such as position changes, mobilisation and presence of pain, as these factors may increase the respiratory rate. A normal breath rate is considered to be between 10 and 17 breaths (Moore 2007). Tachypnoea is defined as rate of 18 or more breaths per minute and bradypnoea is defined as a rate of 12 or less breaths per minute (Doherty et al 2005). As with all vital signs, respiratory rate must be considered within the context of the individual woman's normal values; co morbidities, level of fitness must be considered.

Recognising deterioration

The Portsmouth sign

When the heart rate is higher than the systolic BP it is an early indication of critical illness (Figure 11.4). This phenomenon has been called the 'Portsmouth sign' (Smith 2003), so called as it was first described by physicians in Portsmouth. Patients displaying the Portsmouth sign will require immediate medical attention, as they are likely to be significantly volume depleted and require aggressive fluid resuscitation.

Early warning scores

Early warning scoring (EWS) is a tool commonly used for the assessment of unwell patients in order to identify those at risk of deterioration as soon as possible (Subbe et al 2007). EWS is a simple physiological scoring system suitable for bedside application. EWS are also referred to as Patient Track and Trigger, Patient at Risk scores (PARS) or Modified Early Warning Scores (MEWS).

The early warning score is based on five physiological parameters:

- Systolic BP.
- Pulse rate.
- Respiratory rate.
- Temperature.
- AVPU score (Subbe et al 2001).

Intensive care admissions and cardiac arrests are often preceded for hours or even days by abnormalities in routine observations (Quarterman et al 2005). The purpose of EWS is to attribute scores to these abnormal observations that require health-care professionals to seek expert help when a trigger score is reached. The normal changes in cardiovascular function associated with pregnancy are not reflected in the design of a standard EWS; however, special scoring systems modified for use in the obstetric patient have been developed (Lewis 2007). These have, however, yet to be validated. However, if a standard EWS is utilised on an obstetric patient, the error is on the safe side and women will be referred earlier than may be necessary (Harrison et al 2005, Lewis 2007).

Invasive haemodynamic assessment

Women who have developed a life-threatening illness will require more detailed haemodynamic assessment. Any life-threatening illness whether as

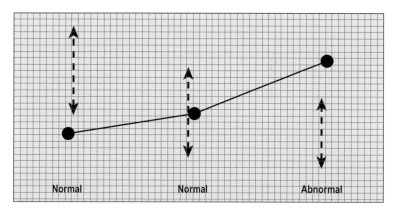

Figure 11.4 ● The Portsmouth Sign (Smith 2003).

a direct result of pregnancy or from a coincidental disease will be aggravated by the physiological demands of pregnancy (Dhond & Dob 2000). Management of life-threatening events in the face of altered maternal physiology, diseases specific to pregnancy and the presence of a fetus provides a great challenge to health-care practitioners (Dhond & Dob 2000). Invasive haemodynamic assessment techniques may be required, therefore, to provide in-depth information on the woman's cardiovascular status to inform clinical decisions and guide and evaluate therapeutic interventions.

Invasive arterial pressure monitoring

Invasive arterial monitoring allows dynamic beat-to-beat monitoring of the systemic circulation. In an unstable circulation the risks are low and the benefits are high (Windsor 1998). Continuous intra-arterial pressure provides more frequent, accurate data than auscultating peripheral BPs (Reynolds 1999). The most common site for arterial catheterisation is the radial artery; other sites include the brachial and femoral, and, more rarely, the posterior tibial and dorsalis pedis. In severe circulatory compromise gaining peripheral access may be difficult and time-consuming. Femoral artery catheterisation may

afford the practitioner with easier access with the added advantage that femoral arterial monitoring reflects the aortic pressure more accurately in low output states (Oh et al 2003). The arterial catheter is connected to pressurised monitoring tubing and a transducer device that transforms changes in pressure within the artery into a pressure waveform that is displayed on a monitor screen (Figure 11.5).

The rapid rise in the arterial waveform follows each QRS complex and is representative of the ventricular contraction. The highest point of the waveform corresponds to the systolic pressure. As the pressure within the ventricle falls, the waveform decreases. A dicrotic notch appears when the aortic valve closes. The lowest point or baseline is the diastolic pressure (Jevon & Ewens 2007).

Complications

There are several complications of arterial catheterisation. Arterial haemorrhage is the most dangerous complication (Garrettson 2005). Haemorrhage may occur during the insertion procedure or may occur due to accidental disconnection of the catheter from the pressurised tubing-transducer set-up (Oh et al 2003). The insertion site should always be easily visible to the health-care professional and not be covered by opaque dressings or bedclothes.

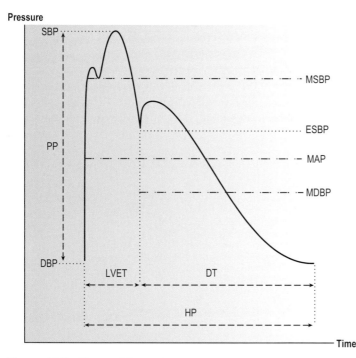

Figure 11.5 • The arterial wave form.

In addition, the integrity of the giving set and transducer setup should be regularly checked with particular attention paid to luer lock connections and stopcock caps.

Retrograde embolisation is another, albeit rare, complication of arterial catheterisation (Oh et al 2003). Small blood clots may form either within the catheter or at the tip, which, if flushed into the systemic system, may compromise blood supply to the hand or limb (Garrettson 2005, Oh et al 2003). Discolouration, mottling, coolness or altered sensation should be observed for. Pulses both proximal and distal to the site of catheter insertion should also be regularly checked (Garrettson 2005).

Infection, as with all vascular catheters is a potential complication of arterial catheterisation. The signs of arterial catheter infection are the same as the venous catheter: redness, inflammation, exudate, and pyrexia (Garrettson 2005). Hand decontamination is suggested as the main defence against nosocomial infection (Hugonnet & Pittet 2000). In addition, arterial catheter insertion, dressing change should be carried out utilising an aseptic technique.

Other more infrequent complications include haematoma, pseudoaneurysm, arteriovenous fistula, and compartment syndrome (Oh et al 2003). The potentially catastrophic complications associated with invasive arterial catheters means that they are only utilised in high-dependency or critical-care areas by appropriately trained health-care professionals.

Central venous pressure monitoring

A central venous catheter is a hollow radio-opaque cannula which is inserted percutaneously, so that the tip lies either in the superior vena cava or within the right atrium (Figure 11.6). Central venous catheters, as well as facilitating venous access allowing rapid drug and fluid administration, may be utilised to measure the central venous pressure (CVP) (Oh et al 2003).

A CVP measurement reflects the filling pressure (or preload) to the right side of the heart. CVP may indicate blood volume, as the CVP reading reflects the pressure within the great veins which hold 60% of the total blood volume (Reynolds 1999). CVP may, therefore, be used to assess blood volume deficits, guide fluid replacement and monitor responses to treatment (Sheppard & Wright 2003).

CVP may be measured either by an electronic transducer system (Figure 11.7) or by a manual water column manometer (Figure 11.8) that is inserted into an intravenous infusion set. The recording should be made with the patient in the same baseline position with the zero point of the manometer level with the patients' right atrium (phlebostatic axis), as illustrated in Figure 11.9. Ideally, the patient should lie flat in a supine position to reflect the right atrial filling pressure. However, this position is not comfortable or tolerable for some patients, particularly during pregnancy. Therefore, measurement may be taken in the recumbent or semi-recumbent position

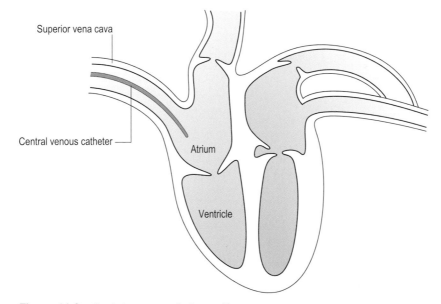

Figure 11.6 • Central venous catheter position.

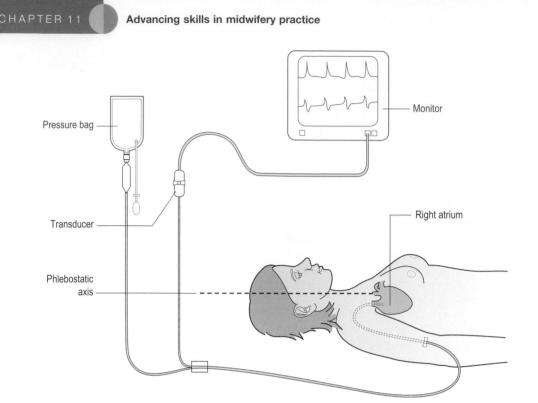

Figure 11.7 • Measurement of central venous catheter utilising an electrical transducer.

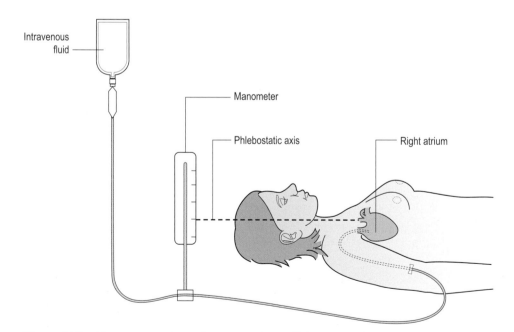

Figure 11.8 • Measurement of central venous catheter utilising a manual water column manometer.

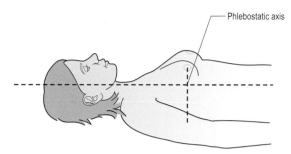

Figure 11.9 ● Phlebostatic axis.

(Dougherty & Lister 2004). It is vital that measurements are carried out in the same position each time. CVP should not be measured when the patient is on their side as this is inaccurate.

The normal CVP range is 3–10 mmHg (5–12 cmH$_2$O), although there is considerable variation in what is considered normal (Sheppard & Wright 2003). During the second half of pregnancy the inferior vena cava, iliac vessels and abdominal aorta may be compressed by the gravid uterus when the mother is in the supine position (Edwards 1998). CVP readings may, therefore, be lower than expected in pregnant women. Ideally, haemodynamic parameters should be obtained with pregnant women in the supine position with the uterus manually displaced to the left. The emphasis on CVP measurements should, therefore, be placed on dynamic change over time rather than absolute values (Oh et al 2003) and readings should be considered within a wider clinical assessment (McGee & Gould 2003). A low CVP indicates fluid loss or hypovolaemia, poor venous return or peripheral vasodilation. A high CVP may be due to hypervolaemia, cardiac failure, pericardial effusion, cardiac tamponade, pulmonary emboli, pneumothorax or artefact (Jevon & Ewens 2007).

As with all invasive procedures there are many complications associated with central venous catheterisation. Potential complications are detailed in Box 11.4.

Professional responsibilities

Invasive haemodynamic monitoring devices are associated with potentially catastrophic complications. Care of such devices should, therefore, only be undertaken by appropriately trained, skilled midwives who have been assessed as competent. Women with such devices require careful observation and

---

Box 11.4

Complications of central venous catheterisation

- Local or systemic infection is one of the most serious complications associated with central venous catheterisation (Cole 2007). Effective hand decontamination and aseptic techniques are critical in prevention of infection.
- Thrombus formation at either the tip of the catheter or its surround is another common complication. Thrombus formation may be prevented by regular flushing with normal saline. If an occlusion occurs flushing is not recommended as it may liberate the clot into the systemic circulation (McGee & Gould 2003).
- Air emboli, a potentially life-threatening condition where air may enter the venous system, may occur if there is accidental disconnection of the infusion giving set or manometer. All connections, taps and caps should be regularly checked (Cole 2007).
- Other complications include: pneumothorax/ haemothorax, cardiac tamponade, arrythmias, catheter misplacement/malposition, pain and discomfort, and haemorrhage.

---

monitoring, therefore, should only be cared for in environments where the technical and staffing resources are available to support this. Accurate and correct documentation of observations is essential to ensure clinical decisions and therapeutic interventions are based on the correct information. All entries must be timed and dated and, where appropriate, initialled.

Key practice points

- Complications of pregnancy are rare.
- Early recognition of clinical deterioration is essential to promote positive patient outcome.
- Non-invasive haemodynamic assessment and monitoring techniques are essential tools in recognising clinical deterioration.
- Invasive haemodynamic monitoring whilst useful has inherent risks and complications associated with it.
- Care of invasive haemodynamic devises requires skill, expertise and competence.
- Expert help should be sought in a timely fashion.
- Careful documentation of observations is vital.

References

Amoore, J.N., Lemesre, Y., Murray, K., Mieke, S., King, S.T., Smith, F.E., et al., 2008. Automatic blood pressure measurement: the oscillometric waveform shape is a potential contributor to differences between oscillometric and auscultatory pressure measurements. J. Hypertens. 26 (1), 35–43.

Armstrong, R., 2002. Nurse's knowledge of error in blood pressure measurement technique. Int J. Nurs. Pract. 8, 118–126.

Broad, J., Wells, S., Marshall, R., Jackson, R., 2007. Zero end-digit preference in recorded blood pressure and its impact on classification of patients for pharmacologic management in primary care – PREDICT–CVD–6. Br. J. Gen. Pract. 57 (544), 897–903.

Carlin, A., Alfirevic, Z., 2006. Time to re-visit the role of haemodynamic monitoring in obstetrics? BJOG 113 (9), 989–991.

Cole, E., 2007. Measuring central venous pressure. Nurs. Stand. 22 (7), 40–42.

Dhond, G.R., Dob, D.P., 2000. Critical care of the obstetric patient. Current Anaesthesia & Critical Care 11 (2), 86–91.

Dimond, B., 2006. Legal aspects of midwifery, third ed. Books for Midwives, Cheshire.

Dougherty, L., Lister, S., 2005. The Royal Marsden Hospital manual of clinical nursing procedures. Blackwell Publishing, Oxford.

Edwards, S., 1998. Haemodynamic monitoring of the pregnant woman in intensive care. Nurs. Crit. Care. 3 (3), 112–121.

Eşer, İ., Khorshid, L., Güneş, Ü.Y., Demir, Y., 2007. The effect of different body positions on blood pressure. J. Clin. Nurs. 16, 137–140.

Garrettson, S., 2005. Haemodynamic monitoring: arterial catheters. Nurs. Stand. 19 (31), 55–64.

Guyton, A., Hall, J., 2005. Textbook of medical physiology, Eleventh ed. Saunders, London.

Harrison, D., Penny, J.A., Yentis, S.M., 2005. Case, mix outcome and activity for obstetric admissions to adult, general critical care units; a secondary analysis of the ICNARC Case Mix Programme Database. Crit. Care 9 (Suppl. 3), S25–S37.

Hugonnet, S., Pittet, D., 2000. Hand hygiene: beliefs or science? Clin. Microbiol. Infect. 6 (7), 350–356.

Jevon, P., Ewens, B., 2007. Monitoring the critically ill patient, second ed. Blackwell Science, Oxford.

Kennedy, S., 2007. Detecting changes in the respiratory status of ward patients. Nurs. Stand. 21 (49), 42–46.

Lewis, G. (Ed.), 2007. The Confidential Enquiry into Maternal and Child Health (CEMACH) saving mothers' lives: reviewing maternal deaths to make motherhood safer – 2003–2005. The seventh report of the Confidential Enquiries into Maternal Deaths in the United Kingdom. CEMACH, London.

Luppi, C., 1997. Cardiopulmonary resuscitation: pregnant women are different. AACN Clinical Issues Advanced Practice in Acute Critical Care 8 (4), 574–585.

McGee, D., Gould, M., 2003. Preventing complications of central venous catheterisation. N. Engl. J. Med. 348 (12), 1123–1133.

Moore, T., 2007. Respiratory assessment in adults. Nurs. Stand. 21 (49), 48–56.

Moreau, D., 2005. Assessment made incredibly easy. Lippincott Williams and Wilkins, London.

Mort, J.R., Kruse, H.R., 2008. Timing of blood pressure measurement related to caffeine consumption. Ann. Pharmacother. 42 (1), 105–110.

National Confidential Enquiry into Patient Outcomes and Death (NCEPOD), 2005. An acute problem? Department of Health, London.

National Institute for Health and Clinical Excellence (NICE), 2007. Acutely ill patients in hospital. Department of Health, London.

Oh, T., Bersten, A., Soni, N., 2003. Oh's intensive care manual, fifth ed. Butterworth Heinemann London.

Oliveira, S., Arcuri, E.A.M., Santos, J.L.F., 2002. Cuff width influence on blood pressure measurement during the pregnant-puerperal cycle. J. Adv. Nurs. 38 (2), 180–189.

Quarterman, C., Thomas, A.N., Mackenna, M., McNamee, R., 2005. Use of a patient information system to audit the introduction of modified early warning scoring. J. Eval. Clin. Pract. 11 (2), 133–138.

Reynolds, A., 1999. Critical and high acuity nursing care. Thompson Learning, New York.

Seeley, R., Stephens, T.D., Tate, P., 2007. Anatomy and physiology. McGraw-Hill Higher Education, London.

Sheppard, M., Wright, M., 2003. Principles and practice of high dependency nursing. Baillière Tindall, Elsevier, London.

Smith, G., 2003. ALERT: acute life-threatening events: recognition and treatment. Learning Media Development, University of Portsmouth, Portsmouth.

Subbe, C., Kruger, M., Rutherford, P. Gemmell, L., 2001. Validation of a modified early warning score in medical admissions. Q. J. Med. 94, 521–526.

Subbe, C., Gao, H., Harrison, D.A., 2007. Reproducibility of physiological track-and-trigger warning systems for identifying at-risk patients on the ward. Intensive Care. Med. 33 (16), 619–624.

Thomas, S., Liehr, P., DeKeyser, F., Frazier, L., Friedman, E., 2002. A review of nursing research on blood pressure. J. Nurs. Sch. 34 (4), 313–321.

Wilson, J., Symon, A., 2002. Clinical risk management in midwifery: the right to a perfect baby? Books for Midwives, Oxford.

Windsor, J., 1998. Haemodynamic monitoring. Care of the Critically Ill 14 (2), 44–49.

Further reading

Cole, E., 2007. Measuring central venous pressure. Nurs. Stand. 22 (7), 40–42.

A good practical, easy-to-read guide to measuring central venous pressure.

Moreau, D., 2005. Assessment made incredibly easy. Lippincott Williams and Wilkins, London.

A very readable and informative text describing patient assessment procedures.

Oh, T., Bersten, A., Soni, N., 2003. Oh's intensive care manual, fifth ed. Butterworth Heinemann, London.

An in depth account of haemodynamic monitoring theory and practice.

Stables, D., Rankin, J., 2005. Physiology in childbearing with anatomy and related biosciences, second ed. Elsevier, Oxford.

Provides a useful background to the physiological changes associated with pregnancy.

Sheppard, M., Wright, M., 2003. Principles and practice of high dependency nursing. Elsevier, Baillière Tindall, London.

A good overview of both the underpinning theory and practice issues of caring for the critically ill.

Chapter Twelve

12

Physiological examination of the neonate

Carole England

CONTENTS

Introduction 135
Examination of the heart 136
  Incidence of congenital heart disease . 136
  Detection 136
  Predisposing factors of congenital
  heart disease 136
  Inspection 136
  Palpation 137
  Auscultation 138
Examination of the eye 141
Examination of the hip for developmental
dysplasia of the hip 142
  Incidence 142
  The modified Ortolani and Barlow
  manoeuvres 143
Conclusion 145
Key practice points 145
References 145
Further reading 146

Before reading this chapter, you should be familiar with:
- Statutory rules, standards and professional codes governing the midwife's practice.
- The anatomy of the heart and the physiological changes occurring in the fetal circulation at birth.
- Congenital heart disease.
- The definition of ophthalmia neonatorum, causative organisms and appropriate management.
- The development and anatomy of the fetal hips.

Introduction

Midwives now perform the medical examination of the newborn alongside their paediatric senior house officer colleagues, neonatal nurses and general practitioners. Performed within the first 72 hours of birth, this examination specifically screens for congenital heart disease (CHD), developmental dysplasia of the hip (DDH), congenital cataract and undescended testes. The examination is not part of the role of all midwives, but is an expanded role for those midwives who wish to learn and maintain new competencies in this area of care (Nursing and Midwifery Council [NMC] 2004). This chapter will focus upon examination of the heart, eyes and hips, and will highlight the need for simple but subtle skills in physical examination, whilst aiming to address the professional issues that the midwife should consider when undertaking the examination of the neonate. This is not a comprehensive guide to examination of the newborn, but a snap shot of some aspects that are commonly challenging to midwife examiners. The need for a relevant knowledge base of each subject area is essential because familiarity with the normal is not sufficient to assume that midwives will know what signs are abnormal (Sellwood & Huertas-Ceballos 2008). Knowing a subject thoroughly enables the midwife to offer appropriately expressed information to parents and to communicate effectively when referring to specialists. Learning and maintaining a skill for an expanded role, takes commitment and perseverance, especially when faced by personal and organisational obstacles (Steele 2007).

Examination of the heart

There is an accepted given that good examiners miss abnormal cases. They will send a baby home who will be admitted with a serious heart defect. Thoroughness of examination technique and documentation is, therefore, vital but no guarantee of total success; a reality that all examiners need to embrace. There is an expectation from parents that their baby's heart will be examined and this is accepted as good practice. It offers a reassurance of normality at the time of the examination. At 24 hours of age and beyond is about the best time for it to be performed, when the physiological adaptations have settled down.

Incidence of congenital heart disease

Congenital heart disease (CDH) incidence is 8:1000 live births and is the most common group of structural anomalies (Lissauer & Fanaroff 2006) and accounts for 30% of all congenital abnormalities (Horrox 2002).

Detection

Half of the known cases of CHD are detected by antenatal ultrasound scan, so the postnatal physical examination is the only other means of early detection, but less than 50% of heart defects are actually detected. However, as O'Callaghan and Stephenson (2004) argue, many heart conditions are asymptomatic and trivial. They further say that conditions that present earliest tend to be more immediately life threatening, although many complex and severe conditions may present later. For this reason they believe a better screen for heart defects would be the additional use of a saturation monitor that would pick up a predicted 75% of cases.

Predisposing factors of congenital heart disease

Reading the case notes for details of the present pregnancy and perinatal history is a necessary prerequisite for any physical examination. Park (2003) asserts that maternal rubella infection in the first trimester commonly results in patent ductus arteriosus (PDA) and pulmonary artery stenosis (PAS). Other viral infections in late pregnancy may cause myocarditis. Maternal medications such as anticonvulsants (phenytoin) and amphetamines are highly suspected teratogens. Excessive maternal alcohol intake may cause fetal alcohol syndrome, in which ventricular septal defect (VSD), PDA and tetralogy of Fallot (TOF) are common. Maternal diabetes increases the prevalence of transposition of the great arteries (TGA), VSD, PDA and cardiomyopathy. Chromosomal aberrations include Trisomy 13, 18, 21 and Turner's syndrome (El Habbal 2007). Other associated system malformations are hydrocephalus, diaphragmatic hernia, duodenal atresia, imperforate anus, omphalocele and gastroschisis. Maternal CHD offers 15% prevalence to her children compared to 1% in the general population. When one child is affected the sibling recurrence risk is 3%, especially for high prevalence defects like VSD, which is the most common variety of CHD and accounts for one-third of all cases (Pang & Newson 2005). The probability of recurrence is substantially higher when the mother rather than the father is the affected parent (Park 2003). Gill and O'Brien (2007) recommend that the approach to cardiovascular examination should be eyes, hands then ears. The heart itself should be left until last and auscultation as the final approach.

Inspection

Is a most important skill and should not be rushed. The midwife should look at the general appearance of the baby and compare gestational age with weight and size. Wilkinson (2006) argues that smallness could indicate growth disruption at the time when major organs were being evolved. The midwife should question whether the baby has any dysmorphic features indicative of chromosomal abnormalities that are associated with heart defects. Key questions asked of the mother provide useful information for assessing the baby holistically. Gill and O'Brien (2007) support the notion that the mother's view is valuable and is treated as correct unless proven otherwise. Using words to describe her baby as 'happy', 'cranky', 'responsive', 'sleepy', can provide useful information on the baby's homeostatic state, especially how her baby responds physically to taking a feed.

Central cyanosis needs urgent management, but assessing the colour of the baby can be most difficult, given that different degrees of skin pigmentation in different light settings may offer different interpretations. For all babies, but especially those with a dark skin, their tongue and mucous membranes will reflect their level of oxygenation. Pallor may precede respiratory disease, but again is difficult to assess and, as O'Callaghan and Stephenson (2004) argue, an oxygen saturation of haemoglobin <95% is abnormal and merits cardiologist assessment. They advise that it is wise to always check saturation levels in the feet. If the baby has a PDA, proximal (upper limb) saturations may be within normal limits. Gill and O'Brien (2007) also comment that prolonged (but undetected) central cyanosis may result in a plethoric appearance due to polycythaemia. In the newborn, polycythaemia may also be mistaken for cyanosis and/or trauma in the form of petechae. In the presence of central cyanosis the midwife will look for other signs of respiratory distress (see Box 12.1).

A capillary refill test of perfusion done on the chest over the sternum assesses the time it takes for the blood to refill the capillaries when finger pressure has been applied. Greater than 2 seconds is abnormal in a baby. Oxygen therapy should be considered cautiously as it may close a patent ductus arteriosus (PDA) which is acting as a life-saving conduit (Horrox 2002).

Palpation

This is the next part of the assessment that is particularly focused on the chest and any palpable sounds or murmurs. The precordium is the area over the sternum and ribs. A palpable murmur is referred to as a thrill. A precordial thrill can be seen or palpated and is characteristic of heart disease with a high volume overload such as a left–right

shunt lesion through the ductus arteriosus. Palpation of a thrill is always significant and often of real diagnostic value. A thrill in the suprasternal notch may suggest coarctation of the aorta (COA). Palpation may reveal whether the heart is active or hyper-dynamic. Right-ventricular enlargement is best sought with the fingertips placed between the 2nd, 3rd and 4th ribs along the left sternal edge. The apex beat is found in the 4th intercostal space along the mid-clavicular or nipple line. A diffuse, forceful and displaced apex beat, usually caused by hypertrophied muscle is relatively rare and described as a heave not to be confused by an ectopic apex beat, which may be displaced to the right according to O'Callaghan and Stephenson (2004), as a result of a left-sided pneumothorax or diaphragmatic hernia. Palpation of the upper abdomen of an enlarged liver (greater than 1 cm below the costal margin) may indicate heart failure.

Palpation of the peripheral pulses for rhythm, strength, volume and character then follows. Rhythms originating in the sinoatrial node are called sinus rhythms. In a regular sinus rhythm, the rhythm and rate of the heart beat are normal for the age of the baby. In sinus tachycardia, with beats above 160 per minute, first consider pyrexia. Gill and O'Brien (2007) contend that the pulse rate will accelerate approximately 10 beats per minute for every $1^{\circ}C$ rise in temperature. Hypoxia, circulatory shock, congestive heart failure (CHF) and thyrotoxicosis are other possible causes. Sinus bradycardia is defined as beats below 80 per minute. Hypothermia, hypoxia, increased intercranial pressure and hypothyroidism may be causative factors. In sinus arrhythmia there is a phasic variation in the heart rate, increasing during inspiration and decreasing during expiration. There is no haemodynamic significance and, therefore, no treatment indicated. A normal heart beat, skips a beat. It is not a metronome.

Palpation of the brachial and femoral pulses will require total concentration. Femoral pulses are often difficult to feel. Many examiners apply too much pressure to the artery which may obliterate it (Gill & O'Brien 2007). Strong arm pulses and weak leg pulses suggest COA. If the femoral pulses are thought to be diminished, evidence of brachio-femoral delay is sought, which is a difficult task when the heart rate is rapid. If the right brachial artery pulse is stronger than the left brachial artery pulse, this could suggest a COA where the constriction is proximal to the left subclavian artery. Bounding brachial pulses are found in PDA with a

---

Box 12.1

Signs of respiratory distress

- Asymmetrical chest-wall movements.
- Tachypnoea (breaths over 60 per minute), nasal flaring.
- Sternal or costal recession.
- The use of respiratory accessory muscles.
- Head bobbing.
- Audible expiratory grunt.

wide pulse pressure in the lower limbs. A weak thready pulse is found in congenital heart failure and in circulatory shock.

Auscultation

By the time inspection and palpation have been performed much of the information the baby can supply has been obtained and auscultation is the proverbial 'cherry on the cake'. Fear of missing a heart murmur tends to be a common anxiety in examiners. The use of a paediatric stethoscope is recommended, and the bell and diaphragm utilised at all auscultation sites. The bell is designed as a resonating chamber and must be applied to the skin lightly or else it will stretch the skin and form a diaphragm (Talley & O'Connor 2006). It is used to amplify low-pitched sounds such as those produced by diastolic murmurs. The diaphragm is better for high-pitched sounds such as a systolic murmur. Some modern stethoscopes do not have a bell so the amount of pressure applied on the skin, creates the bell/diaphragm difference. Variations with respiration should be noted. The baby must not be crying. Attempts to auscultate the heart with one hand on the brachial pulse for timing is good practice, but needs plenty of practise to do well.

Each cardiac cycle has two heart sounds that can be heard through a stethoscope when applied to the chest wall. The first heart sound (S1) is known as 'lub' and is described as long and booming and occurs when the atriventricular (AV) valves, the tricuspid and bicuspid (mitral) valves are closing at the beginning of ventricular contraction (systole). The second heart sound is 'dub'; is short and sharp and reflects closure of the semi lunar valves of the aorta and pulmonary arteries, at the beginning of ventricular relaxation (diastole) (see Figure 12.1).

Wherever the stethoscope is placed on the chest, there will be heart sounds, given the size of the head of the stethoscope and the diminutive size of the neonatal chest. The best place to hear the first heart sound (S1) is at the apex or the lower left sternal border (see Figure 12.2). Splitting of the heart sound where the tricuspid and mitral valves close slightly out of synchrony, is not usually heard in a normal baby.

The second heart sound (S2) is heard in the upper left sternal border. Splitting of closure of the aortic (A2) and pulmonary artery valve (P2) is easily heard with the stethoscope and the degree

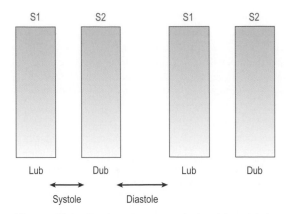

Figure 12.1 ● To show heart sounds 1 and 2 and their phonetic representations.

of splitting normally varies with respiration, increasing on inspiration and decreasing or becoming a single sound on expiration. The third heart sound (S3) represents ventricular filling that starts as soon as the mitral and tricuspid valves open, and the fourth heart sound represents ventricular filling that occurs in response to contraction of the atria. These sounds are not normally heard but can be best auscultated at the apex or lower left sternal border. The fourth heart sound (S4) if heard at the apex is pathological and is seen in conditions with decreased ventricular compliance or CHF. Where there is a combination of a loud S3 or S4 with a tachycardia, common in CHF; this is referred to as a gallop rhythm.

A heart murmur is an additional noise heard during the cardiac cycle and presents two problems to the midwife: firstly, whether one can hear it at all and secondly, distinguishing it as significant or innocent. Absence of a murmur does not exclude CHD. The technique in listening is to wipe out all extraneous and respiratory noise and listen between the first and second heart sounds, very carefully. The location, timing in the cycle, grade, duration or rhythm, quality and radiation of the murmur should be assessed. It is usual to listen to the chest wall in four specific areas (see Figure 12.2). The sternum, clavicles and ribs (costals and intercostal spaces) are important landmarks as well as the heart structures. There are two upper landmarks each side of the upper sternum. The right sternal, 2nd intercostal space is the aortic area. This is sometimes referred to as the upper right sternal border (URSB). The left sternal 2nd intercostal space is the pulmonary area and is known as the upper left sternal border (ULSB). A further two landmarks are both located to the

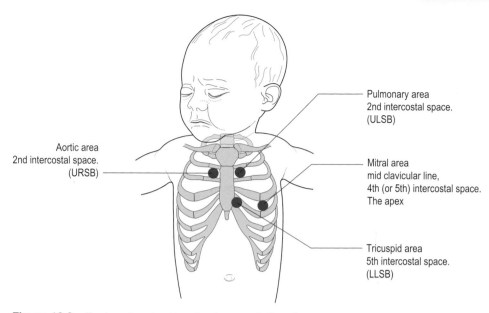

Figure 12.2 ● To show the chest location for auscultation sites.

Aortic area
2nd intercostal space.
(URSB)

Pulmonary area
2nd intercostal space.
(ULSB)

Mitral area
mid clavicular line,
4th (or 5th) intercostal space.
The apex

Tricuspid area
5th intercostal space.
(LLSB)

left of the lower sternum. The left sternal 5th inter-costal space is the tricuspid area and may be called the lower left sternal border (LLSB) and the apex is found below the nipple on the mid-clavicular line, 4th or 5th intercostal space. This is the mitral area.

According to the timing of the heart murmur in relation to the S1 and S2 sounds, the heart murmur is classified as systolic, diastolic or continuous. A systolic murmur occurs between S1 and S2 and is classified as one of two types, either an ejection or regurgitant murmur (see Figure 12.3).

The midwife should pay particular attention to the timing of the onset of the murmur because the onset in relation to S1 is far more important than the duration of the murmur, in determining origin and thus diagnosis. In ejection systolic murmurs there is always an interval between S1 and the onset of the murmur. They are referred to as crescendo–decrescendo murmurs as the murmur is at its maximum, half way through and for this reason are also called a diamond-shaped murmur. A murmur may be short or long in duration and can be caused either by a large volume of blood passing through the semi lunar valves or a normal flow of blood passing through stenosed or deformed semi lunar valves. They can be heard at the base or in the mid precordium and may be innocent or pathological.

By comparison, regurgitant systolic murmurs *begin with* the S1 heart sound which usually lasts

through systole (and even into diastole) and is referred to as pansystolic, meaning from start to finish. They are never crescendo–decrescendo, but sometimes can be decrescendo where they end in middle or early systole. Park (2003) argues that these murmurs are always pathological and are associated with VSD and feature regurgitation of the mitral and tricuspid valves. Gill and O'Brien (2007) believe that examiners should only be concerned with systolic murmurs in the neonate because diastolic murmurs are easier to pick up when the heart rate is slower. A diastolic murmur occurs when the heart is at rest and is between S2 and S1. Continuous murmurs begin in systole and continue without interruption through to S2 into all or part of diastole, e.g. a PDA, disturbances in flow such as COA or a combined systolic and diastolic murmur. Park (2003) asserts that innocent murmurs are accentuated by pyrexia and are associated with normal electrocardiogram (ECG) and X-ray findings. Occasionally in preterm and term babies there is a pulmonary ejection systolic murmur which can be heard specifically at the upper left sternal border. It transmits to the right and left chest, axillae and back. The grade is 1-2/6 in intensity. Innocent murmurs tend not to be louder than 2/6. The intensity of the murmur is customarily graded from 1 to 6 (see Box 12.2).

Quality refers to how the examiner describes the sounds heard, e.g. systolic murmurs of VSD have a

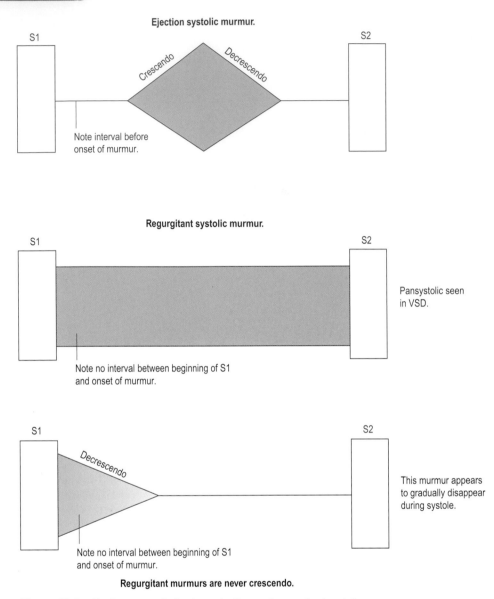

Figure 12.3 • To diagrammatically show ejection and regurgitant systolic murmurs.

uniform high-pitched quality often described as 'blowing' whereas an ejection systolic murmur, where stenosis is featured, has a 'harsh grating' quality. If a murmur radiates from one area to another it is usually pathological, for example a systolic ejection murmur at the base that transmits well to the neck is likely to be aortic and one that transmits well to the sides of the chest and back is likely to arise in the pulmonary valve or pulmonary artery (Park 2003). The key points to consider when examining the heart are listed in Box 12.3.

Thorough documentation will reflect the inspection, palpation and auscultation findings. The details of a cardiac murmur, if present, should be described, e.g. location, timing in the cycle, grade and reflected diagramatically (see Figure 12.3). Parents should be told that *on this occasion* their baby's heart appears normal/or needs referral.

Grading of heart murmurs by intensity on auscultation (Park 2003)

1. Barely audible when using a stethoscope.
2. Soft, but easily audible.
3. Moderately loud but not palpable and no thrill.
4. A loud and palpable murmur and associated with a thrill.
5. Audible with stethoscope barely on the chest. Can be heard with an ear to the chest.
6. Audible at the end of the cot with stethoscope off the chest.

Key points when examining the heart

- The presence of central cyanosis and poor perfusion.
- Tachycardia.
- An abnormal precordium.
- A heart murmur with a gallop rhythm and hepatosplenomegaly.

Examination of the eye

The neonatal eye is 75% of the adult size and it is believed that newborns can see light, colour, shapes and, by evolutionary design, their mother's face. The visual system is immature and their neural connections from eye to brain are incomplete. They have no depth perception because this relies on both eyes working together and neonatal eyes resemble those of chameleons where one eye appears to be functioning independently from the other. During the first 3 months of life there is a need for both eyes to function well because reduced light stimulation to one eye causes the condition amblyopia: a condition where the brain fails to pay enough attention to the poor eye and, as a result, the neural connections for that eye are not created. By 6 months of age, the eyes and brain become 'locked on' to each other and this then sets the stage for the baby's future visual acuity. Amblyopia can occur in one or both eyes and is usually caused by disruption of the light pathways to the retina when there is corneal clouding or scarring, congenital cataract or clouding of the vitreous humour. It is vital to screen for these media opacities within 72 hours of birth and later at 6 weeks of age. The midwife is *not* screening for the requirement of spectacles, reduced vision or squint.

As always, the skills of examination start with inspection. Oedema of the eyelids is common and bruising may be present. The midwife should confirm that any trauma and bruising is commensurate with the birth history and ensure the bruising is not a birth mark like a Salmon patch neavus (stork mark) or something more significant like a port wine stain or strawberry haemangioma. With the baby's eyes closed the midwife can *gently* palpate for the presence of the eyes and compare their size and eyeball pressure. The ocular land marks are the structures that surround the eye and how they appear as part of the face as a whole, are worthy of note. With the ophthalmoscope ready for use, the midwife should be prepared to inspect the eyes should the baby open them. Prising eyelids open may inflict undue pressure, may add to any oedema and may cause some distress from a parental perspective. Sitting the baby up or asking the mother to hold the baby over her shoulder tends to encourage the baby to open its eyes in most cases. The red reflex should be elicited first: the retina is the nervous tissue of the eye which is stimulated by light. Anteriorly, it is in contact with the vitreous humour and is avascular. Posteriorly it is supported by a vascular and lymphatic supply from the underlying choroid. When a light is shone into the eyes, the vascular retina *shines back* and is known on photographs as 'red eye'. If the red reflex can be seen, this should indicate to the midwife that there are no media opacities present. However, the redness of the red reflex may be affected by the colour of the baby's skin. The red eye reflex in Asian, Afro-Caribbean, Chinese and Japanese babies can vary in different hues of redness from brown to grey to purple, which is a reflection of their pigmented choroid and is a normal finding.

The ophthalmoscope dial should be turned to 0 and with the right hand the scope should be held to the midwife's right eye (or vice versa if left handed). Holding the scope close to the midwife's eye is important using the analogy of a hole in a fence. To look through a hole in a fence, it is necessary to get up close to the hole to see through. Each eye is initially examined separately. Thus the midwife, ideally in a darkened room, should shine a white light from the ophthalmoscope at the baby's eye from a distance of 5–10 cm and focus on the pupil margin (O'Callaghan & Stephenson 2004). A red glow from the pupil will be silhouetted against the edge of the iris. To examine both eyes together, the midwife would then hold the ophthalmoscope at a distance of 20 cm from the baby's eyes to simultaneously elicit the red reflex. The absence of a red reflex is called leukocoria. If there is any asymmetry (inequality) of the colour and intensity of the red reflex, or a white papillary reflex is seen, the possibility of a media opacity in one eye should be considered and documented. A congenital cataract is, according to Nischal (2007), the commonest cause of blindness and should be uppermost in the examiners differential diagnosis.

The midwife should then conduct a detailed examination of the front of the eye to detect any abnormalities that are not available to the naked eye. The ophthalmoscope should be set to +9 dioptres and the midwife should focus the scope, using her fore finger, before attempting to closely examine the eye (examiner's right eye to baby's right eye; left to left). The conjunctiva and sclera should be white. Sub-conjunctival haemorrhages are of no clinical significance. A blue sclera is worthy of note as it is indicative of collagen disease, where there is disruption to the production of collagen needed for fibrous, bony structures. The sclera looks blue because it is thin and not supported by collagen, but there are associated collagen diseases, specifically osteogenesis imperfecta, sometimes referred to as brittle bone disease. This finding warrants referral. The cornea should be clear by 2 days after birth and any lacerations or scarring should be noted. Clouding of the cornea could indicate congenital glaucoma. Both pupils should equally respond to light. The lens should look clear. Different coloured eyes at this stage in life is suspicious (Gill & O'Brien 2007) and should be referred. A coloboma, where the iris does not form a complete circle and may be associated with abnormalities that extend to include the ciliary body and choroid, should be referred alongside complete absence of the iris (aniridia).

Assessing whether the eye is infected should be no casual task and the examiner should always consider the gravity of ophthalmia neonatorum. According to Nischal (2007) a sticky eye demands microbiological investigation to rule out gonococcal and/or chlamydial infection, which if untreated can *rapidly* lead to corneal ulceration and blindness. Gonococcal conjunctivitis can present from 1 to 3 days with a profuse purulent discharge with swelling of the conjunctiva and lids. A swab must be taken for microscopy and culture followed by saline irrigation, topical and systemic antibiotics. Treatment of the mother and sexual contact(s) needs to be done sensitively as they may be asymptomatic. Chlamydial conjunctivitis presents later at 5–14 days, but is associated with neonatal pneumonia if the initial systemic antibiotic treatment has been inadequate (O'Callaghan & Stephenson 2004). Nischal (2007) contends that *herpes virus type II* and bacterial infections such as *Staphylococcus aureus* are other causative agents which need immediate treatment. Full documentation of what has been found should be detailed for each eye and the parents informed that *on this occasion*, the eyes are normal (or otherwise).

Examination of the hip for developmental dysplasia of the hip

Developmental dysplasia of the hip (DDH) represents a spectrum of defects where the femoral head is not totally in the acetabulum, but possibly on its border and can only be diagnosed on ultrasound scan (Woolf et al 2007). Dislocation is when the femoral head is outside of the acetabulum. The femoral head continues to grow, but if the femoral head is not in the acetabulum, the acetabulum fails to grow. Secondary adaptive changes occur so that ligaments and muscles shorten and tighten, and the acetabulum fills with filaments, which is a worsening problem.

Incidence

This is 1 in 400 live births and there are two factors which relate to the natural history of DDH, which makes screening difficult. Jones (1998) asserts that as many as 20 babies in every 1000 births have unstable hips, but 90% of these will stabilise spontaneously.

It is not possible to predict which 10% of these hips will remain unstable. Stable hips at birth may later develop DDH. The hip is at its most unstable at the time of term birth. In early gestation, there is nearly total spherical enclosure of the femoral head by the acetabulum, but this becomes less and by term it is shallow by comparison and then deepens again in the postnatal period. The tightness of the uterus and the lack of leg and hip freedom as gestation progresses are the aetiological factors in DDH. The low incident of DDH in preterm babies supports this notion. Predominantly it is a disease of girls with a 9:1 ratio with boys (Lissauer & Fanaroff 2006). The female compared to the male pelvis is structurally shallower, but there are no substantive data that support why girls are more predisposed. It is an anecdotal suggestion that female babies respond to maternal hormonal influences (see Box 12.4 for predisposing factors to DDH).

The ideal time for screening the newborn hip is 7 days; however, for practical reasons the baby is never really available to the midwife. Within 72 hours of birth is, therefore, the best compromise, followed by an examination at 4–8 weeks by

the General Practitioner or Specialist Community Public Health Nurse. Certain examination standards are mandatory because each examination is a part of a process of assessment and unless the following pre-requisites are met, test results will be, at best, unreliable and, at worst, misleading:

- The baby must be warm and comfortable.
- The baby must not be hungry or thirsty.
- The baby should be on a firm flat surface and one of the parents must be present.
- The midwife should have enough room to gain access and to be physically able and comfortable to perform the manoeuvres (Jones 1998).

If the above conditions are not met, it is wise to make an appropriate comment in the record so that the next examiner knows how much reliance to place on the results of the previous examination.

A general inspection followed by a detailed skeletal examination of the baby, may reveal additional risk factors which the history has not elicited. In the *absence* of oligohydramnios, postural foot deformities, plagiocephaly, scoliosis and prominent sacral dimple are all associated with hip abnormalities. Babies who show the effects of intrauterine growth restriction and those with syndromic facies are particularly at risk. With the baby lying on its back and legs bent at the knee with feet on the surface, an initial inspection should look for any asymmetry in the appearance of the legs and groin skin folds. Examination of the knees may show uneven knee height. On the affected side, the knee is lower because the head of the femur has dropped into the soft tissues because it is not being held by the bony acetabulum. However, equal knee height could indicate either normality of both hips or bilateral dislocation of both hips. This examination should never replace the recognised clinical tests. Pulling the legs straight to measure leg length, if performed, should be done *after* the hip examination as the manoeuvre is enough to upset a settled baby. Neonatal legs are often bow-legged and any flexor tone resistance created by the baby, renders the examination useless.

Box 12.4

Predisposing factors to developmental dysplasia of the hip

1. Squashed hips in utero:
   - Breech births (vaginal and caesarean sections).
   - External Cephalic Version performed at term (less important).
   - Oligohydramnios will also cause squashed hips. The midwife should inspect for postural foot deformities ranging from positional talipes to equino-varus and/or calcaneo valgus. Sternomastoid tumour (torticollis) is rare, but can be a coexisting feature (Woolf et al 2007).

2. Genetic predisposition:
   - Higher proportion of identical twins with developmental dysplasia of the hip (DDH) compared to non-identical twins.

3. Family history of dislocation of the hip.

4. Ligament hyper-laxity associated with clicky or clicking hips:
   - On initial examination there may be a tendon/ligament click.
   - A further examination repeated immediately afterwards often results in no click being felt.
   - Hyper-laxity can lead to full abduction in the presence of a dislocated hip (Skaggs & Flynn 2006).

5. Geographical variations/cultural factors:
   - Incidence is 0.25 per 1000 live births.
   - Incidence is 10:1000 where swaddling the legs together, usually for warmth.

6. Any concern by the midwife on examining the hips.

The modified Ortolani and Barlow manoeuvres

Referred to as the combined stress tests (called provocative tests of hip stability by Skaggs and Flynn (2006)), they are performed to make general observations which may put the baby into a high-risk group, to diagnose the subluxatable (dislocatable) or dislocated hip and make it possible to notice the presence or absence of clicks. The range of abduction in flexion is also a useful sign to indicate the degree (if any) of abnormality. There is no set way to examine the hips. Personal technique will develop over time. There are no 'must do's'; however, common sense suggests that giving full attention to one moving joint at a time is preferable and, as Skaggs and Flynn (2006) comment, clicks can also be produced by the knee, so careful assessment is vital. They also recommend that the manoeuvres can be performed multiple times on a single assessment, because they are considered difficult to interpret and examiners need to be confident in their findings. Concerns regarding avascular necrosis of the femoral head are overstated because as a condition of clinical importance, it is relatively rare (Skaggs & Flynn 2006).

Ortolani's manoeuvre

This is the manoeuvre where the midwife reverses the movement of abduction with the baby lying with knees flexed and if there is DDH, a 'click' or popping sensation is felt. When examining the left hip, the midwife should use her right hand to perform the manoeuvre whilst steadying the pelvis between the thumb, placed on the baby's symphysis pubis, and fingers of her left hand, place under the sacrum. With the baby's left leg flexed in the palm of the right hand, the head of the femur is held between the midwife's right thumb, on the inner side of the thigh opposite the lesser trochanter, and the middle longest finger, over the greater trochanter. In an attempt to relocate a posteriorly displaced head of the femur forwards into the acetabulum, the middle finger applies gentle pressure upon the greater trochanter. The baby's thighs are flexed *forward* (to the head of the baby) onto the abdomen and rotated and *abducted* through an angle of 70–90° towards the examining surface. If the hip is dislocated, a clunk will be felt as the head of the femur slips *into* the acetabulum. Skaggs and Flynn (2006) comment that usually a positive finding can be appreciated by others in the room. A high-pitched click is probably a product of soft-tissue structures moving over bony prominences. This manoeuvre is then repeated for the right hip. Remember **ORTOLANI** – **O**ut to **I**n (Baston & Durward 2001).

Barlow's manoeuvre

The Barlow's manoeuvre is a modification of the Ortolani manoeuvre and can also be used to detect DDH. The manoeuvre is described for examination of the left hip using the midwife's right hand. From a position of abduction, the hip is *adducted* to 70° and gentle pressure is exerted by the midwife's right thumb on the lesser trochanter in a *backward* and lateral direction. If the thumb is felt to move backwards over the labrum (the fibro-cartilaginous rim of the acetabulum) onto the posterior aspect of the joint capsule, a clunk may be heard as the head of femur dislocates *out* of the acetabulum. Skaggs and Flynn (2006) describe the noise as not a high-pitched tissue click, but a deeper clunk with significant motion rather like going over a speed bump. The dislocatable hip can feel strangely soft with little or no resistance. The Ortolani manoeuvre will then be performed to return the head of femur to the acetabulum. To examine the right hip the role of the midwife's hands is reversed. In the case of bilaterally dislocated hips, abduction is symmetrical though decreased. One would be suspicious of DDH, if the hips do not abduct more than 60–70°. The baby must be naked and on a flat surface. Subtle asymmetry may be missed if the midwife attempts to perform the examination on the mother's knee in an attempt to comfort an irritable baby. It is better to abandon the examination for another day than to compromise the test conditions.

The Barlow and Ortolani tests involve gentle manoeuvres. The gentler the examination, the more information is secured. Indeed, very little pressure is needed to dislocate the head of femur because the acetabulum is so shallow. A heavy-handed approach will often make the baby stiffen and resist; crying and agitation may follow. In this circumstance the midwife needs to abandon the examination, talk to the baby (and parents) to aid relaxation and restore calm before attempting a further examination with a much lighter touch. A useful analogy is a rigid gear stick in a car. Gentle manipulation of the baby's legs in a circular rotation helps to reduce muscle and nerve tension. Likewise, the lightest of touch can help that gear stick. Tension in the driver, can result in a crunched gear – ouch! Learners often associate this examination with the added comment *'I'm not good with bones'* or *'I am frightened of hurting the baby'*.

Documentation of findings in the personal child health record should offer details and be explained to the parents. Dove et al (2004) assert that it is not enough to place a tick against the word hips. An entry that communicates normality must reflect that both hips abduct fully in flexion and there is no apparent shortening on knee height inspection. It should be clear that both hips are stable and the combined stress test Ortolani and Barlow manoeuvres are negative for both hips. The parents should be told that *on this examination/occasion*, their baby's hips are normal.

Conclusion

There are key issues that emerge from examining newborn hearts, eyes and hips. It is essential to take a thorough family, present pregnancy and perinatal history by reading the case notes and checking out information with parents, where applicable. Inspection is a vital skill and cannot be overemphasised. Assessing the baby's holistic behaviour can provide valuable information and should not be hurried. Palpation, auscultation and the performance of specific manoeuvres call for specialised knowledge and skills that initially need to be overlearned and then continually practised. Feedback to parents when no abnormalities have been found, should express that *'today's examination is one in a process of many and on this occasion, everything appears normal'*. The midwife will inevitably build an extensive knowledge of the normal which in time will enable her to instinctively know when the abnormal is present. Asking for a second opinion is both recommended and part of maintaining ongoing competency. Detailed accurate record keeping and follow-up on referrals will help to reinforce sound practice (NMC 2004).

Key practice points

- Read the history before approaching the baby and its family.
- Listen to the mother; she is the expert on her baby.
- Concentrate on inspection, before palpation. Most information can be ascertained *before* auscultation is attempted.
- If a heart murmur is discovered: draw it.
- Central cyanosis, poor perfusion, an abnormal precordium and hepatospenomegaly are significant findings that need urgent attention.
- Always perform the Ortolani–Barlow combined stress tests when examining hips for DDH.
- Eye infections should not be underestimated: some can seriously damage an eye in hours.
- Record keeping should offer enough detail to provide a sound starting point for the following examination within the screening process.
- When reporting normality, the midwife should inform the parents that *'on this occasion everything appears normal'*.
- Seeking a second opinion from the multi-professional team is good practice and an invaluable aid to ongoing learning.
- Maintaining skills for an expanded role calls for strength of character as the midwife's peer support may be in the next ward or county.
- Midwives must recognise knowledge/practice limitations and always work within their professional responsibilities/boundaries to protect themselves and the families they provide care to.

References

Baston, H., Durward, H., 2001. Examination of the newborn. A practical guide. Routledge, London.

Dove, R., Bennett, J., Hunter, J., Twining, P., 2004. Nottingham guidelines for screening for developmental dysplasia of the hip. Nottingham University Hospital NHS Trust, Nottingham.

El Habbal, M.H., 2007. Cardiology. In: Strobel, S., Marks, S.D., Smith, P.K., El Habba, M.H., Spitz, L. (Eds.), The Great Ormond Street colour book of paediatrics and child health. Manson Publishing, London, 110–130.

Gill, D., O'Brien, N., 2007. Paediatric clinical examination made easy. Churchill Livingstone, London.

Horrox, F., 2002. Manual of neonatal and paediatric heart disease. Whurr Publishers, London.

Jones, A.J., 1998. Hip screening in the newborn. A practical guide. Butterworth Heinmann, Oxford.

Lissauer, T., Fanaroff, A.A., 2006. Neonatology at a glance. Blackwell Publishing, London.

Nischal, K.K., 2007. Ophthalmology. In: Strobel, S., Marks, S.D., Smith, P.K., El Habbal, M.H., Spitz, L. (Eds.), The Great Ormond Street colour book of paediatrics and child health. Manson Publishing, London, 161–204.

Nursing and Midwifery Council, 2004. Midwives rules and standards. NMC, London.

O'Callaghan, C., Stephenson, T., 2004.
Pocket paediatrics. Churchill
Livingstone, London.

Pang, D., Newson, T., 2005. Paediatrics.
Mosby, London.

Park, M.K., 2003. The pediatric
cardiology handbook. third ed.
Mosby, Philadelphia.

Sellwood, M., Huertas-Ceballos, A.,
2008. Review of NICE guidelines on
routine postnatal infant care. Arch.
Dis. Child Fetal Neonatal Ed. 93,
10–13.

Skaggs, D.L., Flynn, J.M., 2006.
The paediatric orthopaedic

physical exam. In: Skaggs, D.L.,
Flynn, J.M. (Eds.), Staying out of
trouble in paediatric orthopaedics.
Lippincott Williams and Wilkins,
London, 296–307.

Steele, D., 2007. Examining the
newborn: why don't midwives use
their skills? Br. J. Midwifery 15 (12),
748–752.

Talley, N.J., O'Connor, S., 2006.
Clinical examination. A systematic
guide to physical examination.
Churchill Livingstone, London.

Wilkinson, J., 2006. Assessment of
the infant and child with suspected

heart disease. In: Roberton, D.M.,
South, M. (Eds.), Practical
paediatrics. Churchill Livingstone,
London, 517–525.

Woolf, V.J., Fixsen, J.A., Hill, R.A.,
Jones, D.H.A., 2007. Orthopaedics
and fractures. In: Strobel, S., Marks,
S.D., Smith, P.K., El Habba, M.H.,
Spitz, L. (Eds.), The Great Ormond
Street colour book of paediatrics and
child health. Manson Publishing,
London, 565–599.

Further reading

Park, M.K., 2008. Pediatric cardiology
for practitioners. Mosby,
Philadelphia.
*This text offers more detailed information
on congenital heart disease and
physical examination than the 2003
pocketbook referred to in the text. It is
suitable for those who wish to deepen
their knowledge in cardiac
assessment.*

National Health Service Quality
Improvement Scotland, 2008.
Routine examination of the newborn.
Available online: www.
nhshealthquality.org
*A useful document that provides best
practice statements underpinned by
key principles to guide health-care
professionals who undertake routine
examination of the newborn within
their scope of practice.*

UK National Screening Committee,
2008. Newborn and infant physical
examination: standards and
competencies. Available online:
www.screening.nhs.uk
*Provides national guidance on the
standards and competencies to
achieve best practice utilising a
consistent approach.*

Chapter Thirteen

13

Infant massage

Robina Aslam

CONTENTS

Introduction 147
The geography and history of infant
massage 148
Scientific claims and evidence 149
Demonstrable benefits of infant massage . 149
   Better sleep patterns 149
   Weight gain, especially noticed
   in preterm infants 149
   Improved general development
   of the infant 149
   Lower stress levels and greater well
   being hormones 149
   Improved relationship 149
Type of massage 150
Areas for further testing of claimed
benefits 150
Comment on the Cochrane reviews 151
Professional issues 151
   Respect 151
   Inappropriate situations for massage . . 152
Practical infant massage 154
   Massage oils 154
   Types of massage 154
   The strokes 154
Establishing classes for parents
and carers 157
   Accreditation and insurance 157
   Health and safety 157
   Data protection issues 157
   Abuse 158
Conclusion 158
Key practice points 158
References 158
Further reading 159
Professional bodies 159

Before reading this chapter, you should be familiar with:
* The digestive system, nervous system circulatory, respiratory and immune systems of the neonate.
* Professional Rules and Standard 23 relating to the administration of complementary and alternate therapies (NMC 2004, 2008).
* Issues of consent regarding minors.
* The use of midwifery supervision to develop competency in new skills.
* Legislation regarding child protection issues and awareness of local supportive agencies/ networks.

Introduction

Midwifery practice includes the promotion of the welfare of both mother and baby and the improved interaction between parent and baby. This chapter will examine one technique for improving the welfare of infant and the attachment of parent to infant, namely infant massage.

Infant massage is a 'complementary therapy'. It does not presume to offer an alternative to traditional therapy, but is supportive of it. The House of Lords Science and Technology Committee's Sixth Report (House of Lords 2000) suggested that knowledge of such therapies should become a competency in undergraduate courses, and that, where practitioners sought to undergo specialist training in such therapies, this should be recognised at the post-registration stage.

This chapter will not provide the midwife with the specialist practical skills to teach or perform infant massage. This can most readily be achieved by completing a course from a recognised institution such as the International Association of Infant Massage (IAIM). The purpose of this chapter is to enable the midwife to appreciate what is offered by infant massage.

Infant massage has attracted many adherents. However, unsupported claims are often made for the benefits of infant massage and a sense of proportion is required. Many respectable research articles suggest that infant massage gives rise to objectively measurable clinical benefits. As will be discussed below, the Cochrane systematic reviews in this area (Underdown 2006, Vickers et al 2004) recognise that benefits do flow from massage; they are, however, somewhat reserved in some areas.

Young babies obviously have limited verbal powers; non-verbal communication, particularly the use of touch, is all important. Skin sensitivity is one of the first senses to develop. Touch can convey emotion and the type of touch can convey very specific emotions, including love, empathy and security (Walker 1998). The primacy of touch for a baby to understand its world and its relations with people means that it is essential for it to learn and hence for organic and psychological development. The possible effect of touch deprivation can be seen in a number of settings, e.g. Romanian orphanages from the days of Ceausescu (Field 2001, Sinclair 1992). For all these reasons it is essential that a baby is stimulated to interact with his or her world and, hence, infant massage enables this need to be met in an enjoyable way both for parent and for baby.

Infant massage seeks to promote four primary groups of benefits, see Box 13.1.

The geography and history of infant massage

Infant massage is an ancient technique practised by many cultures. In countries such as India, where it traces its roots to Ayurvedic medicine, it dates back as far as 1800 BC (Field et al 1996a). It is still

---

Box 13.1

Primary benefits which infant massage seeks to promote

- Positive interaction between infant and parent/carer.
- Positive relationship between parent/carer and infant.
- Acts as a stimulant for the baby's respiratory, digestive and circulatory systems.
- Offers manual assistance in the treatment of colic, wind, constipation and mucous.

---

commonly practised amongst all classes and backgrounds. The author, born in the sub-continent, experienced this technique personally, watching, observing and participating as a young child. She also used it on her own children. She is pictured in the Dorling Kindersley book *Infant Massage* in 1999 (Heath & Bainbridge, 2004) with her daughter demonstrating the techniques widely used in India and Pakistan.

But infant massage is not specific to one location. For instance, the use of massage for babies was described in China during the 2nd century AD and soon after in Egypt. Today, the Ibo tribe in Nigeria and the Kwakiatis of North America – on the other side of the Atlantic Ocean – massage their babies from birth to stimulate survival mechanisms and help them resist disease. It seems that the practice developed independently in many cultures, places and times, suggesting that it can realistically be described as 'natural'.

Unfortunately, in some Western cultures, including the United Kingdom (UK), touch is often avoided. However, the role of Indian techniques is becoming particularly well-known and has acted as a stimulus to the development (or more probably re-introduction) of the practice in contemporary Western cultures. The founder of the International Association of Infant Massage, for instance, is quite candid in stating that she developed her interest in infant massage whilst watching mothers in India – and contrasted it with touch-aversion societies such as the United States of America (USA) where she lives. She was impressed by the importance placed by Indian mothers on touch and physical contact in developing and maintaining a respectful intimacy between carer and child, and providing reassurance when resources, such as those taken for granted in the West, were scarce (McClure 2001).

Scientific claims and evidence

It is important for midwives to treat all claims for the alleged benefits of infant massage critically. A number of prestigious universities around the world have established work in the area of touch therapy. Amongst the most significant in infant massage are through the Touch Institute at the University of Miami School of Medicine, Imperial College London School of Medicine and the University of Warwick. However, the level of research into this area remains limited.

Demonstrable benefits of infant massage

Areas of benefit evidenced in the published literature are set out in Box 13.2. The sections below investigate the evidence.

Better sleep patterns

Infants who received massage therapy versus those who were rocked to sleep were reported to experience more organised sleep/wake behaviours and soothability (Field et al 1996a). It was found that preterm infants who were massaged before sleep, fell asleep more quickly and slept more soundly with better sleep patterns.

Weight gain, especially noticed in preterm infants

It has been reported in a number of studies that preterm infants gained more weight following massage. In one article (Field et al 1986) it was reported that

---

preterm infants gained 47% more weight and were discharged 6 days earlier. In other studies it has been found that the effect is significant over a short period. Dieter et al (2003) found that preterm infants gained more weight following as few as 5 days of massage therapy; in another earlier study Scafidi et al (1993) found that when preterm infants received three daily 15-minute massages for 10 days, the massage-therapy infants gained significantly more weight per day than did the control infants.

The mechanisms by which these benefits arise are still the subject of debate. One hypothesis for increased weight is that massage promotes increase in vagal activity (related to the vagus nerve, which innervates the intestine) and, in turn, an increase in gastric motility (Diego et al 2005), but this remains speculative.

Improved general development of the infant

Massage is reported in a number of publications to improve alertness and interaction behaviour (Field et al 1996b). It was found in one research programme that preterm infants exhibited improved development following massage therapy, including improved cognitive and motor development 8 months later (Field et al 1987).

Lower stress levels and greater well being hormones

Infants who received massage therapy versus those who were rocked/comforted were reported to have lower cortisol (a stress-related hormone) and increased serotonin (well being) levels (Field et al 1996a).

Improved relationship

In relation to babies of depressed mothers, the results provided improvements in mother–baby relationship. In one study, mothers with depression attending mother–infant massage classes were compared with a similar group who attended a support group. At the end of the test period the massage group had significantly less depression and very significantly better interactions with their babies, than the control group. This is the first time that a method has been found for improving the relationship between

---

Box 13.2

Some areas of benefit evidenced in the literature

- Better sleep patterns.
- Weight gain, especially noticed in preterm babies.
- Improved general development of the infant.
- Lower stress levels and greater well being hormones.
- Improved relationships between parent/carer and infant.

a depressed mother and her baby (Onozawa et al 2001). The relationships of fathers were also improved as a result of infant massage (Cullen et al 2000, Scholtz & Samuels 1992).

Type of massage

It is unrealistic to assume that all massage therapies deliver identical results or, indeed, that all are equally relevant across the range of situations that may exist. In one study the researchers compared the effect of tickling and poking versus the effect of stroking on babies between 2 and 4 months in age (Pelaez-Noguera et al 1997). They concluded that rhythmic stroking more effectively reinforced continuous eye contact. However, there was no measure of pressure or a rigorous separation of poking and tickling which seem to be different types of stimulus. Intensities of touch were explored in a later study by Perez and Gewirtz (2004) where the researchers monitored the effect of various stimuli on leg-kicking, which was assumed to express a positive outcome. Each kick was recorded automatically. It was found that intense stroking produced the most significant response.

A particular problem arises in the case of fragile infants, such as early preterm neonates. Thus, whilst it is reported that this is one key area where tangible clinical benefits are significant, there is some concern that massage as it is ordinarily understood may be inappropriate where the baby is fragile. One possibility here is what is sometimes called 'gentle human touch' (GHT) therapy. In a number of studies (e.g. Harrison 2004, Jay 1982, Tribotti 1990) it has been reported that benefits arise from still, gentle touch, typically for periods of 10–20 minutes, including increased respiratory regularity, decreased levels of active sleep and behavioural distress.

Areas for further testing of claimed benefits

The research appears to indicate that infant massage provides demonstrable clinical benefits as well as being an enjoyable way to improve attachment with babies. Its impact on areas such as weight gain in infants also suggests that it may be a cost-effective approach. However, as always, a sense of proportion is required.

The Cochrane Database gives two reviews which need to be considered when weighing up the evidence. In 'Massage intervention for promoting mental and physical health in infants aged under six months', Underdown et al (2006) offers an assessment of 23 published reports. The review accepts that there are benefits, particular in some social settings, but considers that further research is required before universal provision is recommended – a fuller exposition is found in Box 13.3, taken from the summary of the review. In 2004, Vickers et al updated their earlier systematic review 'Massage for promoting growth and development of preterm and/or low birth-weight infants' (see Box 13.4), which dealt

---

Box 13.3

Cochrane systematic review by Underdown et al (2006)

Main results

Twenty-three studies were included in the review. One was a follow-up study and thirteen were included in a separate analysis due to concerns about the uniformly significant results and the lack of dropout. The results of nine studies providing primary data suggest that infant massage has no effect on growth, but provides some evidence suggestive of improved mother–infant interaction, sleep and relaxation, reduced crying and a beneficial impact on a number of hormones controlling stress. Results showing a significant impact on number of illnesses and clinic visits were limited to a study of Korean orphanage infants. There was no evidence of effects on cognitive and behavioural outcomes, infant attachment or temperament. The data from the 13 studies regarded to be at high risk of bias show uniformly significant benefits on growth, sleep, crying and bilirubin levels.

Authors' conclusions

The only evidence of a significant impact of massage on growth was obtained from a group of studies regarded to be at high risk of bias. There was, however, some evidence of benefits with regard to mother–infant interaction, sleeping and crying, and hormones influencing stress levels. In the absence of evidence of harm, these findings may be sufficient to support the use of infant massage in the community, particularly in contexts where infant stimulation is poor. Further research is needed, however, before it will be possible to recommend universal provision.

Box 13.4

Cochrane systematic review by Vickers et al (2004)

Main results

Massage interventions improved daily weight gain by 5.1 g (95% CI [Confidence Interval] 3.5, 6.7 g). There is no evidence that gentle, still touch is of benefit (increase in daily weight gain 0.2 g; 95% CI–1.2, 1.6 g). Massage interventions also appeared to reduce length of stay by 4.5 days (95% CI 2.4, 6.5) though there are methodological concerns about the blinding of this outcome. There was also some evidence that massage interventions have a slight, positive effect on postnatal complications and weight at 4–6 months. However, serious concerns about the methodological quality of the included studies, particularly with respect to selective reporting of outcomes, weaken credibility in these findings.

Authors' conclusions

Evidence that massage of preterm infants is of benefit for developmental outcomes is weak and does not warrant wider use of preterm infant massage. Where massage is currently provided by nurses, consideration should be given as to whether this is a cost-effective use of time. Future research should assess the effects of massage interventions on clinical outcome measures, such as medical complications or length of stay, and on process-of-care outcomes, such as care-giver or parental satisfaction.

more specifically with preterm infants and acknowledged the potential benefits. However, the reviewers raised the question whether it was cost-effective for health service staff to carry out massage. This underscores the fact that the review examined primarily the objective medium-term medical benefit rather than seeing infant massage as a multi-faceted exercise, the benefits of which include positive interactions between carer and baby, and generating a sense of well being and togetherness.

Comment on the Cochrane reviews

The Cochrane reviews considered above acknowledge that benefits do arise. For example, in Underdown et al's (2006) review, it is acknowledged that there was some evidence of benefits on mother–infant

interaction, sleeping and crying patterns, and on hormones influencing stress levels. Where they are critical is in the methodological approaches of a number of writers which do not thus permit the results to be accepted uncritically. For example, Vickers et al (2004) states that massage interventions appeared to also reduce length of stay by 4.5 days (95% CI 2.4, 6.5), though there are methodological concerns about the blinding (i.e. the process whereby the subject is unaware of the treatment offered) of this outcome.

On the University of Warwick website (University of Warwick 2006), the emphasis is very much on the positive aspect of infant massage. This is set out in Box 13.5. In conclusion what appears to be uncontroversial is that infant massage provides demonstrable benefits in terms of sleeping and crying, the impact on hormone levels, as well as improved dynamics in the parent–infant relationship. Infant massage appears to have no negative side-effects. It may, in fact, produce significant benefits, e.g. in terms of duration of stay in hospital for preterm babies, but further research is required to validate this assertion.

Professional issues

Respect

Although modern Western society has arguably become too touch averse, it is important also to recognise that there are proper boundaries. A baby is unable to resist behaviour practised on it by an adult. It is essential, therefore, that any touching is done with respect. One way of making sure that this remains in the carer's mind at all stages is to ensure that two facets of the process are acknowledged.

Many organisations, such as the IAIM, emphasise that the child's permission should be sought formally before commencement. Whilst this may seem at first sight an empty formality, it serves an important function. It ensures that the adult actively considers that he or she must act with respect. With slightly older infants it also emphasises the distinction between positive and negative touch, and may help a child in later life to recognise and perhaps fend off negative or unwanted touch.

The second facet is that the parent/carer, during massage, should be alive to signals seeking to disengage; and that if the baby continues to exhibit signs of distress for any period of time, the adult should end the session.

Box 13.5

Adapted summary of the University of Warwick's review of the systematic review undertaken by Underdown et al (2006)

Research says massage may help infants sleep more, cry less and be less stressed

New research by a team at the University of Warwick states that massage may help infants aged under 6 months sleep better, cry less and be less stressed.

The team of researchers from Warwick Medical School and the Institute of Education at the University of Warwick was led by Angela Underdown. They examined nine studies of massage of young children covering a total of 598 infants aged under 6 months. They found the various studies showed a range of significant results including indications that infants who were massaged cried less, slept better, and had lower levels of stress hormones such as cortisol compared to infants who did not receive massage. One of the studies examined also claimed that massage could affect the release of the hormone melatonin, which Underdown et al (2006) also stated was important in aiding infants' sleeping patterns. She added that it was not surprising to find some evidence of an effect on sleep and crying.

One study also provided evidence that massage could help build better relationships between infants and mothers who had postnatal depression, although the reviewers said more research is needed to confirm this effect.

Another study indicated that massage, eye contact and talking had a significant effect on growth and a significant reduction in illnesses and clinic visits for infants receiving little tactile stimulation in an orphanage, but this was an unusual set of circumstances and the other studies, where infants were receiving normal levels of tactile stimulation, found no effect on growth.

The studies mainly involved infant massage by parents who were trained by health professionals in appropriate technique. Parents who wish to massage their babies can learn how to do this at locally run classes.

The review entitled 'Massage intervention for promoting mental and physical health in infants under six months (review)' appears in The Cochrane Library, a publication of The Cochrane Collaboration, an international organisation that evaluates medical research.

Inappropriate situations for massage

One valuable feature of infant massage is that it has no apparent adverse side-effects in the normal case. However, there are settings where massage may be harmful, for example in the case of injury and illness, or contraindicated. These can be considered to fall into the following categories as shown in Box 13.6.

Legal inappropriateness

Where the adult performing the massage is the child's own parent or legal guardian no issue as to consent arises. Where any other person carries out massage, full informed consent from the parent/guardian and adequate supervision is required.

Fragile infants

There is some concern that massage, as it is ordinarily understood, may be inappropriate where the baby is fragile; here 'gentle human touch' (GHT) therapy may be appropriate.

Situations where the infant is not receptive to massage

It is important that the baby is receptive to massage. Otherwise, massage will be inappropriate and may lead to distress and to negative feelings. Careful attention should, therefore, be paid to a child's response before, during and after massage. The parent/carer should note the infant's response and be prepared to alter touch accordingly or discontinue altogether, depending on the behavioural cues exhibited.

Box 13.6

Contraindications to infant massage

- Legal inappropriateness.
- Fragile infants.
- Situations where the infant is not receptive to massage.
- Situations where illness or injury makes massage inappropriate.
- Recent immunisation.

According to McClure (2001) it is not possible to establish definitively a universal language of cues: 'Not all babies mean the same thing when they hiccough, hold up a hand or look away' (McClure 2001, p. 134). On that basis developing cues for engagement and disengagement will be more of an art than a science, although clearly crying and smiling are basic indicators. Typically used cues are set out in Table 13.1.

Whenever it is evident that the infant perceives the stimulation to be unpleasant, parents/carers should react by modifying the massage experience – either by responding to immediate physiological needs or by changing location, pressure and direction of massage strokes. It may be necessary to discontinue entirely if negative cues persist for longer that 1 minute. Gentle stroking may help return infant to a calmer state, but again should be stopped if there is no obvious change in behaviour.

Note that one common mistake is to assume that drowsiness represents a relaxed state; therefore, the baby is enjoying the massage. Falling asleep is a change in state and indicates that the infant is seeking to withdraw from the interaction. Massage should not be performed when the infant is sleeping, although in certain circumstances it may be appropriate to start when the infant is in a drowsy state and, therefore, move to a quiet alert state.

Situations where illness or injury makes massage inappropriate

Massage should obviously be avoided where there is an acute condition that requires immediate medical attention, such as open wounds, burns, systemic contagious or infectious conditions, acute or unstable circulatory, respiratory, renal conditions, recent surgery or certain orthopaedic conditions such as congenital dislocation of the hips or osteogenesis imperfecta.

In the case of local infections, such as impetigo, massage has the potential to spread infection and should be avoided. Even in cases where the child appears simply to be 'feeling under the weather' it may be inappropriate to massage. Children may have a lower tolerance of touch when unwell and massage may lead to discomfort.

In some cases, the massager will have to use their judgment. Where there is acute colic, eczema or

Table 13.1 Some engagement and disengagement cues (University of Nottingham 2005)

Engagement cues – showing that the baby is ready to interact	Disengagement cues – indicating that the baby is trying to reduce environmental stress
Eyes widening	Autonomic signs: Hiccoughing. Yawning. Startled response.
Hands open with relaxed fingers	Motor signs: Frantic activity of limbs. Grimacing. Frowning. Eyes closing. Turning away. Rigid posture.
Giggling and smiling	State changes: Moving from quiet to fussy to crying. indicates wishing to disengage.
Sustained eye contact	
Reaching towards the parent/carer	
Quieting/restful legs	

psoriasis, massage may produce benefits. However, this will have to be judged at the time. It is clearly inappropriate to impose massage with a view to long-term benefit at the cost of short-term distress.

Recent immunisation

Massage therapy may stimulate the circulation and lymphatic drainage; therefore, some therapists recommend that massage should be avoided on the day and about 4 days following immunisation as it may intensify the reaction.

Practical infant massage

Massage oils

The use of oil can enhance the massage experience. As a lubricant, the oil reduces the friction between hand and skin and gives a smoother flow with less traction and, hence, it is more comfortable. Oils can also be of benefit in moisturising the skin.

Scented oils

Scented oils are discouraged as they have unknown additives and also mask the natural smells of the parent/carer.

Toxicity

To avoid any problem with toxicity, edible vegetable oils are preferable for use in infant massage.

Allergies

Sensitive newborns may experience allergy to particular oils. Allergens in oils are protein-bound and, therefore, usually too large a molecule to enter the bloodstream via the skin; however, there is concern that in new babies in particular there may be some transmission and there is a risk in the case of broken skin. Nut allergies are on the increase with peanut allergy being potentially fatal. Parents/carers should be advised to watch out for allergic reactions and counselled to avoid ingestion if there is any indication of allergy. If there is an indication, avoid the relevant oil and use refined oil that was made using heat and, hence, the allergenic properties are reduced. It may also be sensible to advise using a

patch test in advance to check whether there is any adverse reaction.

Typical oils used for infant massage are:
* Coconut oil.
* Grapeseed oil.
* Olive oil.
* Sunflower oil.
* Wheatgerm oil.

A useful review with more detailed information on oils is available on the IAIM website (Bond 2007). This includes references to articles of interest. As Bond (2007) points out:
* There is concern that manufacturers do not always reveal all relevant facts about the oils they supply and it is often difficult to secure a supply which can be considered totally safe.
* The literature on allergies is constantly shifting and the latest research findings should be consulted.

Types of massage

There are a number of techniques for infant massage, including Swedish, Indian and Chinese. The overall principles for all of the above remains that touch/massage is not harmful, but assists circulation, elimination, drainage, well being, bonding, muscle tone and common ailments, such as colic, constipation, wind and muscle fatigue. The strokes commonly used in northern Europe are based on a combination of both Swedish and Indian massage.

The strokes

The intention of this section is to introduce some of the strokes that may be used for infant massage. A number of approaches can be used and the strokes are referred to by a variety of names. In this section, the approach developed at the University of Nottingham is generally followed (University of Nottingham 2005). Before starting the massage, permission is sought from the baby by gently using the whole hands from head down both sides of the body.

Legs

Start the massage, one leg at a time. Legs are receptive to touch and are handled easily and confidently. Use long, firm, milking strokes down the legs to ankles. Let the hands overlap. Take care over joints,

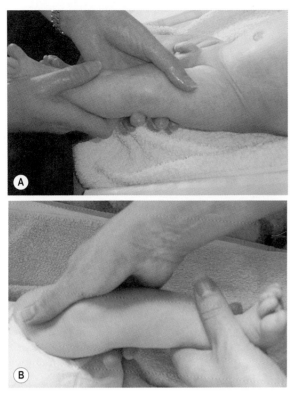

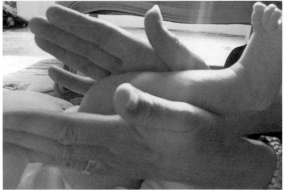

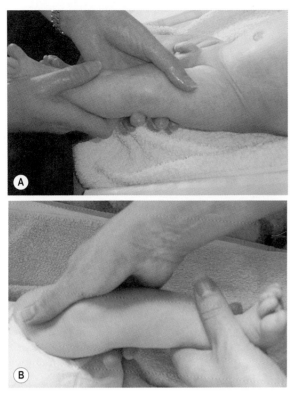

Figure 13.1 • A and B Leg massage milking strokes.

especially the knee. Be firm but do not pull hard (Figure 13.1A and B).

Feet

Support the ankle in your hands. Use your thumbs to make small circles up the sole of the foot to the toes. Apply pressure under toes with the forefinger and then slide finger down foot so it rests on the ball of the heel (Figure 13.2).

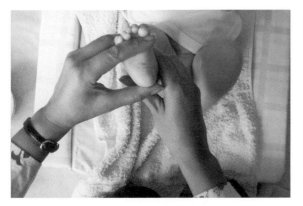

Figure 13.2 • Infant foot massage.

Solar plexus reflexology

A reflexology point on the sole of the foot is said to release tension in the diaphragm/solar plexus. Apply pressure with your thumb for a few seconds (Figure 13.3).

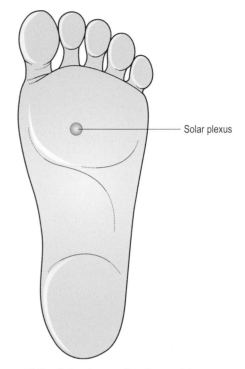

Solar plexus

Figure 13.3 • Solar plexus reflexology point.

Rolling leg

Using both hands roll the leg between the palms working from the top of the leg down (Figure 13.4). Do not twist.

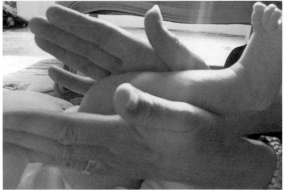

Figure 13.4 • Rolling leg massage.

Abdomen

This is a sensitive area and some babies may not enjoy this on their first attempt. Avoid massage after feeds. There are a number of different strokes for the abdomen. Used singularly or together they can assist with colic, constipation, and wind. They work on the large intestine, ascending, transverse and descending colon. The following technique combines three strokes (Figure 13.5):

1. Follow descending colon move hand down to form letter I.

2. Place hand on infant's right side, bring hand across right to left and then downwards follow transverse and descending colon.

3. Place hand on infant's right hip move hand up and across and then down the abdomen. Follow ascending, transverse and descending colon.

Windy paddle

Hand over hand stroke like paddles. One hand should always stay in contact with the abdomen (Figure 13.6). This movement aids peristalsis, moves trapped gases and aids relaxation of abdominal area.

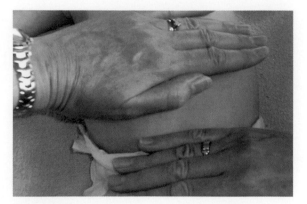

Figure 13.6 • 'Windy paddle' abdominal massage.

Knee lift

Lift legs together supporting heels with your hands. Bend knees towards chest to bring thighs together onto stomach (Figure 13.7). Hold for a few seconds; can be repeated 3–4 times.

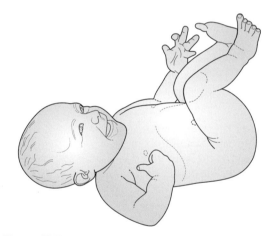

Figure 13.7 • Knee lift.

Sinus stroke

There is no need to apply oil to the face as the skin produces its own natural oils. Apply the flats of your thumbs on either side of the top of the nose. Apply gentle pressure and stroke down the sides of the nose and around the cheekbone towards the ears. Repeat this 3–4 times (Figures 13.8 and 13.9).

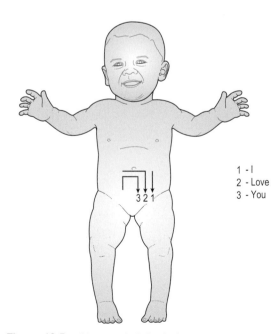

1 - I
2 - Love
3 - You

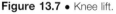

Figure 13.5 • 'I love you' abdominal massage.

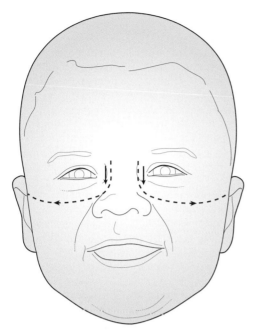

Figure 13.8 • Sinus stroke.

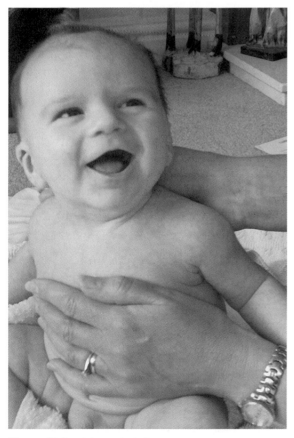

Figure 13.9 • A happy baby!

Establishing classes for parents and carers

Prior to establishing classes for parents and carers there are a series of matters to be borne in mind, whether one is acting as a professional midwife within a hospital setting or offering classes to the public. These include the factors set out in Box 13.7.

Accreditation and insurance

Any professional teaching massage should have completed and passed a recognised course, such as one offered by the IAIM, and have full insurance. Professionals working in the National Health Service (NHS) should ensure that their employment covers indemnity insurance and that they are members of a professional body.

Health and safety

There are two factors with regard to infant massage. First, wherever classes are held, all appropriate health and safety requirements must be in place; for example, evacuation procedures must be in place. Second, the course content must emphasise safe massage. Presenters should ensure that health and safety issues are clearly spelled out to carers; for example, the need to ensure that massage is not done at a height if there is any risk of a fall, allergy advice.

Data protection issues

Any database of client's details may have to be registered, e.g. in the UK in accordance with the Data Protection Act.

Box 13.7

Issues to be addressed when setting up classes

- Accreditation and insurance.
- Health and safety.
- Data protection issues.
- Abuse.

Abuse

Because babies will be in a state of undress during massage care must be taken to ensure privacy. From time to time the midwife may observe evidence on a child which suggests abuse and should, in those circumstances, advise the relevant authorities. It is not recommended that a midwife or other health professional perform the actual massage on an infant when demonstrating the skill or observing parents learning the skill. Life-like models, which are available, are effective teaching aids.

Conclusion

This chapter provides the midwife with an introduction to the concept of infant massage, its origins and the scientific evidence. The discussion of techniques and some of the practical issues are touched on briefly.

As infant massage is becoming ever more popular with the public, midwives need to understand it; not least so that they can discuss it with parents and carers who seek guidance on it. This chapter sets out the key factors that a midwife will need to know when discussing the option of infant massage.

Key practice points

- Competency in teaching infant massage to parents/carers should be gained through accredited courses (see professional bodies listed at the end of the chapter).
- Infant massage is a complementary therapy and does not seek to compete with or offer an alternative to traditional therapies.
- There is evidence that infant massage promotes better sleep patterns, weight gain, especially noticed in preterm babies, in addition to improved general development of the infant, lower stress hormone levels, increased well being and improved relationships.
- Midwives should be aware of situations where infant massage is inappropriate, such as lack of parental/guardian consent, fragile babies, lack of infant response, and any illness or injury, including any recent immunisation that the baby has received.
- Setting up infant-massage classes requires planning and preparation. Allergies/toxicities associated with massage oils must be considered, as must legal issues such as consent, insurance, data protection and protection of infants from abuse.
- Although infant massage is recognised as producing benefits to both parent/carer and infant, the health and well being of the infant must be considered paramount throughout.

References

Bond, C., 2007. Using oils for infant massage. Available online: http://www.iaim.org.uk/oils.html Accessed 1 March 2008.

Cullen, C., Field, T., Escalona, A., Hartshorn, K., 2000. Father–infant interactions are enhanced by massage therapy. Early Child Dev. Care 164, 41–47.

Diego, M.A., Field, T., Hernandez-Reif, M., 2005. Vagal activity, gastric motility, and weight gain in massaged preterm neonates. J. Pediatr. 147, 50–55.

Dieter, J.N., Field, T., Hernandez-Reif, M., Emery, E., Redzepi, M., 2003. Stable preterm infants gain more weight and sleep less after five days of massage therapy. J. Pediatr. Psychol. 28 (6), 403–411.

Field, T., 2001. Massage therapy facilitates weight gain in preterm infants. Curr. Dir. Psychol. Sci. 10, 51–54.

Field, T., Schanberg, S.M., Scafidi, F., Bauer, C.R., Vega-Lahr, N., Garcia, R., et al., 1986. Tactile/kinesthetic stimulation effects on preterm neonates. Pediatrics 77 (5), 654–658.

Field, T., Scafidi, F., Schanberg, S., 1987. Massage of preterm newborns to improve growth and development. Pediatr. Nurs. 13, 385–387.

Field, T., Grizzle, N., Scafidi, F., Abrams, S., Richardson, S., 1996a. Massage therapy for infants of depressed mothers. Infant Behav. Dev. 19, 109–114.

Field, T., Schanberg, S., Davalos, M., 1996b. Oils versus no oil massage.

Pre and Perinatal Psychology Journal 11, 73–78.

Harrison, L., 2004. Tactile Stimulation of Neonatal Intensive Care unit preterm infants. In: Field, T. (Ed.), Touch and Massage in Early Child Development. Johnson and Johnson Pediatric Institute, USA, pp. 139–162.

Heath, A.R., Bainbridge, N., 2004. Baby massage: the calming power of touch. second ed. Dorling Kindersley, London.

House of Lords, 2000. Report into Complementary and Alternative Medicine, November 2000. Available online: http://www.publications.parliament.uk/pa/ld199900/ldsel/ldsctech/123/12302.htm Accessed 1 March 2008.

Jay, S., 1982. The effects of gentle human touch on mechanically ventilated very-short-gestation infants. Matern. Child. Nurs. J. 11, 199–259.

McClure, V., 2001 Infant massage a handbook for loving parents. Third ed. Souvenir Press, London.

Nursing and Midwifery Council, 2004. Midwives rules and standards. NMC, London.

Nursing and Midwifery Council, 2008. Standards for medicines management. NMC, London.

Onozawa, K., Glover, V., Adams, D., Modi, N., Kumar, C., 2001. Infant massage improves mother-infant interaction for mothers with postnatal depression. J. Affect. Disord. 63, 201–207.

Pelaez-Noguera, M., Field, T., Gewirtz, J.L., 1997. The effects of systematic stroking versus tickling and poking on infant behaviour. Journal of Applied Developmental Psychology 18, 169–178.

Perez, H., Gewirtz, J.L., 2004. Maternal touch effects on infant behaviour.

In Field, T. (Ed.), Touch and massage in early child development. Johnson and Johnson Pediatric Institute, USA, pp. 39–48.

Scafidi, F., Field, T., Schanberg, S., 1993. Factors that predict which preterm infants benefit most from massage therapy. Dev. Behav. Pediatr. 14, 176–180.

Scholtz, K., Samuels, C., 1992. Neonatal bathing and massage intervention with fathers. International Journal of Behavioural Development 15, 67–81.

Sinclair, M., 1992. Massage for healthier children. Wingbow Press, Oakland California.

Tribotti, S.J., 1990. Effects of gentle touch on the premature infant. In Gunzenhauser, N. (Ed.), Advances in touch: new implications in human development. Johnson and Johnson Baby Sillman, New Jersey, pp. 80–89.

Underdown, A., Barlow, J., Chung, V., Stewart-Brown, S., 2006. Massage intervention for promoting mental and physical health in infants aged under six months. Cochrane

Database Syst. Rev.2006 Issue 4. Art. No.: CD005038. DOI: 10.1002/14651858.CD005038. pub2.

University of Nottingham, 2005. Introduction to Infant Massage Module DM2200/DMIIM. University of Nottingham, Nottingham (contact the author for further information).

University of Warwick, 2006. Online news and events. Available online: http://www2.warwick.ac.uk/newsandevents/pressreleases/ne1000000231138 Accessed 1 March 2008.

Vickers, A., Ohlsson, A., Lacy, J.B., Horsley, A., 2004. Massage for promoting growth and development of preterm and/or low birth-weight infants. Cochrane Database Syst. Rev. 2004 Issue 1. Art. No.: CD000390. DOI: 10.1002/14651858.CD000390. pub2.

Walker, P., 1998. Baby massage – a practical guide to massage for babies and infants. Judy Piarkis Publishers Ltd, London.

Further reading

Field, T. (Ed.), 2004. Touch and massage in early child development. Johnson and Johnson Pediatric Institute, USA.
This book is a useful resource for midwives wishing to gain a deeper understanding of the research surrounding infant massage.

Each chapter is written by a specialist from various countries.
McClure, V., 2001. Infant massage: a handbook for loving parents. Souvenir Press Ltd, London.
This book is written by the founder of the IAIM who was instrumental in

bringing touch therapy into the public domain. It aims to provide the reader with the knowledge and benefits of infant massage. The book provides some easy-to-follow instructions demonstrating each massage stroke.

Professional bodies

International Association of Infant Massage
This was founded in 1986 and is the main international body for Infant Massage. It offers training courses and accreditation, with the accredited person known as a Certified Infant Massage Instructor (CIMI). The UK Chapter (office) is based at 26 Chigwell Road, South Woodford, London, E18 1LS and the website can be accessed at http://www.iaim.org.uk

The Guild of Infant and Child Massage
This body provides accredited courses and information for carers and health professionals and is based at Fyfield, Greenhill Park Road, Evesham, Worcestershire WR11 4NL. http://www.gicm.org.uk

Chapter Fourteen

14

Postnatal physiological examination of the mother

Debra Bick

CONTENTS

Introduction 161
Framework for postnatal care 162
The context of care 163
Maternal morbidity 163
Physiological examination to detect
major maternal morbidity 164
   Uterine involution and abnormal
   blood loss 164
   Detection of infection 165
   Blood pressure 165
Physiological examination to identify
common maternal health problems 166
   Urinary incontinence 166
   Bowel problems 167
   Perineal care 167
   Headache 168
   Backache 168
   Fatigue 169
Other postnatal health needs 169
   Obesity 169
   Social and psychological needs 170
Key practice points 170
References 170
Further reading 172

- Impact of morbidity on women's lives and relationships.
- Recommendations of NICE postnatal care guideline (NICE 2006).
- Recommendations of CEMACH (Lewis 2007).
- Skills for health competencies for postnatal care.

Key skills to implement effective, timely and appropriate postnatal physiological examination.
- Communication and listening.
- Clinical judgement to know when physiological examination is required, to accurately perform, interpret and act on findings.
- Awareness of local referral pathways and protocols to manage maternal health problems.
- Planning and implementing individualised care based on findings of physiological examination.

Introduction

During the course of the last century, instigated by the first Midwives Act of 1902, postnatal physiological examination of a mother became the core focus of midwifery care following a birth. Not only was the content of the physiological examination prescribed, but also the postnatal 'period' was defined by the number of days during which a midwife should attend a woman.

Before reading this chapter, you should be familiar with:
- Maternal physical and psychological morbidity after birth.

Midwives have continued to be trained and educated to implement postnatal care which places great emphasis on monitoring and documenting maternal physiological changes following birth, including monitoring temperature, uterine involution and vaginal blood loss. Observation and examination may also include measuring a woman's blood pressure (BP) and checking for signs and symptoms of deep vein thrombosis. A century ago, this ritualistic approach to physiological examination was viewed as essential to reduce the then high maternal mortality rate. Physiological care was implemented during a prescriptive pattern of midwifery contacts which included visiting a woman twice a day for the first 3 days after birth, followed by daily visits until the tenth postnatal day. Current guidance for midwives is that the postnatal period should take place for 'not less than 10 days and for such longer period as the midwife considers necessary' (Nursing and Midwifery Council [NMC] 2004, p. 7). In reality, most midwifery visits will end between 10 and 14 days after birth (Beake & Bick 2007) and few midwives will continue to visit women for the remainder of the 6–8 week postnatal period, unless there is a specific indication for this. Other than dropping the need for visits twice a day for 3 days and introduction of 'selective visits' in 1986 (United Kingdom Central Council for Nursing, Midwifery and Health Visiting [UKCC] 1992), the content of physiological care has been subject to minimal revision. This is despite the dramatic decline in maternal mortality in the United Kingdom (UK), the progressive move of birth from the home to the hospital and the drive for evidence-based care.

In the first decade of the 21st century, the traditional components of the physiological examination and duration of midwifery contacts persist, with little consideration for the emotional health and well being of women (Beake et al 2005, Singh & Newburn 2000) or identification of widespread and persistent maternal physical morbidity such as backache, urinary and faecal incontinence, and fatigue now known to be experienced after giving birth (Bick et al 2002, MacArthur et al 2002). It is debatable that routine physiological examination meets the needs of women today and the priority accorded to postnatal services, given competing demands on finite resources, has declined to such an extent it is frequently referred to as the 'Cinderella' service (Neale 2007). Ironically, given the increased use of medical interventions during labour and birth, and growing concerns related to changing public health priorities including obesity, drug, alcohol and domestic abuse, women may be in poorer health and in more need of supportive, directed and prolonged postnatal midwifery care than at any time during recent decades. In this chapter, evidence of the effectiveness of the components of the physiological examination will be explored, as will the need to consider the importance of providing care and support tailored to individual need. It will also reflect concerns about the increasing complexity of women's lives and consequences for their immediate and longer-term postnatal health.

Framework for postnatal care

Although there is limited evidence of the benefit and effectiveness of the content and timing of the routine physiological examination, midwives do need to consider the aim of the observations and examinations they perform and the information they can offer about a woman's health and recovery. The increasing number of women who have a caesarean section will also impact on skills necessary to optimise postnatal outcomes, with implications for postoperative as well as postnatal care. Skills and approaches to care will also have to reflect changes in socio-demographic, economic and psychosocial aspects of women's lives. Midwives are likely to be caring for more women giving birth at an older age, who are obese and who are from diverse social and cultural backgrounds (King's Fund 2008).

The publication of the National Institute for Health and Clinical Excellence (NICE) guideline for routine postnatal care of women and their babies which was published in 2006 forms the framework for this chapter, as this is the standard of care all women and their babies should now receive. Whilst the guideline was written to inform National Health Service (NHS) care in England and Wales, the evidence and recommendations for practice can be adapted for other parts of the UK and internationally. This is the first time that evidence to inform the provision and content of postnatal care, including maternal physiological examination, has been presented. The guideline refers to the level of competency a health-care professional should have in order to provide an appropriate and informed level of care at each postnatal contact. These are based on the competencies developed by Skills for Health (www.skillsforhealth.org.uk) and it is advisable that readers of this chapter, who are likely to be both providing direct care and managing postnatal areas, are familiar with the levels of competency required.

The context of care

It is important that care takes place in a context which is welcoming and supportive. The majority of women in the UK give birth in the hospital setting and will spend the first few hours and days after giving birth on the postnatal ward. For many, this will be their first experience of being admitted to hospital and, as such, they will be unfamiliar with routines and unaware of the roles and responsibilities of the staff caring for them (Yelland et al 2007). The NICE (2006, p. 7) guideline stipulates:

> ...women and their families should always be treated with kindness, respect and dignity. The views, beliefs and values of the woman, her partner and her family in relation to her care and that of her baby should be sought and respected at all times.

It is important to consider how this ethos could be implemented into practice. Women are most likely to complain about care in hospital, which includes dissatisfaction with the level of communication they experienced with midwives and other clinicians, often in contrast to their experiences during antenatal and intrapartum care (Redshaw et al 2007). On arrival onto the postnatal ward, it is important for the midwife to introduce herself and consider her communication skills as detailed in Box 14.1.

Box 14.1

Important communication skills when welcoming a woman to the postnatal ward

- Has the woman been congratulated on her birth?
- Is there acknowledgement that she may be tired or in pain?
- Is her partner or another relative with her?
- Is there acknowledgement of the support a woman's partner and/or relative can offer and how valuable this is to her?
- Have the woman's immediate needs been met by pointing out where bathrooms, toilets and call bell are located?

Communication may seem a very basic level of 'skill' to describe, but it is an essential first step to building an effective relationship with a woman and her partner. Studies have shown that effective communication between a woman and her midwife or other health professional can impact on a number of aspects of maternal well being and satisfaction during pregnancy (Hegarty et al 2007, Rowe et al 2002) and it is likely that postnatal outcomes could also be enhanced with improved communication skills.

Maternal morbidity

One of the main aims of postnatal care is to detect deviation from expected normal recovery (Bick & MacArthur 1997) and the physiological examination remains an important component of this. What needs to be considered is, however, whether the assessment is appropriate to meet the needs of the woman at each point of contact and whether the clinician performing the examination is aware of the implications of findings, particularly if they deviate from expected normal recovery. Baseline assessment of a woman's immediate recovery from birth is extremely important to inform the level of care she may require during the immediate and later postnatal period. Although the value of the routine physiological examination has been questioned in recent years (Marchant et al 1996) and few studies have provided evidence to support optimal performance of the examination, NICE (2006) recommends health-care professionals remain alert to life-threatening conditions particularly within the first 24 hours of birth. To detect signs and symptoms of major morbidity, key components of the physiological examination should include those detailed in Box 14.2.

Based on NICE (2006) guidance, the signs and symptoms highlighted in Box 14.3 should remain at the forefront of care and, if appropriate, inform the content of the physiological examination. If signs or symptoms of the following potentially life-threatening conditions are detected, **emergency action** must be taken.

Robust evidence to inform some of the above signs and symptoms is lacking and, as a consequence, some recommendations are based on 'best practice' as decided by the Guideline Development Group (NICE 2006). Findings of the physiological examination should be explained and discussed with the woman and information used to inform

Key components of the postnatal physiological examination of the mother

- Assessment of uterine involution.
- Observation of lochia.
- Maternal temperature.
- Maternal BP.
- Perineal observation.
- Examination of the woman's legs.
- The guideline also recommends that within 24 hours of giving birth women receive information on signs and symptoms of major maternal morbidity in order that they and their partners are aware of when they should immediately contact a health-care professional or seek emergency help.

Box 14.3

Signs and symptoms that must be taken into account when conducting the postnatal physiological examination of the mother

- Sudden or profuse blood loss and signs and symptoms of shock.
- Fever, shivering, abdominal pain and/or offensive vaginal loss. If a woman's temperature exceeds 38°C, it should be repeated in 4–6 hours. If the temperature remains high and/or there are other signs and symptoms of infection, the woman should be referred immediately.
- Severe or persistent headaches.
- A diastolic BP greater than 90 mm Hg accompanied by other signs of pre-eclampsia, such as a severe or persistent headache, vomiting, abdominal discomfort. If the diastolic is greater than 90 mm Hg with no other signs or symptoms, repeat the BP in 4 hours. If it remains above 90 mm Hg after 4 hours, the woman should be referred immediately.
- Shortness of breath or chest pain (potential pulmonary embolism) or unilateral calf pain, redness or swelling (potential deep vein thrombosis).

subsequent management, including timing and content of contacts. Not all women will require all components of a physiological examination to be performed at each contact, but *all women should*

be asked at each contact, including at 6–8 weeks, how they are feeling. Prompting with questions to identify potential problems, the midwife then should decide which, if any, observations or assessments are required to monitor health and well being.

Physiological examination to detect major maternal morbidity

Uterine involution and abnormal blood loss

It is important to reflect on why aspects of physiological examination to detect life-threatening conditions remain relevant to maternal health in current practice. A core component of the routine physiological examination during the last century has centred on daily measurement of uterine involution to detect signs and symptoms of haemorrhage and infection. Deaths among women in the UK from haemorrhage have declined dramatically over the last 50 years. The maternal mortality rate during 2003–2005 was 7 per 100 000 maternities (Lewis 2007). Primary and secondary PPH are defined as severe blood loss occurring within the first 24 hours (primary) or after the first 24 hours of birth, and up to 6 weeks postpartum (secondary). The NICE (2006) postnatal guideline defines primary and secondary PPH as 'excessive' vaginal blood loss, but does not include a precise definition of this.

Whether delay or failure of involution is a risk factor for potentially life-threatening haemorrhage or infection is unclear. Involution describes the return of the uterus to a pelvic organ and the progress of involution is usually assessed by measurement of the symphysio-fundal distance (S-FD). Delayed uterine involution (sub-involution) is diagnosed by perceived delay in the reduction of the size of the uterus. There is limited information about the number of women diagnosed as having sub-involution, the relationship between sub-involution alone and subsequent outcome, the referral rate and the most appropriate management of sub-involution as a solitary sign (Bick et al 2002). The most commonly used methods to assess involution are anthropometry (simple abdominal palpation) or a tape measure. Midwifery textbooks vary in their description of the rate at which uterine involution occurs and lack detail of how measurement of fundal height should be obtained (Cluett et al 1995). Nevertheless, failure of the uterus to involute could indicate the presence of retained products of conception.

Cluett et al (1997) studied uterine involution among a small sample of primiparous women who had a normal vaginal birth ($n = 28$) and found considerable variability in not only the pattern of uterine involution between women, but also the daily rate of decline experienced by individual women. Twenty-two women had at least one episode of 'slow decline' (defined as a decline in the S-FD of < 1 cm over 3 or more days) at various times during the puerperium. As there was no evidence to suggest midwives could measure S-FD with precision, an earlier study by the same researchers investigated intra-observer and inter-observer variability (Cluett et al 1995). Results showed a significant degree of error in measurement of the S-FD when measurements for the same women were taken repeatedly by the same midwife. The degree of error was even greater when measurements from the same women were taken by different midwives. Study findings suggested that routine assessment of involution using a tape measure was not precise enough to enable clinical judgments to be made about the progress of uterine involution. On the basis of evidence presented NICE (2006) concluded that there was no evidence to support routine measurement of fundal height or how often uterine assessment should be undertaken within routine postnatal care. The guideline does stress that uterine assessment can be used to discount or confirm morbidity when performed in combination with observation of symptoms such as fever, uterine or abdominal tenderness. Better evidence is needed to inform this area of care.

Detection of infection

Observation of signs and symptoms of infection should remain a high priority for physiological examination in the postnatal period. It is important to ensure midwives not only have the skills to perform clinical assessments and elicit information from a woman, but to know when to act on findings. Concern was expressed in the most recent Confidential Enquiry (Lewis 2007) that clinical staff, including midwives, failed to identify signs and symptoms of maternal sepsis and critical illness, including raised respiratory rate and tachycardia.

Of the 22 women who died in the last triennial period from sepsis, three died following an uneventful pregnancy and normal vaginal birth, and 10 from genital-tract sepsis after a caesarean section (Lewis 2007). The Enquiry team found that in some cases clinical staff failed to check the women's baseline observations or did not appreciate the significance of their findings and the importance of early postnatal observation and examination was highlighted.

The source of puerperal sepsis is likely to be the genital tract, but the term could include any cause of sepsis during the postnatal period. The terms genital tract sepsis, uterine infection and endometritis are all used in the literature. There is no defined range for what constitutes pyrexia during the postnatal period and a transient elevation in maternal temperature is not uncommon, for example, among women who experience breast engorgement on or about the third postpartum day (Royal College of Midwives [RCM] 2002), although the aetiology of this is unclear. World Health Organisation (WHO) (2006) identifies symptoms of uterine infection as a temperature of $>38^{\circ}C$ and any of the following: feeling very weak, abdominal tenderness, foul-smelling lochia, profuse lochia, uterus not well contracted, lower abdominal pain or history of heavy vaginal bleeding. NICE (2006) guidelines as outlined above state sepsis may be suspected in the presence of two or more of these signs and symptoms. The level of evidence for this recommendation is a best-practice point based on the experience of the Guideline Development Group. As there is no definition of surgical or perineal wound infection in postnatal populations, local guidelines for diagnosis of wound infection should be adhered to. Given the much earlier transfer home of women from hospital, community midwives and general practitioners (GPs) have to remain vigilant to the potential development of genital-tract sepsis and wound infection.

Blood pressure

With regard to some components of the physiological examination, NICE (2006) guidance recommends when, in relation to the birth, some baseline observations and assessments should be undertaken. The guideline recommends **all** women have their BP measured within 6 hours of the birth and the result documented. The true prevalence of postpartum hypertension is difficult to ascertain, but the importance of this aspect of care was highlighted by the Confidential Enquiry which reviewed 18 maternal deaths from eclampsia or pre-eclampsia between 2002 and 2005 (Lewis 2007); three women died after postnatal transfer. Pre-eclampsia is considered to occur when pregnancy-induced hypertension (PIH) is associated with significant proteinuria (300 mg/l in 24 hours) (Davey & MacGillivray 1988), although the precise relationship remains unclear. The most common definition of eclampsia is convulsions, accompanied by signs and symptoms of pre-eclampsia such as headache, vomiting, visual disturbances and epigastric discomfort, where other causes of convulsion have been excluded (Douglas & Redman 1994). It is vital BP measures are obtained by someone competent to perform the measurement accurately, who can interpret increases in and absolute values of systolic and diastolic measurement. Midwives delegating performance of a BP assessment to a student midwife or a health-care assistant should ensure they have the competency to obtain accurate measurements and report on findings.

Physiological examination to identify common maternal health problems

The first observational studies to present evidence that for many women, health did not return to 'normal' within 6–8 weeks of giving birth also led to questions about the benefit and effectiveness of traditional midwifery care with its focus on routine physiological examination (Bick & MacArthur 1995a, MacArthur et al 1991) and the timing and content of the routine 6–8 week GP consultation (Bick & MacArthur 1995b). Studies found a wide range of persistent maternal morbidity, including backache, urinary and faecal incontinence, depression and perineal pain, much of which had not been reported to or identified by midwives or GPs within routine care.

Of three randomised controlled trials undertaken in the UK to assess the outcome of revisions to routine postnatal care to enhance maternal health outcomes (MacArthur et al 2002, Morrell et al 2000, Reid et al 2002), only one trial found a positive impact on women's health, although confined to psychological and not physical outcomes (MacArthur et al 2002). Of note is that this was the only trial to revise the content and duration of midwifery care, rather than develop and evaluate an intervention as an addition to routine care (MacArthur et al 2002). The trial implemented a 'package' of midwifery-led community-based care focused on the identification and management of common maternal-health problems. The duration of midwifery contact was extended for all women to 28 days, with an additional visit at 10–12 weeks to replace the routine GP visit at 6–8 weeks. A symptom checklist was administered by midwives at 10 and 28 days and at 10–12 weeks to ask women about their experience of common health problems, with evidence-based guidelines to inform the management of these (Bick et al 2002).

Based on evidence of widespread and persistent maternal morbidity, NICE (2006) guidance includes recommendations for systematic assessment of women's well being and care including advice on when identification of common health problems should be implemented. Of note is that the guideline recommends all women have a review of their physical, social and emotional well being at 6–8 weeks, which should include aspects of physiological health described here. However, rather than recommending which health professional should undertake this contact, the guideline refers to the role of a co-ordinating health professional with the competencies necessary to perform the consultation. This suggests the potential for midwives to take responsibility for discharging women on completion of their maternity episode, which should be arranged in liaison with the GP, as responsibility for infant immunisation and payment for maternity services would have to be addressed.

It is important that midwives ask women about symptoms during all postnatal contacts to identify problems in the first instance and prompt appropriate observation and assessment. The following sections refer to identification of some common health problems within the physiological examination; psychological and psychiatric health problems are not described as the focus of this chapter is physiological examination.

Urinary incontinence

NICE (2006) recommend **all** women are asked within 6 hours of giving birth if they have voided, to identify women at risk of developing urinary retention. The exact incidence of postpartum retention is difficult to ascertain since it has received little research attention and has been variably defined. Yip et al (2002) in a review article noted that a commonly used symptom-based clinical definition is the absence of spontaneous voiding within 6 hours of vaginal birth and for caesarean sections, no spontaneous voiding within 6 hours following removal of an indwelling catheter (more than 24 hours after birth). Retention can be covert, being detected by elevated post-void residual measurements with ultrasound or catheterisation. Epidural analgesia, instrumental birth and prolonged labour have been associated with retention after birth (Ching-Chung et al 2002) and women exposed to these factors should be closely monitored. Bladder care should remain a high priority until women have been able to void spontaneously. If symptoms of retention do not resolve following advice to assist micturition, NICE (2006) recommends as **urgent** action, that bladder volume is assessed and catheterisation considered.

Stress incontinence can be used to describe a symptom or a diagnosis (Bick et al 2002). When describing a symptom, stress incontinence refers to the involuntary leakage of urine, usually on exertion (Abrams et al 2002). As a diagnosis it refers to involuntary loss of urine when the intravesical pressure exceeds that of the urethra, with no simultaneous detrusor contraction. It is an extremely common symptom in the general female population, with a high prevalence among women after birth. A UK postal questionnaire survey of 11 701 women contacted 1–9 years after birth, found that 20.6% reported stress incontinence which started for the first time within 3 months of giving birth and lasted beyond 6 weeks (MacArthur et al 1991). Three-quarters of the symptomatic women reported symptoms lasting for at least 1 year. A large multi-centre longitudinal study recruited 7879 women at 3 months postpartum, 4214 of whom were followed up at 6 years (MacArthur et al 2006). Of the women contacted at 6 years, 24% had urinary incontinence at both times: of women who were symptomatic when first contacted at 3 months, 73% still had symptoms. As part of planned postnatal care, women should be regularly asked throughout the postnatal period about symptoms of stress incontinence. Women may not volunteer symptoms as they may expect to experience stress incontinence as a 'normal' consequence of giving birth (Bick & MacArthur 1995a). Evidence from RCTs to support the benefit of postnatal pelvic floor muscle exercises

(PFME) to manage symptoms of stress incontinence is inconclusive (Chiarelli & Cockburn 2002, Glazener et al 2001, Wilson & Herbison 1998); however, it is likely that if benefit is to accrue, PFME should be taught by someone trained to teach the technique.

Bowel problems

The guideline also stipulates that women should be asked if they have had their bowels opened within 3 days of giving birth (NICE 2006). Although evidence of the prevalence and risk factors for constipation is limited, reduced dietary and fluid intake during labour may lead to the development of postnatal symptoms. Women may also feel reluctant to open their bowels if they have experienced perineal trauma, with baseline examination of the perineal area useful not only to monitor healing of trauma, but also to identify the presence of haemorrhoids. If a woman has not had her bowels opened after receiving advice on diet and fluid intake, a gentle laxative may be necessary to relieve symptoms.

Faecal incontinence has only recently been identified as a problem experienced by women following birth. Data on prevalence and risk factors have been obtained from epidemiological studies and pathophysiological studies of symptom occurrence following occult anal sphincter injury (MacArthur et al 1997, Oberwalder et al 2003, Saurel-Cubizolles et al 2000, Sultan et al 1993). Some data have also been obtained from studies primarily examining other problems, for example urinary incontinence (Sleep & Grant 1987). Two main risk factors for the development of faecal incontinence and occult anal sphincter damage have been identified; instrumental vaginal birth and third/fourth-degree perineal tears. NICE (2006) guidance is that women who are symptomatic should be asked about the severity, duration and frequency of symptoms. Furthermore, if symptoms do not resolve, women should be referred for further assessment and evaluation, with **urgent** action recommended.

Perineal care

Women should receive information on perineal hygiene within 3 days of giving birth and asked at each contact about the healing of their perineum (NICE 2006). This is important as the majority of women who have a vaginal birth will experience perineal trauma, with second-degree trauma most commonly sustained (Kettle et al 2002). Perineal pain is one of the most commonly reported symptoms in the postnatal period (Sleep 1995), and for some women symptoms persist for many weeks and months after birth. Studies from the UK and overseas have shown that at least 8–10% of women experience perineal pain beyond discharge from maternity care at 6–8 weeks (Brown & Lumley 1998, Glazener et al 1995, Macarthur & Macarthur 2004). The aim of the physiological examination of the perineum should include identification of signs and symptoms of wound infection, inadequate repair and other morbidity, for example haematoma, as well as ascertaining women's perceptions of the level of pain they are experiencing. Care should be taken to ensure that the whole perineal area is observed, to enable any problems to be identified. Paracetamol is usually recommended as first line of pain management; however, if this is not providing adequate pain relief, oral or rectal non-steroidal anti-inflammatory drugs should be prescribed, after confirming that these are not contraindicated for the woman.

Evidence from methodologically robust studies of practices associated with reduced levels of perineal pain is accruing. A Cochrane systematic review of suturing materials (Kettle & Johanson 2000) concluded that the use of absorbable synthetic suture material (polyglycolic acid and polyglactin sutures) appeared to decrease short-term perineal pain, although the length of time taken for synthetic material to be absorbed was a concern. The effects of continuous subcuticular versus interrupted transcutaneous sutures for closure of perineal skin on long and short-term perineal pain and dyspareunia (difficult or painful sexual intercourse) was examined in a recently updated Cochrane systematic review (Kettle et al 2007). Seven trials which provided data on 3822 women were included. Meta-analysis showed that continuous suture techniques (all layers or perineal skin only) were associated with less pain for up to 10 days postpartum (relative risk (RR) 0.70, 95% confidence interval [CI] 0.64 to 0.76) when compared with interrupted sutures for perineal closure. These finding highlight that minimisation of health problems after birth should be a priority for practice through the continuum of maternity care. NICE (2006) recommend that women are offered information on contraception and asked about the resumption of sexual intercourse within 2–6 weeks of the birth. Resumption of sexual intercourse should also be discussed at the 6–8 week contact, given the association between perineal trauma and dyspareunia (Glazener 1997). For further information, please refer to Chapter 10.

Headache

Migraine and tension headache are commonly reported in the general population, with more women than men experiencing symptoms. It is unclear if these types of headache (sometimes referred to as primary headaches) are more commonly reported in the postnatal population than among women who have not recently given birth as there are no comparative studies. There is information, however, about some conditions which are more common among postnatal women and which can present with, or result in, secondary headaches. These are: post-dural puncture headaches (PDPH) following spinal or epidural anaesthesia and headache associated with postpartum hypertension, pre-eclampsia or eclampsia (Bick et al 2002). The incidence of PDPH is around 1–4% (Chan et al 2003, Goldszmidt et al 2005), although the incidence could be higher, as women may have been transferred home from hospital prior to developing symptoms. Epidural analgesia is a common intervention in labour, with most units now offering lower-dose infusions which enable women to be more mobile. A recent Cochrane review of combined spinal-epidural (CSE) versus epidural analgesia in labour which included data on 2658 women from 19 trials found no difference between CSE and epidural techniques and incidence of PDPH (Simmons et al 2007). Women who have had spinal or epidural analgesia should be asked about their experience of headaches and informed that if they experience 'classic' symptoms of a PDPH they should contact their midwife. If a woman is experiencing headaches accompanied with other symptoms of pre-eclampsia/eclampsia, she should be referred immediately.

Backache

Backache is also common in the general population and among pregnant and postnatal women. Prevalence studies of backache in postnatal populations have found between 20% and 50% of women experience backache, depending on definition of symptoms and how and when symptoms were assessed. For some women, backache can impact on aspects of their daily lives, particularly physical activities related to taking care of their baby (Bick & MacArthur 1995).

Risk factors for the development of backache include a previous history of symptoms, with some risk factors also identified from maternal or obstetric characteristics. Breen et al (1994) found younger maternal age and greater maternal weight predictors of postpartum backache in a study from Boston, USA. Glazener et al (1995) found backache more likely to be reported by women who had instrumental or caesarean births, although a study from Australia which found proportionally more backache reported following these births did not find a statistically significant difference (Brown & Lumley 1998). MacArthur et al (1991) found an association with ethnic group, with Asian women much more likely to report backache and other musculo-skeletal symptoms, although postulated that this may have been due to cultural differences in the reporting of morbidity (MacArthur et al 1993). As no studies have specifically investigated the management of backache in postnatal women, primary management should be based on general population guidance for acute low back pain (NICE 2006).

Fatigue

Fatigue after giving birth is to be expected given demands of caring for a newborn infant, but evidence from large observational studies of maternal morbidity show that symptoms of fatigue can persist and affect aspects of physical and psychological well being (Bick & MacArthur 1995, Glazener et al 1997, MacArthur et al 1991). In a study to examine the extent, severity and effect of postnatal health problems, fatigue was commonly reported (Bick & MacArthur 1995). Of 1278 women who completed a postal questionnaire, 523 (40%) reported fatigue, and of these, 77% (n = 405) reported that it impacted on their lives in some way. This included women reporting an inability to concentrate, a reluctance to socialise and feeling bad-tempered for no apparent reason. Postnatal fatigue was associated with problems resuming sexual intercourse in a large study of postnatal health in the Grampian region of Scotland (Glazener 1997) which followed women up at 8 weeks after birth and a sub-sample of women at 12–18 months.

Independent risk factors for fatigue identified in the study by MacArthur et al (1991) included multiple pregnancy, longer first stage of labour,

inhalation anaesthesia and postpartum haemorrhage. Milligan and Pugh (1994) found a significant association between caesarean section and fatigue in a group of 259 women surveyed before transfer from hospital, but when the same women were surveyed at 6 weeks and 3 months, no significant effect was seen. Tiredness was more common in women who had a caesarean section when surveyed at 6–7 months after the birth in Brown and Lumley (1998) large Australian study of postnatal health, but the effect was not statistically significant.

Paterson et al (1994) investigated the impact of low (<10.5 g/dl) haemoglobin (Hb) on the health of 1010 postnatal women. Hb tests were obtained at the first antenatal visit, 34 weeks, 3 days and 6 weeks postpartum. Women completed questionnaires about their health at 10 days, 4 weeks and 6 weeks after birth. Full data including Hb were only obtained for half of the original sample. A low Hb on day three was more likely to be diagnosed in women aged under 25, among primiparae; women who had had an operative or instrumental birth; women who had a low Hb at 34 weeks' gestation; and those with a blood loss of over 250 ml recorded at birth. Some of these variables are interrelated, but statistical analysis to determine independence of effect was not undertaken. Levels of fatigue should be asked about during postnatal contacts and at the 6–8 week contact (NICE 2006). Women who report persistent fatigue should be offered advice on diet, gentle exercise and planning activities (for example, to sleep when the baby sleeps). If symptoms do not improve, a Hb check should be performed with management based on local policy if the Hb is low. This is particularly important if women feel unable to undertake day-to-day activities because of fatigue.

Other postnatal health needs

Obesity

An area of health currently giving cause for concern is the increasing number of women who are obese. Obesity which is usually defined as a body mass index (BMI) of ≥30 (Lewis 2007) has significant implications for maternal and infant mortality and morbidity, including a major risk factor for thromboembolism. During 2003–2005, 14 of 31 women with a recorded BMI who died of a thromboembolic event were obese (Lewis 2007). Obesity was also reported by the Enquiry team as a risk factor for maternal deaths from sepsis and cardiac disease that they reviewed. In addition to maternal mortality, maternal morbidity associated with obesity includes gestational diabetes, hypertension, pre-eclampsia and postpartum haemorrhage; it is also associated with increased risk of stillbirth (Dixit & Girling 2008). A woman who is obese will need postnatal care planned not only to reduce the risk of thrombosis, but to identify signs and symptoms of hypertension and infection, with plans prepared in discussion with relevant members of the multidisciplinary team. Ideally, planning for her postnatal management should be commenced during her pregnancy.

Social and psychological needs

In addition to considering physiological examination to detect deviation from immediate physical recovery, an assessment of a woman's social and psychological needs should also be undertaken. These aspects of well being should not be separated from aspects of women's physical health. With respect to psychological care, there should be an opportunity for women to talk about their birth and ask questions about their experiences, although routine debriefing should not be undertaken, as this may be harmful (NICE 2007, Small et al 2002). If there has not been an opportunity during the woman's hospitalisation to discuss her birth experiences, it should be noted on her transfer records and initiated as soon as possible during a community-based contact. Recent policy and guidance has recommended midwives are aware of signs and symptoms of maternal mental health problems and a woman's psychiatric history is identified at her antenatal booking visit (DH 2004, Lewis & Drife 2004, NICE 2008). Levels of support available to a woman on transfer home could impact on her health, and women identified with low levels of support may benefit from referral to community-based parenting or peer support groups.

Key practice points

- Postnatal care should take place in a welcoming and supportive environment.
- Physiological examination should aim to identify potential major maternal morbidity within the immediate postnatal period and more commonly experienced health problems in the days and weeks after birth.
- Each postnatal contact should be undertaken by someone with the appropriate skills and competence.
- The content and timing of postnatal contacts should reflect a woman's individual health needs and include information to enable her to take care of her own health.
- In addition to physiological health, consideration should also be given to psychological and social health needs.

References

Abrams, P., Cardozo, L., Fall, M., Griffiths, D., Rosier, P., Ulmsten, U., et al., 2003. Standardisation of terminology of lower urinary tract function: report from the Standardisation Sub-committee of the International Continence Society. Neurology and Urodynamics 21, 167–178.

Beake, S., Bick, D., 2007. Maternity service policy: does the rhetoric match the reality? Br. J. Midwifery 15 (2), 89–93.

Beake, S., McCourt, C., Bick, D., 2005. Women's views of hospital and community–based postnatal care: the good, the bad and the indifferent.

Evidence-Based Midwifery 3 (2), 80–86.

Bick, D., MacArthur, C., 1995a. The extent, severity and effect of health problems after childbirth. Br. J. Midwifery 3 (1), 27–31.

Bick D, MacArthur C., 1995b Attendance, content and relevance of the 6 week postnatal examination. Midwifery 11, 69–73.

Bick, D., MacArthur, C., Winter, H., Knowles, H., 2002. Postnatal care: guidelines and evidence for practice. Churchill Livingstone, Edinburgh.

Bick, D.E., MacArthur, C., 1997. Common health problems after childbirth. In: Henderson,

C., Jones, K. (Eds.), Essential midwifery. Mosby, London, 285–318.

Breen, T.W., Ransil, B.J., Groves, P.A., Oriol, N.E., 1994. Factors associated with back pain after childbirth. Anesthesiology 81 (1), 29–34.

Brown, S., Lumley, J., 1998. Maternal health after childbirth: results of an Australian population based survey. Br. J. Obstet. Gynaecol. 105, 156–161.

Carley, M.E., Carley, J.M., Vasdev, G., Lesnick, T.G., Webb, M.J., Ramin, K.D., et al., 2002. Factors that are associated with clinically overt postpartum urinary retention after vaginal delivery. Am. J. Obstet. Gynecol 187, 430–433.

Chan, T.M.L., Ahmed, A., Yentis, S.M., Holdcroft, A., 2003. Postpartum headaches: summary report of the National Obstetric Anaesthetic Database (NOAD) 1999. International Journal of Obstetric Anaesthesia 12, 107–112.

Chiarelli, P., Cockburn, J., 2002. Promoting urinary continence in women after delivery: randomised controlled trial. Br. Med. J. 324, 1241–1246.

Ching-Chung, L., Shuenn-Dhy, C., Ling-Hong, T., Ching-Chang, H., Chao-Lun, C., Po-Jen, C., 2002. Australian and New Zealand. J. Obstet. Gynaecol. 42, 365–368.

Cluett, E.R., Alexander, J., Pickering, R.M., 1995. Is measuring the symphysis fundal distance worthwhile? Midwifery 11 (4), 174–183.

Cluett, E.R., Alexander, J., Pickering, R.M., 1997. What is the normal pattern of uterine involution? An investigation of postpartum uterine involution measured by the distance between the symphysis pubis and the uterine fundus using a tape measure. Midwifery 13, 9–16.

Davey, D.D., MacGillivray, I., 1988. The classification of the hypertensive disorders of pregnancy. Am. J. Obstet. Gynecol. 158 (4), 892–898.

Department of Health, 2004. National Service Framework for children, young people and maternity services. Department of Health, London.

Dixit, A., Girling, J.C., 2008. Obesity and pregnancy. J. Obstet. Gynaecol. 28 (1), 14–23.

Douglas, K.A., Redman, C.W.G., 1994. Eclampsia in the United Kingdom. Br. Med. J. 309, 1359–1400.

Glazener, C., Herbison, G., Wilson, P., MacArthur, C., Lang, G.D., Gee, H., et al., 2001. Conservative management of persistent postnatal urinary and faecal incontinence: randomised controlled trial. Br. Med. J. 323, 593–596.

Glazener, C.M.A., 1997. Sexual function after childbirth: women's experiences, persistent morbidity and lack of professional recognition. Br. J. Obstet. Gynaecol. 104, 330–335.

Glazener, C.M.A., Abdalla, M.I., Stroud, P., Naji, A., Russell, I.T., 1995. Postnatal maternal morbidity: extent, causes, prevention and treatment. Br. J. Obstet. Gynaecol. 102, 282–287.

Goldszmidt, E., Kern, R., Chaput, A., Macarthur, A., 2005. The incidence and etiology of postpartum headaches: a prospective cohort study. Canadian Journal of Anesthesia 52, 971–997.

Hegarty, K., Brown, S., Gunn, J., Forster, D., Nagle, C., Grant, B., et al., 2007. Women's views and outcomes of an educational intervention designed to enhance psychosocial support for women during pregnancy. Birth 34 (2), 155–163.

Kettle, C., Johanson, R.B., 2000. Absorbable synthetic versus catgut suture material for perineal repair (Cochrane Review). Cochrane Database Syst. Rev. Issue 3.

Kettle, C., Hills, R.K., Jones, P., Darby, L., Gray, R., Johanson, R., 2002. Continuous versus interrupted perineal repair with standard or rapidly absorbed sutures after spontaneous vaginal birth: a randomised controlled trial. Lancet 359, 2217–2223.

Kettle, C., Hills, R.K., Ismail, K.M.K., 2007. Continuous versus interrupted sutures for repair of episiotomy or second degree tears. Cochrane Database Syst. Rev. Issue 4.

King's Fund, 2008. Safe births: everybody's business. Independent inquiry into the safety of maternity services in England. King's Fund, London.

Lewis, G., (Ed.), 2007. The Confidential Enquiry into Maternal and Child Health (CEMACH) saving mothers' lives: reviewing maternal deaths to make motherhood safer – 2003–2005 The seventh report of the Confidential Enquiries into Maternal Deaths in the United Kingdom. CEMACH, London.

Lewis, G., Drife, J., (Eds.), 2004. Confidential Enquiry into Maternal and Child Health: why mothers die – 2000–2002. 6th report of the Confidential Enquiries into Maternal Deaths in the United Kingdom. RCOG, London.

Macarthur, A.J., Macarthur, C., 2004. Incidence, severity and determinants of perineal pain after vaginal delivery: a prospective cohort study. Am. J. Obstet. Gynecol. 191 (4), 1199–1204.

MacArthur, C., Lewis, M., Knox, E.G., 1991. Health after childbirth. HMSO, London.

MacArthur, C., Lewis, M., Knox, E.G., 1993. Comparison of long-term health problems following childbirth in Asian and Caucasian women. Br. J. Gen. Pract. 42, 519–522.

MacArthur, C., Bick, D.E., Keighley, M.R.B., 1997. Faecal incontinence after childbirth. Br. J. Obstet. Gynaecol. 104, 46–50.

MacArthur, C., Winter, H., Bick, D.E., Knowles, H., Lilford, R., Henderson, C., et al., 2002. Effects of redesigned community postnatal care on women's health 4 months after birth: a cluster randomised controlled trial. The Lancet 359, 378–385.

MacArthur, C., Glazener, C.M.A., Wilson, P.D., Lancashire, R.J., Herbison, G.P., Grant, A.M., 2006. Persistent urinary incontinence and delivery mode history: a six-year longitudinal study. Br. J. Obstet. Gynaecol. 113, 218–224.

Marchant, S., Alexander, J., Garcia, J., 1996. Postnatal observations. Letter Midwives 109 (1302), 204.

Milligan, R.A., Pugh, L.C., 1994. Fatigue during the childbearing period. Annu. Rev. Nurs. Res. 12, 33–49.

Morrell, C.J., Spiby, H., Stewart, P., Walters, S., Morgan, A., 2000. Costs and effectiveness of community postnatal support workers: randomised controlled trial. Br. Med. J. 321, 593–598.

National Institute for Health and Clinical Excellence, 2006. Routine postnatal care of women and their babies. NICE, London.

National Institute for Health and Clinical Excellence, 2007. Antenatal and postnatal mental health. NICE, London.

National Institute for Health and Clinical Excellence, 2008. Antenatal care: routine care of the healthy pregnant woman. NICE, London.

Neale, C., 2007. Personalised postnatal care. New Digest 37, 19–21.

Nursing and Midwifery Council, 2004. Midwives rules and standards. NMC, London.

Oberwalder, J., Wexner, S.D., 2003. Meta-analysis to determine the incidence of obstetric anal sphincter damage. Br. J. Surg. 90, 1333–1337.

Paterson, J.A., Davis, J., Gregory, M., Holt, S.J., Pachulski, A., Stamford, D.E., et al., 1994. A study of the effects of low haemoglobin on postnatal women. Midwifery 10, 77–86.

Redshaw, M., Rowe, R., Hockley, C., Brocklehurst, P., 2007. Recorded delivery: a national survey of women's experiences of maternity care 2006. National Perinatal Epidemiology Unit, University of Oxford, Oxford.

Reid, M., Glazener, C., Murray, G.D., Taylor, G.S., 2002. A two-centred pragmatic randomised controlled trial of two interventions of social support. BJOG 109, 1164–1170.

Rowe, R.E., Garcia, J., Macfarlane, A.J., Davidson, L.L., 2002. Improving communication between health professionals and women in maternity care: a structured review. Health Expect. 5, 63–83.

Royal College of Midwives, 2002. Successful breastfeeding. third ed. Churchill Livingstone, Edinburgh.

Saurel-Cubizolles, M.J., Romito, P., Lelong, N., Ancel, P.Y., 2000. Women's health after childbirth: a longitudinal study in France and Italy. Br. J. Obstet. Gynaecol. 107, 1202–1209.

Simmons, S.W., Cyna, A.M., Dennis, A.T., Hughes, D., 2007. Combined spinal-epidural versus epidural analgesia in labour. Cochrane Database Syst. Rev., Issue 3.

Singh, D., Newburn, M., 2000. Access to information and support. Women's needs and experiences before and after giving birth. National Childbirth Trust, London.

Sleep, J., Grant, A., 1987. Pelvic floor exercises in postnatal care. Midwifery 3, 158–164.

Sleep, J., 1995. Postnatal perineal care revisited. In: Alexander, J., Levy, V., Roch, S. (Eds.), Aspects of midwifery practice. A research based approach. Macmillan Press, London, Chapter 7, pp. 132–153.

Small, R., Lumley, J., Donohue, L., Potter, A., Waldenstrom, U., 2000. Randomised controlled trial of midwife led debriefing to reduce maternal depression after operative childbirth. Br. Med. J. 321 (7268), 1043–1047.

Sultan, A.H., Kamm, M.A., Hudson, C.N., Thomas, J.M., Bartram, C.I., 1993. Anal-sphincter disruption during vaginal delivery. N. Engl. J. Med. 329 (26), 1905–1911.

United Kingdom Central Council for Nursing, Midwifery and Health Visiting, 1992. Registrar's Letter no. 11. UKCC, London.

Wilson, P.D., Herbison, G.P., 1998. A randomised controlled trial of pelvic floor muscle exercises to treat postnatal urinary incontinence. In. Urogynecol. J. 9, 257–264.

World Health Organisation, 2006. Pregnancy, childbirth, postpartum and newborn care: a guide for essential practice. World Health Organisation, Geneva.

Yelland, J., McLachlan, H., Forster, D., Rayner, J., Lumley, J., 2007. How is maternal psychosocial health assessed and promoted in the early postnatal period? Findings from a review of hospital postnatal care in Victoria, Australia. Midwifery 23, 287–297.

Yip, S.K., Sahota, D., Chang, A.M.Z., Chung, T.K.H., 2002. Four-year follow-up of women who were diagnosed to have postpartum urinary retention. Am. J. Obstet. Gynecol. 187, 648–652.

Further reading

Bick, D., MacArthur, C., Winter, H., Knowles, H., 2002. Postnatal Care: Guidelines and Evidence for Practice. Churchill Livingstone, Edinburgh, Chapter 3, pp. 39–58; Chapter 4, pp. 59–88.
These chapters provide evidence on risk factors and management of a range of commonly experienced maternal health problems and recommendations for practice not explored indepth within this book.

Wiley, V.C.H., Hofmeyr, J., Neilson, J., Alfirevic, Z., 2008. Pregnancy and childbirth. A Cochrane Pocket Book. Wiley and Sons, Chichester.
Presents summaries of relevant reviews from the Cochrane Library, a range of useful information on systematic review protocols and format of results in Cochrane reviews.

Chapter Fifteen

Working in new ways to advance midwifery skills in practice

Maureen D. Raynor

CONTENTS

Introduction 173
Advancing skills versus 'extended' role . . . 173
   Team work 174
   Protecting the social model of care 175
Continuity of care: opportunities and
challenges 176
Meeting the education needs of midwives . 176
Role changes and leadership: midwives
as change agents 177
   Role of the consultant midwife 178
   A vision of midwifery supervision 178
The future 179
Key practice points 179
References 180
Further reading 180

Introduction

Over recent years the seismic shift in the balance of power between women and health-care professionals has been driven by socio economic reforms in the National Health Service (NHS) and by women themselves. There are, therefore, compelling reasons to advance skills in midwifery practice for the good of mother and baby, such as improving continuity of care. Moreover, changes influenced by the choice agenda (Department of Health [DH] 2004, 2007a, 2007b, 2008a) should be seen as a strategy and opportunity to be creative and innovative in order to drive changes for a more midwifery-led and woman-centred maternity service. As outlined in the introduction, the book is concerned with strengthening the role of the midwife, not undermining it. Thus, emphasis has been placed on role development. The premise and guiding principle behind this book has been to highlight the opportunities available to midwives to enhance practice and improve care for mothers and babies. Further, it is concerned with protecting the social model of care in order to provide quality and a more cost-effective service in what has increasingly become a cash-strapped NHS. Bringing the book to its conclusion, this final chapter has at its core the following:

- The key themes which have emerged within the preceding chapters.
- The implications of advancing skills in midwifery practice and how midwives can influence the future of maternity care.
- Recognition that in order to lead change, midwives need effective role models, such as the consultant midwife and supervisor of midwives.
- An acknowledgement that the midwife's role must be imbued with the power and authority to realise autonomous practice and deal with the often complex and diverse challenges in the work environment.

Advancing skills versus 'extended' role

Lavender (2003) provides an interpretation of what it means to extend the role of the midwife and the implications of midwives undertaking skills

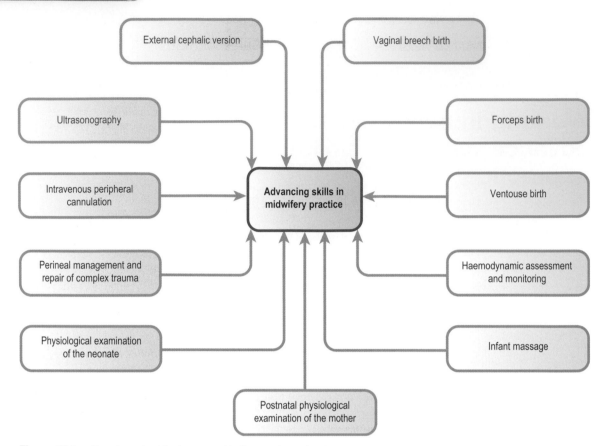

Figure 15.1 • Overview of subjects covered in the previous chapters.

previously carried out by other health-care professionals namely doctors. Most of these skills are addressed in the previous chapters and summarised in Figure 15.1.

However, Lavender (2003) identifies a number of consequences of acquiring skills that take midwives into the realms of what some may construe as *quasi-obstetric*; the implications of which are outlined in Figure 15.2. Acknowledging the contradictions in the quest to achieve woman-centred care, Kirkham (2000) urges a note of caution, especially in the NHS where hierarchical structures are entrenched. Care should be exercised to ensure that another tier of midwives is not developed – *the experts*. There is a danger that this could lead to unfair competition, resentment and alienation within the workforce.

Team work

Shifting paradigms has resulted in increased roles and responsibilities, interprofessional working and the skill mix being magnified (DH 2001a). Sidebotham (2001) states that it is pivotal to harness midwifery skills so that midwives can focus on fulfilling their role and responsibilities, and staff from other disciplines, such as obstetrics, can focus their attention and expertise on the women who need such specialist attention. Good team work requires effective communication. A central theme within a number of key reports (Health Care Commission [HCC] 2008, Redshaw et al 2007, Royal College of Anaesthetists et al 2007) is the need to improve communications not only between health-care professionals, but also between professionals and women. Maternity units should foster a team approach based on mutual respect, a shared philosophy of care and a clear organizational structure for both midwives and doctors, with explicit and transparent lines of communication.

Traditional models of maternity care in the United Kingdom (UK) have involved an array of different health-care professionals, namely the general practitioner (GP), midwife and obstetrician. At times this has resulted in power struggles and confusion regarding the understanding of

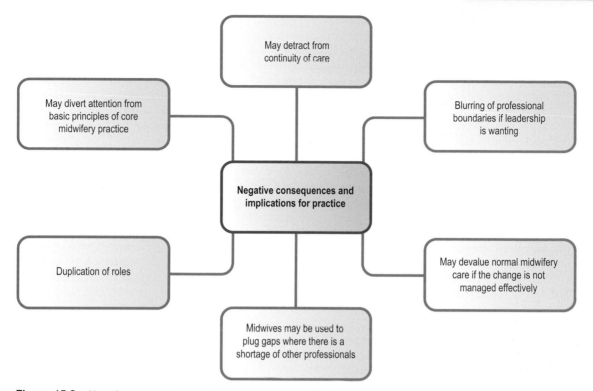

Figure 15.2 • Negative consequences of viewing advancing skills for midwives as an extended role.

professional roles. There should be mutual respect for professional boundaries and professional autonomy. Kirkham (2007) recalls the hierarchical structure of the NHS in which most midwives work, and how the current political and managerial climate has resulted in a rigid power structure and relentless demand to get things done. The net result of which often negate midwives feelings and culminate in the devaluing of midwives. The whole business of professionalization and the pressures to be knowledgeable doers and specialist midwives, she argues, also impacts negatively on midwives. At best this breeds contempt and at worst leads to a bullying culture. Much of this resonates with the evidence from a report on maternal deaths by the HCC (2006) which concluded that a dysfunctional team is often the result of poor communication, lack of support and a bullying culture. Four key factors that emerge from this report are:

- Poor leadership.
- Lack of a visionary approach and shared philosophy.
- Reactive rather than proactive supervision.
- Inadequate training.

These factors are often triggers to midwives leaving the profession (Ball et al 2002). Spiers (2008, p. 26) attests that 'cultural change requires structural change'. With this in mind, advancing skills in midwifery practice require critical thinkers, enablers, innovators, proactive supervision, and strong and effective leaders. Effort and vision is also needed to seize opportunities and embrace new ways of working, whilst remaining true to the philosophy of midwifery care, reflective of the social model of care.

Protecting the social model of care

To advance skills in midwifery practice the social model of care must remain sacrosanct and at the core of maternity care. Deeply rooted in the ethos of normality, this model is a woman's and midwife's charter, as it is concerned with protecting the dignity and sanctity of pregnancy/childbirth as well as respecting the heterogeneity of women within their socio-cultural setting. This approach to care is committed to continuity of care. Advancing midwifery skills, it could be argued, is one way of achieving just that for every woman. However, this raises a paradox and questions how expanding the role of the midwife into the realms of interventions, customarily regarded as the domain of doctors, can safeguard the social model of care. Some may construe it as a polemic argument and a vexed issue as the Royal College of Midwives (RCM 2005, 2006) points out that midwives are required to take on increasing responsibilities without any extra remuneration, adding to their already burgeoning workload. Diametrically opposed are the protagonists who view much of the skills outlined in the preceding chapters as an opportunity to champion change and provide continuity of care for women. Sceptics on the other hand will be less enthused and convinced by the argument that midwives can make a worthwhile difference to women and maintain their professional integrity by acquiring pseudo-obstetric skills. It is easy to align oneself with either viewpoint but the restructuring and redesign of the National Health Service as outlined by the Darzi report (DH 2008a) requires midwives to break the mould and think outside the box. Thus as a consequence of this report, the DH (2008b) has published a strategy previously highlighted in the introduction to the book, called *Framing the nursing and midwifery contribution*. This bold report signals the key actions that are needed to help transform nursing and midwifery over the ensuing years.

Whilst caution should be exercised, prudence does not mean to not engage with change nor does it mean precipitous action by poor clinical judgement and flawed decision making (Spiers 2008). To this end the RCM (2006, p. 1) states that 'reforming a role, or introducing new practices and responsibilities', can have ramifications that do not come to light immediately. Consequently, they recommend that any innovations in practice should be subjected to a rigorous process of scrutiny and evaluation pre and post implementation. Emphasizing that this guiding principle is even more crucial where midwives are expected to take on new or altered responsibilities. This includes new delegation and shared responsibilities.

Continuity of care: opportunities and challenges

As great strides are made into the 21st century midwives face a number of changes and challenges, not least being the depletion of midwives. This in part

is brought about by a number of factors including, an aging workforce, mobilization through emigration and inflexible working conditions (RCM 2005). Midwives are increasingly being put under pressure to take on more responsibilities and expected to prove their cost-effectiveness with very little reward. Despite the challenges, there are many new and exciting opportunities for midwives to advance their skills in practice.

Central themes to women's satisfaction with their care are continuity of care, choice and communication (DH 2007b, Hodnett et al 2007, Redshaw et al 2007). There is high level of evidence to support continuity of care or midwife-led care. It is also clear that the potential for the midwife to be the primary carer in both community and hospital setting should be maximised (DH 2007b). This framework of care provides great opportunities for advancing the midwife's skills and providing enhanced control and achieving professional autonomy. Thus, within the choice agenda (DH 2001b, 2003a, 2007a, 2007b, 2008a) it is recognised that midwives play a key role in providing women with continuity of care and social support: a great leverage that benefits both women and midwives.

Birth centres it seems could be one way of heralding change. Walsh (2006) and Kirkham (2003) highlight the benefits of birth centres where intervention is minimised, the family is included and birth is experienced as a social rather than a medical event. Midwifery care such as that experienced in birth centres is well placed to provide quality economically sustainable services to childbearing women. Although the midwifery model of care rightly focuses on the normal, midwives are well equipped to identify deviations from normal and implement life-saving interventions through mutually agreed upon guidelines. Skills such as perineal repair, intravenous cannulation, facilitation of vaginal breech and uncomplicated forceps and ventouse birth can assist in avoiding unnecessary transfers to consultant- (i.e. obstetric) led care.

Meeting the education needs of midwives

The key themes emerging from the chapters are detailed in Figure 15.3. One of which is the continuing education needs for midwives undertaking clinical skills. Midwives must be supported in

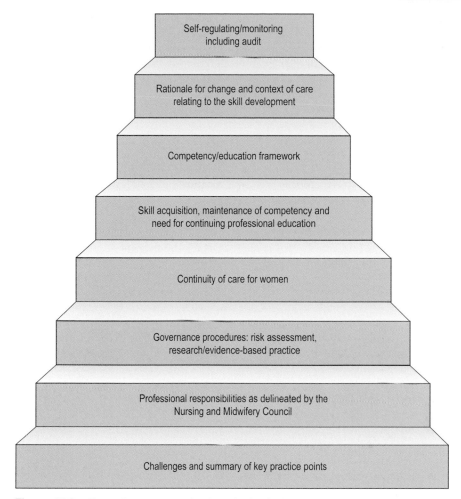

Figure 15.3 • Thematic steps emerging from the book chapters.

practice with time and paid study days to update their knowledge and skills in order to maintain their competence. Supervisors of midwives should advocate for midwives to ensure that the care received by mothers and babies is not compromised.

Role changes and leadership: midwives as change agents

The book has alluded to the financial imperatives and streamlining of the NHS, such as the reduction in junior doctors hours, that have resulted in an increased workload for midwives. To advance skills in midwifery practice midwives will need to develop and improve upon their leadership abilities,

negotiation skills, research skills and communication skills. The review of the NHS by Lord Darzi (DH 2008a) has resulted in national debates to find ways to make the NHS more effective and cost efficient in developing and delivering quality. This is necessary to meet the diverse and complex needs of the population it serves. However, the report by Lord Darzi (DH 2008a) also highlights that more could be done in the NHS to improve leadership. To have an impact, change needs to be driven from the grassroots and led by midwives committed to change. Therefore, the report also placed emphasis on leadership and the importance of initial pre-registration education and training to cultivate and nurture leadership skills. Midwife educationalist are charged with the task of ensuring that pre-registration midwifery programmes equip the next generation of midwives to be fit for both practice and purpose. *Making a difference* (DH 2001b) challenges midwives to expand their role and change practice to include wider responsibilities for women's health. The previous chapters of this book have demonstrated that some midwives have taken up the gauntlet to advance their skills in a range of areas. However, key leaders are needed to sustain change.

Role of the consultant midwife

Against a backdrop of a financially driven modernizing health service agenda, the role of the consultant midwife was created by the DH (1999) as a means of unification. It was meant to signal a new career opportunity to help retain experienced, dynamic and visionary midwives willing to act as key leaders and catalysts for change. It was also meant to diffuse the power dynamics between obstetricians and midwives, bringing about a more levelling and sharing of power. However, according to O'Loughlin (2001), whilst real equity between midwives and obstetricians is more apparent, a direct result of consultant midwives being introduced into practice, there is a paradox. She argues that the implementation of consultant midwives has in some ways made midwifery even more hierarchical. This has happened at a time when the profession is working towards flattening hierarchy in order to diffuse inherent tensions that accompany such structures.

Depicted as a role model, the consultant midwife remit is meant to represent a bridge between education, practice development and research/evidence-based care. Sidebotham (2001) argues that through having a portfolio of expertise and a strategic vision, consultant midwives, like supervisors of midwives, are expected to be innovators, enablers, and strong and effective leaders. It is necessary that these paragons of virtue do not only lead change but help to avert adversity and implement change without destabilising the workforce. The aim of the role should also be to refocus normality throughout pregnancy and childbirth. Sadly, a number of consultant midwives have left their posts to become heads of midwifery. This is despite evaluative studies, such as that conducted by Coster et al (2006), that relate the positive impact the implementation

of such posts have had. In conjunction with educationalists, consultant midwives have contributed to improved staff education. Additionally they have influenced service reconfiguration and practice development (Coster et al 2006). This means that consultant midwives have played a pivotal role in supporting women and midwives to reclaim normal childbirth. It is a pity, then, that despite the government's effort to make the appointment of consultant midwives less bureaucratic (DH 2003b), the visibility of consultant midwife's posts nationally is now less apparent. There is a real need for continued and sustained evaluation of the efficacy of consultant midwife's posts as they have not been implemented long enough to get a true sense of the scale of difference they have made nationally to NHS reforms. This will become more transparent over time given that it is less than a decade since such posts were introduced. To this end, Lavender (2003) points out that a thorough evaluation of the role of the consultant midwife is needed and the contribution they have made through improvements within the workforce.

A vision of midwifery supervision

In its publication *Modern supervision in action*, the Nursing and Midwifery Council [NMC] (2008) provides useful guidance, but more work is needed at national level to continue to establish clear guidance for supervisors. As a statutory mechanism supervision of midwifery is a legal requirement. Not only is it enshrined in statute to protect the welfare of mothers and babies against unsafe practice, but it also serves to strengthen the midwifery commitment to the development of practice initiatives. In so doing, supervision in midwifery practice actively promotes safe standards of care and represents professional self-regulation. In this way midwifery supervision is committed to quality assurance reflected by the clinical governance agenda. By working in partnership with other members of the multiprofessional team, supervisors of midwives should ensure that midwifery practice is never compromised. This is particularly important given the increasing complexities of care that midwives currently face in contemporary practice. Development of guidelines, for example, must assist midwives in carrying out their role autonomously

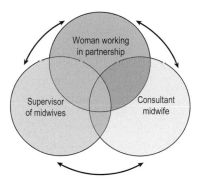

Figure 15.4 • Woman centered care: a framework for partnership.

seize every opportunity to work in new and different ways that challenge the status quo. Midwives need to champion changes that improve quality of care for mothers and babies. This means constantly striving to go the extra mile to influence, manage and lead change. However, in order to support women in their choice, midwives need to be supported to continue to develop their knowledge, skills and competence. This can be done by regular updating and a commitment and drive to continue to build a critical mass of research evidence and influence guideline development that protects and safeguards women. Advancing skills in midwifery practice should be the business of ***every*** practising midwife.

without jeopardizing their position or the standard of care received by mothers and babies. Cognisance of professional boundaries and the legislative framework of supervision should serve to clarify professional roles. Proactive rather than reactive supervision is also needed. In other words supervisors must be strong advocates for women and midwives, and help midwives to build their skills of networking and negotiation.

Figure 15.4 identifies a schematic framework with overarching values and interface between consultant midwives and supervisors of midwives working in partnership with women.

The future

The complexity of care precipitated by socio political and demographic changes provides opportunities and challenges. It has never been more crucial to have unification between midwives and women. However, the nexus for advancing skills in midwifery practice and transforming professional practice more generally lies with midwives and not with other professional groups. Commitment and investment in midwives is needed if midwifery skills and practice are to be advanced in areas that have been highlighted in the preceding chapters. Midwives need to remain focused and connected to the principles of 'normality', but at the same time still collaborate rather than compete with peers and colleagues. Progression through the new millennium signals greater choice and the current climate of choice provides scope for midwives to

Key practice points

- Reaffirm the role of the midwife by clarification of role and responsibilities that acknowledges:
  - professional accountability.
  - the right to autonomy in the exercise of clinical judgement and informed decision making.
- A robust database is needed to demonstrate commitment to evidence-based care. Midwifery-led care will only be valued and measured with a firm commitment to research.
- Strong, visionary and skilled leaders are needed in midwifery practice to drive change and influence care whilst supporting and nurturing midwives to provide best care for mothers and babies.
- Midwives in the front line, consultant midwives, heads of midwifery, supervisors of midwives, midwives working as educationalists are all at the vanguard of change and should collaborate to ensure an emboldened and cost effective service.
- A culture in midwifery that is both facilitative and supportive will be open to new ideas and weed out bullying.
- A systematic midwifery career pathway that is fit for purpose is needed. One that enriches the midwifery experience and provides midwives with rewarding and innovative opportunities. This should allow for:
  - better work and pay conditions.
  - flexibility.
  - protected time to update and attend to continuing professional development needs beyond registration.

References

Ball, L., Curtis P., Kirkham M., 2002. Why do midwives leave? RCM, London.

Coster, S., Redfern, S., Wilson-Barnett, J., Evans, A., Peccei, R., Guest, D., 2006. Impact of the role of nurse, midwife and health visitor consultant. J. Adv. Nurs. 55 (3), 352–363.

Department of Health, 1999. Nurse, midwife and health visitor consultants – establishing posts: making appointments. Health Service Circular 1999/217 Available online: www.dh.gov.uk Accessed 31 August 2008.

Department of Health, 2001a. Working together – learning together. A framework for lifelong learning for the NHS. Available online: www.dh.gov.uk accessed 2 August 2008.

Department of Health, 2001b. Making a difference: the nursing, midwifery and health visiting contribution – the midwifery action plan. Available online:www.dh.gov.uk Accessed 2 August 2008.

Department of Health, 2003a. Building on the best: choice, responsiveness and equity in the NHS. HMSO, London.

Department of Health, 2003b. Approval of nurse, midwife and health visitor consultant posts; PLCNO (2003). Available online: www.dh.gov.uk Accessed 31 August 2008.

Department of Health, 2004. National service framework for children, young people and maternity services. HMSO, London.

Department of Health, 2007a. Our health, our care, our say: making it happen. Available online: www.dh.gov.uk Accessed 29 July 2008.

Department of Health, 2007b. Maternity matters: access and continuity of care in a safe service. HMSO, London.

Department of Health, 2008a. High quality care for all: NHS next stage review final report (Chair Lord A Darzi). Available online: www.dh.gov.uk Accessed 8 August 2008.

Department of Health, 2008b. Framing the nursing and midwifery contribution: driving up the quality of care. HMSO, London.

Health Care Commission, 2006. Investigation into 10 maternal deaths at, or following delivery at Northwick Park Hospital, Northwest London Hospitals NHS Trust between April 2002 – April 2005. Available online: www.cqc.org.uk. Accessed 8 May 2009.

Health Care Commission, 2008. Towards better births: a review of maternity services in England. Available online: www.cqc.org.uk. Accessed 8 May 2009.

Hodnett, E.D., Gates, S., Hofmeyr, G.J., Sakala, C., 2007. Continuous support for women during childbirth. The Cochrane Library of Systematic Reviews. Available online: http://www.thecochranelibrary.com Accessed 31 July 2008.

Kirkham, M. (Ed.), 2003. Birth Centres: a social model for maternity care. Elsevier, Oxford.

Kirkham, M., 2000. How can we relate. In: Kirkham, M. (Ed.), 2000 The midwife–mother relationship. Palgrave Macmillan, London, pp. 227–254.

Kirkham, M., 2007. Traumatised midwives. AIMS Journal 19(1). Available online: http://www.aims.org.uk/Journal/Vol19No1/traumatisedMidwives.htm Accessed 1 August 2008.

Lavender, T., 2003. The extended role of the midwife. J. Hosp. Med. 64, 134–135.

Nursing and Midwifery Council, 2008. Modern supervision in action: a practical guide for midwives. NMC, London.

O'Loughlin, C., 2001. Will the consultant midwife change the balance of power? Br. J. Midwifery 9 (3), 151–154.

Redshaw, M., Rowe, R., Hockley, C., Brocklehurst, P., 2007. Recorded delivery: a national survey of women's experience of maternity care 2006. National Perinatal Epidemiology Unit, Oxford.

Royal College of Anaesthetists, Royal College of Midwives, Royal College of Obstetricians and Gynaecologists, Royal College of Paediatrics and Child Health, 2007. Safer childbirth: minimum standards for the organisation and delivery of care in labour. RCOG, London.

Royal College of Midwives, 2005. Evidence to the pay review body. Available online: www.rcm.org.uk Accessed 8 August 2008.

Royal College of Midwives, 2006. Guidance paper: refocusing the role of the midwife; position paper 26. RCM, London.

Sidebotham, M., 2001. The consultant midwife role: will it make a difference? Available online: www.midwives.co.uk Accessed 8 August 2008.

Spiers, J., 2008. Who decides who decides? Enabling choice, equity, access, improved performance and patient guaranteed care. Radcliffe, Oxon.

Walsh, D., 2006. Improving maternity service: small is beautiful – lessons from a birth Centre. Radcliffe, London.

Further reading

Curtis, P., Ball, L., Kirkham, M., 2006. Bullying and horizontal violence: cultural or individual phenomena? Br. J. Midwifery 14 (4), 218–221. *This article highlights the effects of working in an unsupportive and bullying culture and how this can lead to midwives feeling vulnerable and unhappy.*

Raynor, M.D., Marshall, J.E., Sullivan, A., (Eds.), 2005. Decision making in midwifery practice. Churchill Livingstone, Edinburgh. *Provides a framework of effective decision making to assist midwives in fulfilling their autonomous role.*

Index

NB: page numbers in **bold** refer to boxes and figures

A

Abdomen, infant massage, 156, **156**
Abdominal circumference (AC), fetus, 36, **36**, 43
Abdominal shape/content, fetus, 39–40, **39**
Abdominal situs, fetal heart, **40**
Aberdeen knot, 112
Aberdeen Maternity Hospital (AMH), 78, 79, 85
Abortion Act (1967), 7
Abuse
  infant massage and, 158
  sexual, 105
Accountability
  Bergman's preconditions to, 8, **8**
  breech birth and, 97, 99
  Kitson's dimensions of, 8, **9**
  peripheral intravenous cannulation (PIVC) and, 60
  record keeping and, 63, **63**
  ventouse births and, 72
Accreditation, 157
Acts of Parliament, 7
Acupuncture, 20, 22, 24, 52
Advanced midwife practitioners (AMP), 2
Advancing skills, 2, 173–180, **174**, **177**
  change agents, 177–179
  continuity of care, 176
  education needs, midwife, 176–177
  future trends, 179
  key points, 179
  overview, 4
  vs 'extended' role, 173–176, **175**
Afterload, 122–123
ALARA (as low as reasonably achievable),
    sonography and, 31
'All fours' position, 93, **94**, 95, 97, **98**
ALSO® training course, 70
Alternative therapies, 20
Amblyopia, 141
Amphetamines, 136
Anal incontinence, 110
Anal sphincter injury
  legal implications, 118
  occult, 167
  trauma repair, 110, **111**, **112**

  see also External anal sphincter (EAS); Internal anal
      sphincter (IAS)
Aniridia, 142
Anterior posterior abdominal diameter (APAD), 36, **36**
Anthropometry, 164
Anticonvulsants, 136
Anti-D immunoglobulin, 51
Anus, imperforate, 136
  see also entries beginning Anal
Aristotle, 49
Arms, extended, 94, 96, **96**
Aromatherapy, 20, 21–22
Arterial blood pressure *see* Blood pressure (BP)
Arterial catheterization, 128–129
Arterial haemorrhage, 128
Assisted birth midwife practitioner, key principles of, 80, **80**
Assisted birth programme, 81
  distance learning, 78
Audit programme, midwife ventouse practitioner
    (MVP) and, 70
Autonomous practice, 99–100
Autonomy, respect for, 13, **13**
AVPU level of consciousness scale, 123, **123**
Ayurvedic medicine, 20, 22, 148

B

Bach flower remedies, 22
Backache, postnatal, 162, 168–169
Beneficence, respect for, 13–14, **13**
Bergman's preconditions to accountability, 8, **8**
Biparietal diameter (BPD), 35, 36
Birth centres, 176
Birth programme, midwife assisted, 79
Blackboard Virtual Learning Environment (VLE), 81
Bladder 67 acupoint, 22–23, **22**, 52
Bladder care, 167
Blood loss, abnormal, 164–165
Blood pressure (BP), 123
  auscultatory measurement, 125–126
  automated oscillatory measurement, 126
  invasive measurement, 128–129, **128**
  maternal, 165–166
  non-invasive measurement, 125, **126**

Body mass index (BMI), 169
Bolam principle, 11, 62, 99
Bowel problems, 167
Brachial pulse, 137
Breech birth, 48, **48**, 89–102
  complications, 92, **92**
  evidence, 90–91
  incidence, 90
  indications/contraindications, 91, **91**
  intrapartum checklist, 93, **95**, 100
  key points, 100
  manoeuvres to assist, 94–97, **96**, **98**
  overview, 3
  place of birth, 92–93
  position for birth, 93, **94**
  professional responsibility, 97, 99–100
British Acupuncture Council, 53
British Medical Ultrasound Society (BMUS), 30
Bulletin, NHS maternity statistics (Richardson and
    Mmata), 78
Burns Marshall manoeuvre, 96, **96**

C

Caesarean section, 162, 165, 167
  avoiding planned, 48–49
  unnecessary *see* external cephalic version (ECV)
Calman Report (DH), 1, 7, 78, 79
Canadian Institute of Health Research, 49
Capillary refill, 124
  test of perfusion, 137
Cardiac cycle, 138
Cardiac disease, 170
Cardiac output (CO), 122
Cardiomyopathy, 136
Cardiotocography (CTG), 49, 50–51
Care
  continuity of, 176
  holistic midwife-led and woman-focused model, 14
  medico-technocratic model, 14
  social model of, 175–176
Care Quality Commission, 12, 63, 100, 174, 175
  maternal deaths and, 175
Catheterization, 167
'Cat-lick' manoeuvre, 95
Cavum septum pellucidum (CSP), 36, 37
Central cyanosis, 124, 136–137
Central Delivery Suite (CDS) (Bath), 70
Central venous pressure (CVP)
  complications, 131, **131**
  monitoring, 129, **129**, **130**, 131, **131**
Cerebellum, fetus, 38, **38**
Cerebral ventricles, fetus, 37–38
Cerebrospinal fluid (CSF), 37, **38**

Cervical length, ultrasound, 42, **42**
Cervix, transvaginal measurement of, **42**
Change
  agents, midwives as, 177–179
  management theory, 14
Changing childbirth (DH), 68, 74
Chinese massage, 154
Chinese medicine, traditional (TCM), 22, 23, 25
Chiropractic, 22
Chlamydial conjunctivitis, 142
Choice, women and, 176
Choroid plexus cysts (CPC), 38
Chromosomal abnormalities, 136
'Cinderella' service, 162
Circulatory shock, 137, 138
Circumcision, female, 114
Cleft lip, 38, **39**
Clinical Governance, 14
Clinical Negligence Scheme for Trusts (CNST), 15, 62, 99
Clinical risk, 15
Clinics, perineal care, 117–118
Clitoridectomy, **115**
Coarctation of aorta (COA), 137, 139
Cochrane Database, 150, **150**, **151**
Cochrane systematic reviews, 77, 108, 110
  infant massage, 148, **150**, 151, **151**, **152**
  suturing materials, 168
*The Code: Standards of conduct, performance and ethics for
    nurses and midwives* (NMC), 10, 12, 59, 60, 69
Colic, acute, 153
Collagen disease, 142
Coloboma, 142
Colour
  eye, 142
  haemodynamic assessment and, 124
  neonate, 136–137
Combined spinal-epidural (CSE), 168
Combined stress tests, 143–145
Communication
  postnatal ward, 163, **163**
  skills, 163, **163**
  women and, 176
Competence
  beyond registration, 10, **10**
  in breech birth, 97
  competencies, 162–163, 166
  defined, 9
  five levels of, 2
  in new skills, 58–59, **59**
Complementary therapies (CTs), 19–28
  contraindication/precautions, 23–25
  evidence-based practice, 25–26
  infant massage, 147
  key points, 26

mechanism of action, 21–23
overview, 3
responsibility, midwife, 20–21
see also Moxibustion
Confidential Enquiry into Maternal and Child Health
(CEMACH), 42, 48, 92, 122, 165, 166, 170
Confidential Enquiry into Stillbirths and Deaths in Infancy
(CESDI), 91
Congenital cataract, 135, 142
Congenital diaphragmatic hernia (CDH), 39
Congenital Disabilities (Civil Liability) Act (1976), 12
Congenital heart disease (CHD), 135, 136, 138
detection, 136
predisposing factor, 136
Congestive heart failure (CHF), 137, 138
Consciousness, level of, 123, **123**
Consent, 11–12, **12**
breech birth and, 99
external cephalic version (ECV) and, 50, 52
infant massage and, 152
midwives and, 52
peripheral intravenous cannulation (PIVC) and, 61, **61**
Consultant midwife, 2
role of, 178
Continuing professional development (CPD), 10, **10**, 20, 21
Continuous suturing techniques, 108, **109**, 117, 168
non-locking, 108, **109**, 112, 117
Contraception, 168
Contractility, 123
Cornea, 142
Cortisol, 149
Crown rump length (CRL), 32–33, **33**
Crystal therapy, 20
Cultures, infant massage and various, 148
Curve of Carus, 83, 93, 97
Cyanosis, 124, 136–137
Cystic hygroma, 35, **35**

D

Dandy Walker Malformation, 38
Darzi Report (DH), 1, 8, 176, 177
Data Protection Act, 157
Deaths *see* Maternal mortality
Department of Health (DH), 12, 178
Development dysplasia of the hip (DDH), 135, 142–145, **143**
Barlow's manoeuvre, 143–144, 144–145
incidence, 142–143
Ortolani's manoeuvre, 143–144
predisposing factors, **143**
Development, infant, 149
Diabetes, 136
gestational, 170
Diaphragmatic hernia, 136, 137

Diastolic murmur, 139
Dichorionic diamniotic (DC/DA) twin pregnancies, 33–34, **34**
Disengagement cues, engagement and, 153, **153**
Dislocation, 142
Distance learning, 78, 79
Distress
fetal, 83
incontinence, 167
levels, infant, 149
management, 22
Dizygotic twins, 33
Documentation, 136
blood pressure (BP), **126**
eyes, 142
of observations, 131
pulse rate, 125, **125**
temperature, 124, **124**
see also Record keeping
Doppler waveforms, 43–44, **43**
Down's syndrome, 34–35, 38, 136
Dowsing, 20
Drug prescribing, midwives and, 51
Duodenal atresia, 136
Dysmorphic features, 136
Dyspareunia, 108, 110, 168
Dysplasia of the hip *see* Development dysplasia
of the hip (DDH)

E

Early ECV Pilot Trial, 49
Early warning scoring (EWS), 127
Eastern therapies, 22
Eclampsia, 166, 168
ECV *see* External cephalic version (ECV)
Eczema, 153
Education, 58
classes, parent/carer, 157–158, **157**
distance learning, 78, 79
EU Directive, 97
external cephalic version (ECV), 51–52
forceps-assisted birth and, 80, 81–82, **81**, 83, 85
midwife needs, 176–177
perineal management, 104–105
peripheral intravenous cannulation (PIVC), 59–60, **60**
standards (NMC), 9–10
see also Training
Ejection systolic murmurs, 139–140, **140**
Electronic transducer system, 129, **130**
Elgin District General Hospital, 82, 85
Emergency
action, postnatal physiological examination, 163
breech birth as, 90, 100
Employer responsibility, 14–16

Endometritis, 165
Engagement and disengagement cues, 153, **153**
'English pray' (all fours) position, 93, **94**, 95, 97, **98**
Epidural, 105
    analgesia, 167
    combined spinal- (CSE), 168
Episiotomy, 108
Ethical responsibility, 12–14, **13**
European Union (EU), midwifery education/training, 97
European Working Time Directive (DH), 1, 7
Examination
    rectal, 105
    see also Physiological examination, mother; Physiological
        examination, neonate
Exercises
    as alternative to external cephalic version (ECV), 52
    pelvic floor muscle (PFME), 167
Extended role, 1, 173–176, **175**
    NMC and, 135
External anal sphincter (EAS), 105, **106**, **107**
    suture material, 110
    suture techniques, 110, **111**
External cephalic version (ECV), 20, 24–25, 47–55
    alternatives to, 52–53
    breech presentations, 48, **48**
        avoiding, 48–49
    case study, 53–54, **54**
    complications, 50
    contraindications, 49, **49**
    cost effectiveness, 51
    information for women, 52, **52**
    key points, 53
    optimal gestation time, 49
    overview, 3
    procedure, 50–51, **51**
    professional issues, 51–52
    success factors, 49–50, **50**
    training for, 51–52
Eye, neonate examination, 141–142

F

Faecal incontinence, 110, 167
    postnatal, 162
Fatigue, postnatal, 162, 169
Feet, infant massage, 155, **155**
Female circumcision, 114
Female Genital Mutilation Act (2003), 114
Female genital mutilation (FGM), 105, 114, 116
    assessment/care planning, 116–117, **116**
    classification/prevalence, 114, **115**
    evidence, 116
    legal context, 114, 116
    perineal suturing and, 117

Femoral pulse, 137
Femur length (FL), fetus, 36, 43
Fetus
    abdominal shape/content, 39–40, **39**
    abnormality, 36–37, **37**, 90
        chromosome, 34–35
    blood sampling, 78
    distress, 83
    estimated weight (EFW), 43
    growth, 42–43
        restriction (FGR), 43, 44
    head
        and face, 38, **39**
        shape/internal structures, 37–39, **37**
    heart examination, 40, **41**
    limbs, 40–41
    measurements, 35–36, **36**
    spine, 38–39
Fibroids, 90
Fitness to Practise Committee (NMC), 12, 63, 100
Flatus incontinence, 110
Forceps-assisted birth, 67–68, 77–87
    best practice, 79, **80**
    case study, 85, **85**
    clinical practice, 79–80, **80**
    complications, 83
    education, 80
        challenges, 83, 85
        implementation, 81
        management, 81–82
        training requirements, **81**
    guidelines, **82**
    overview, 3
    procedure, 82–83, **84**
        instrument choice, 83
    rationale, 78–79
    supervisor role, **82**
Four-chamber view, fetal heart, **40**, **41**
Fragile infants, 152
*Framing the nursing and midwifery contribution: driving up
    the quality of care* (DH), 1, 8, 176

G

Gastroschisis, 136
Genital tract sepsis, 165
Gentle human touch (GHT) therapy, 150, 152
Gestational age
    large for (LGA), 44
    small for (SGA), 43
Gestational diabetes, 170
Gonococcal conjunctivitis, 142
Governance, clinical, 14
Green-top Guideline No 29 (RCOG), 110, 111

Growth, fetus, 42–43
    restriction (FGR), 43, 44
Guideline Development Group (NICE), 163, 165
Guidelines, 69
Guidelines for records and record keeping (NMC), 12, 62, 99

H

Haematoma, perineal, 114, **114**
Haemodynamic assessment, 121–133
    changes, pregnancy, 123
    invasive, 127–129, 131
    key points, 131
    non-invasive, 123–127, **123**
    overview, 3–4
    physiology, 122–123
    pregnancy complications, 121–122, **121**, **122**
    professional responsibility, 131
    skills, 121
Haemoglobin (Hb) tests, 169
Haemorrhage, 128
Head, fetus, 38, **39**
    circumference (HC), 33, 36, **36**, 37, 38, 43
    shape, 37–39, **37**
Headache, 168
Health needs, maternal, 169–170
Health problems, common maternal, 166–169
Health and safety, 15, 157
Health and Safety at Work Act (1974), 15
Health and Safety Commission, 15
Health Care Commission, 174, 175
    maternal deaths and, 175
Heart examination
    fetus, 40, **41**
    neonate, 136–140
        auscultation, 138–140, **138**, **139**, **140**, **141**
        inspection, 136–137
        key points, **141**
        palpation, 137–138
Heart murmurs, 139, **140**, **141**
Heart sounds, 138, **138**
Herpes virus type II, 142
Hip, dysplasia of neonate, 142–145, **143**
Holistic midwife-led and woman-focused model of care, 14
Homeopathy, 22
Hormones, well being, 149
House of Commons Health Committee, 68
House of Lords Science and Technology Committee Sixth
        Report, 147
Hydrocephalus, 38, **38**, 136
Hydrocephaly, 90
Hymenal remnants, 112, **113**
Hypertension, 125, 170
Hypnosis, 22
Hypotension, 125

Hypothermia, 124, 137
Hypothyroidism, 137
Hypovolaemia, 124
Hypoxia, 137

I

'I love you' abdominal massage, 156, **156**
Illness, infant, 153–154
Immunization, infant massage and, 154
Imperforate anus, 136
Imperial College London School of Medicine, 149
Incontinence, 105, 110, 162, 166–167
Indian Ayurvedic medicine, 20, 22, 148
Indian massage, 154
Infant massage, 147–159
    benefits, **148**, **149**, 149–150, 150–151, **150**, **151**
    classes, parent/carer, 157–158, **157**
    Cochrane reviews, 148, **150**, 151, **151**, **152**
    contraindications, 152–154, **152**, **153**
    evidence, 149
    geography/history of, 148
    key points, 158
    overview, 4
    practical, 154–156
    professional issues, 151–154
    types of, 150, 154
Infant Massage (Heath & Bainbridge), 148
Infant morbidity, 169
Infant mortality, 169
Infection, 129
    eye, 142
    postnatal, 165
Infibulation, **115**
    procedure for de-infibulation, 117
Information Centre for England (NHS), 78
Informed consent *see* Consent
Injury, infant, 153–154
Instrumental birth, 167
Insurance, 157
Internal anal sphincter (IAS), 105, **106**, **107**
    suture materials, 110
Internal structures, fetus, 37–39, **37**
International Association of Infant Massage (IAIM), 148, 151,
        154, 157
International Consultation on Incontinence, 105
Interprofessional Team Objective Structured Clinical
        Examination (ITOSCE), 97
Interrupted sutures, 108, 168
Intracranial haemorrhage, 97
Intrapartum asphyxia, 92
Intrapartum care, 68, 116–117, **116**
    check list, 93, **95**, 100
Intrauterine growth restriction, 143
Iris, 142

J

Japanese shiatsu, 22
Justice, respect for, 13, **13**

K

Keillands forceps, 83
Kidneys, 39
  deficiency, 23
Kitson's dimensions of accountability, 8, **9**
Knee lift, infant, 156, **156**
Knee-chest position, 90
Knowledge and skills framework (KSF) (NHS), 14
Korotkoff sounds, 126

L

Labia majora, removal of, **115**
Labia minora
  removal of, **115**
  tears to, 112, **113**
Labour
  preterm, 90
  prolonged, 167
Large for gestational age (LGA), 44
Last menstrual period (LMP), 32
Law of tort, 61
Leadership, 177–179
Learner capacity, advanced skill development and, 12
Leeds Teaching Hospitals NHS Trust, 78, 79, 85
Left ventricle (LV), **41**
Left ventricular outflow tract (LVOT), fetal heart, **40**, **41**
Legal responsibility, 11–12, 58
  breech birth and, 99–100
  female genital mutilation (FGM), 114, 116
  infant massage, 152
  obstetric/sphincter injury, 118
  peripheral intravenous cannulation (PIVC), 60–62
Legislation
  Abortion Act (1967), 7
  Congenital Disabilities (Civil Liability) Act (1976), 12
  Data Protection Act, 157
  Female Genital Mutilation Act (2003), 114
  Health and Safety at Work Act (1974), 15
  Midwives Act (1902), 161
  Prohibition of female circumcision (1985), 114
Legs
  extended, 94, **96**
  infant massage, 154–155, **155**
Lens, 142
Leukocoria, 142
Liability *see* Vicarious liability
Life force, 22
Life-threatening conditions *see* Maternal morbidity

Lithotomy
  poles, 105
  position, 96, 97, **98**
Litigation Authority (NHS), 15, 62
Loop knot, 112
Løvsets manoeuvre, 94, 96, **96**
Lower left sternal border (LLSB), 139

M

McMaster University (Canada), 49
Making a difference (DH), 69, 178
Manual water column manometer, 129, **130**
Massage, 21, 22
  see also Infant massage
Maternal congenital heart disease (CHD), 136
Maternal, Infant and Reproductive Health Research Unit
    (Toronto), 49
Maternal morbidity, 163–164, 164–166, **164**, 169
Maternal mortality, 169, 175
Maternity matters (DH), 68, 71, 72, 74
Mauriceau-Smellie-Veit manoeuvre, 96–97, **98**
Mean arterial pressures (MAP), 123
Mean sac diameter (MSD), 32–33
Medical conditions, pre-existing, **122**
'Medicalisation', 79
Medico-legal matters *see* Legal responsibility
Medico-technocratic model of care, 14
Mid-cavity Forceps, 83
Midwife ventouse practitioner (MVP) *see* Ventouse births
Midwives Act (1902), 161
Midwives Rules and Standards (NMC), 60
  Rule 6, 9–10, 58–59, 85, 97
  Rule 9, 12, 62, 85, 99
  Rule 12, 11
Migraine, 168
Mitral area, 139
Modern supervision in action (NMC), 178
Modernising medical careers (DH), 78
Modified Early Warning Scores (MEWS), 127
Monochorionic diamniotic (MC/DA) twins, 34, **34**
Monochorionic monoamniotic (MC/MA) twins, **34**
Monozygotic twins, 33, **34**
Morbidity
  infant, 169
  maternal, 163–164, 164–166, **164**, 169
Mortality
  infant, 169
  maternal, 169, 175
  perinatal, 42, 92
Moxa sticks, 20, 22
Moxibustion, 20, 22–23, 25, 52–53
  contraindications/precautions, 24–25, **24**
  mechanism of action, 22–23, **22**

overview, 3
skill of, 23
Müllerian fusion of uterus, 90
Multiple pregnancy, 90

N

National Confidential Enquiry for Patient Outcome and
    Death (NCEPOD), 122
National Council for the Professional Development of
    Nursing and Midwifery (Eire), 2
National Health Service (NHS)
    accreditation and insurance, 157
    midwives and, 58
    NHS Plan (DH), 61
    reforms in, 173, 178
    restructuring, 176
    streamlining, 177
    Trusts, 7, 14, 15–16, 60, 77, 86
        vicarious liability and, 99
National Institute for Health and Clinical Excellence
    (NICE)
    acute illness, 122
    breech presentation, 93
    female genital mutilation, 114
    perineal tears classification, 105, **105**
    placental guidelines, 41
    postnatal care, 117, 162, 163, 165
    see also Physiological examination, mother
*National service framework for children, young people and
    maternity services* (DH), 68
Negligence, 11, **11**, 15, 61, **61**
    breech birth and, 99
    case study, **61**
    necessary elements, 62
    proof of, 61–62
Neonatal pneumonia, 142
Neonates *see* Physiological examination, neonate
Neville-Barnes Forceps, 83
NHS *see* National Health Service (NHS)
NICE *see* National Institute for Health and Clinical
    Excellence (NICE)
NMC *see* Nursing and Midwifery Council (NMC)
Non-locking continuous suture technique, 108,
    109, 112, 117
Non-maleficence, respect for, 13–14, **13**
Non-steroidal anti-inflammatory drugs (NSAIDS),
    168
Nottingham University Hospitals NHS Trust, 49, 58
Nuchal pad/fold (NP), 38
Nuchal translucency, 34, 35
Nursing and Midwifery Council (NMC)
    CTs and, 21
    key functions, 9, **9**

postnatal period and, 162
post-registration education, 10, **10**
professional responsibility and, 1, 20
record keeping, 91
statutory supervision and, 11

O

Obesity, 169–170
Obstetric and Gynaecology Committee, 81
Occipital frontal diameter (OFD), 36
Oedema, 124
    of eyelids, 141
Oils, massage, 154
Oligohydramnios, 143
Omphalocele, 136
Ophthalmia neonatorum, 142
Osteogenesis imperfecta (brittle bone
    disease), 142
Osteopathy, 20
Our health, our care, our say (DH), 68
Outlet Forceps, 83
Ovarian cysts, 90
Oxygen therapy, 137

P

Pallor, 137
Patent ductus arteriosus (PDA), 136, 137,
    138, 139
Patient at Risk scores (PARS), 127
Patient Group Direction (PGD), 52
Patient Track and Trigger, 127
Peel Report, 90
Pelvi calcaceal dilation (PCD), 40, **40**
Pelvic floor muscle exercises (PFME), 167
Pelvic masses, 90
Perinatal Mortality
    2005 (CEMACH), 92
    2006 (CEMACH), 42
Perineal haematoma, 114, **114**
Perineal management, 103–120
    background, 104
    care clinics, 117–118
    education/training, 104–105
    evidence, 106–108
    key points, 118
    medico-legal implications, 118
    overview, 3
    pain, 110, 168
    postnatal, 117, 167–168
    practitioners, 111–112, **112**
    risk factors, 110
    sphincter trauma repair, 110, **111**, **112**

Perineal management (*Continued*)
  spontaneous tear classification, 105, **105**
  sutures
    materials, 108, **109**, 110
    techniques, 108, 110, 117
  trauma
    assessment, 105, **106**
    management of complex, 110
    tears, 167
Peripheral cyanosis, 124
Peripheral intravenous cannulation (PIVC), 57–66
  indications for, **58**
  key points, 65
  legal/professional responsibility, 58–64
  midwife's role, 58
  overview, 3
  skills checklist, 64, **64**
Peripheral pulses, 137
Periurethral lacerations, 113–114
Phenytoin, 136
Phlebostatic axis, 129, **131**
Physiological examination, mother, 161–172
  common health problems, 166–169
  context of care, 163, **163**
  health needs, 169–170
  key components, **164**
  key points, 170
  morbidity, maternal, 163–164, 164–166, **164**
  overview, 4
  postnatal care, framework, 162–163
  signs and symptoms, **164**
Physiological examination, neonate, 135–146
  eye, 141–142
  heart, 136–140, **141**
  hip, 142–145, **143**
  key points, 145
  overview, 4
Placenta praevia, 90
Placental presentation, 41
Plagiocephaly, 143
Pneumothorax, 137
Polycythaemia, 137
Polydiaxanone suture material (PDS), 110
Polyglactin (coated Vicryl®) suture material, 108, 110, 168
Polyglycolic acid, 168
Polyhydramnios, 90
Popliteal fossa, 94, **96**
Portsmouth sign, 127, **127**
Post-dural puncture headaches (PDPH), 168
Postnatal care
  context of, 163, **163**
  framework, 162–163
  perineal, 117, 167–168
  see also Physiological examination, mother

Postpartum haemorrhage (PPH), 164, 170
Postpartum hypertension, 168
Post-Registration Education and Practice (PREP)
    requirements (NMC), 10, **10**
Postural foot deformities, 143
Precordial thrill, 137
Pre-eclampsia, 125, 166, 168, 170
Pregnancy
  complications, 121–122, **121**, **122**
  first trimester ultrasound, 32–35, **32**, **33**
    multiple, 33–34, **34**
  haemodynamic changes, 123
  multiple, 90
  second trimester ultrasound, 35–42
  third trimester ultrasound, 42–44
Pregnancy-induced hypertension (PIH), 166
Preload, 122
PREMODA study, 91
Prescribing drugs, 51
Pressure waveform, 128
Preterm labour, 90
Primary Care Trusts (PCT), 16
Princess Anne Wing (PAW) (Bath Hospital), 70
Professional responsibility *see* Responsibility
Prohibition of female circumcision legislation (1985),
    114
Prominent sacral dimple, 143
Provocative tests of hip stability, 143–145
Psoriasis, 154
Psychological needs, 170
Pulmonary artery stenosis (PAS), 136
Pulsatility index (PI), 44
Pulse
  haemodynamic assessment, 125, **125**
  palpation of, 137
Pupils, 142
Pyrexia, 139

Q

Quality, 14
Quality Assurance Agency for Higher Education
    (QAAHE), 81
  Code of Practice, 80

R

Randomized controlled trials (RCTs), 25
  early external cephalic version (ECV), 49
  pelvic floor muscle exercises, 167
  perineal management and, 106, 107–108, 110
  postnatal period, 166
Reasonable care, 62
  breech birth and, 99

legal responsibility and, 60
Record keeping, 12
  breech birth and, 91, 99–100
  development dysplasia of the hip (DDH) and, 144–145
  forceps-assisted birth and, 85, **86**
  key points, 86
  NMC guidelines, 12, 62, 99
  perineal injury and, 110
  peripheral intravenous cannulation (PIVC) and, 62–64, **63**
  ventouse births and, 72, **73**
  see also Documentation
Rectal examination, **105**, **107**
Rectal mucosa (buttonhole) tear, 112
Red eye reflex, 141–142
Reference guide to consent (DH), key principles, 61
Reflexology, 22
Regurgitant systolic murmurs, 139, **140**
Reiki, 20
Relationship, mother-baby, 149–150
Resistance index (RI), 44
Respect, 151
Respiratory system
  disease, 137, **137**
  distress, signs of, **137**
  haemodynamic assessment, 126–127
Responsibility, 7–17
  competence in breech birth, 97
  complementary therapies (CTs) and, 20–21
  employer, 14–16
  ethical, 12–14, **13**
  four pillars of, **9**
  framework of, 8–9, **8**, **9**
  haemodynamic assessment, 131
  key points, 16
  legal, 11–12, 60–64
  overview, 3
  peripheral intravenous cannulation (PIVC) and, 58–64
  professional, 9–11, **9**
  Royal College of Midwives (RCM) and, 176
Retention, urinary incontinence and, 167
Retina, 141
Retrograde embolization, 129
Rhesus-negative women, 51
Right-ventricular enlargement, 137
Right-ventricular outflow tract (RVOT), fetal heart, **40**, **41**
Risk
  assessment, vaginal breech birth and, 91, 93
  management, 15–16
Role changes, midwife, 177–179
Rolling leg massage, 155, **155**
Rotational Forceps, 83
Royal College of Midwives (RCM), 13, 78, 165, 176

Royal College of Obstetricians and Gynaecologists (RCOG), 20, 36–37, 49, 97, 105
  Green-top Guideline No 29, 110, 111
  Scottish Committee, 78

S

Safety
  health and, 15, 157
  moxa and, 25–26
  ultrasound, 30
  ventouse births, 69
Salmon patch neavus, 141
Sclera, blue, 142
Scoliosis, 143
Scottish Executive, 78
Secretary of State for Work and Pensions, 15
Selective postnatal visits, 162
Self regulation, ultrasound, 30–31, **30**, **31**
Senior house officer (SHO) training, 83, 85
Sepsis, 165, 170
Serotonin, 149
Sexual abuse, 105
Sexual intercourse, 168
Shock
  circulatory, 137, 138
  skin temperature and, 124
Signs and symptoms, physiological examination, 163, **164**
Sinus bradycardia, 137
Sinus stroke, 156, **157**
Sinus tachycardia, 137
Size (neonate), 136
Skills *see* Advancing skills
Skills for Health (DH), 162
Skin
  colour, 124, 136–137 (neonate)
  condition, 136, 136–137
  temperature, 124
Sleep patterns, infant, 149, 153
Small for gestational age (SGA), 43
Social enterprise scheme (DH), 16
Social model of care, 175–176
Social needs, 170
Solar plexus reflexology, 155, **155**
Spencer Wells forceps, 117
Sphygmomanometer, 126
Spina bifida, 38
Standards, professional, **59**
Staphylococcus aureus, 142
Statutory supervision, 11
Stillbirth, 42, 170
Strokes, massage, 154–156
Sub-conjunctival haemorrhages, 142

Supervision
  midwifery, 178–179, **179**
  statutory, 11
Suture materials, 168
  external anal sphincter (EAS), 110
  internal anal sphincter (IAS), 110
  polyglactin, 108, 110, 168
  vicryl, 108, 110, 112, 113, **113**, 117
Suture techniques
  continuous, 108, **109**, 117, 168
    non-locking, 108, **109**, 112, 117
  external/internal anal sphincter (EAS/IAS), 110
  interrupted, 108, 168
  perineal management, 108, 110, 117
Swedish massage, 154
Symphysio-fundal distance (S-FD), 164–165
Syndromic facies, 143
Systolic murmurs, 139, **140**

T

Tachycardia, 165
Teamwork, 174–175
Temperature
  documentation, 124, **124**
  skin, haemodynamic assessment and, 124
Teratogens, 136
Terbutaline, 52
Term Breech Trial, 53, 90–91
Testes, undescended, 135
Tetralogy of Fallot (TOF), 136
Three-vessel view, fetal heart, **40**
Thrill, 137
Thromboembolism, 169
Thyrotoxicosis, 137
Tort, law of, 61
Touch
  deprivation, 148
  therapy, 21
Touch Institute, University of Miami School of Medicine, 149
Traditional Chinese Medicine (TCM), 22, 23, 25
Training, 58
  anal sphincter repair, 111
  assisted births, 79
  classes, parent/carer, 157–8, **157**
  distance learning, 78, 79
  EU Directive, 97
  external cephalic version (ECV), 51–52
  fetal blood sampling, 79
  House of Lords Report, 147
  perineal management, 104–105
  peripheral intravenous cannulation (PIVC), 59–60, **60**
  senior house officer (SHO), 83, 85
  standards (NMC), 9–10

ultrasound, 51
ventouse births, 70, 72, **72**
  see also Education
Trans cerebellum diameter (TCD), 38
Transabdominal ultrasound (TA), 32
Transposition of great arteries (TGA), 136
Transvaginal measurement of cervix, **42**
Transvaginal ultrasound (TVS), 32, **32**, 41, 42
Transverse abdominal diameter (TAD), 36, **36**
Tricuspid area, 139
Trisomy
  13, 136
  18, 136
  21 (Down's syndrome), 34–35, 38, 136
*Trust, Assurance and Safety: the Regulation of Health
    Professionals in the 21st Century* (DH), 2
Tsubo, 22
Tuina, 22
Turner's syndrome, 35, 136
Twins, 33–34, **34**
Twin-to-twin transfusion syndrome (TTTS), 34, 41–42

U

Ultrasonography, 29–45
  basic technology, 31
  external cephalic version (ECV) and, 50
  first trimester
    chromosome abnormalities, 34–35
    multiple pregnancies, 33–34, **34**
    pregnancy, 32–35, **32**, **33**
  key points, 44
  machines, controls, 31
  overview, 3
  safety, 30, **31**
  second trimester, 35–42
    abdominal shape/content, 39–40, **39**
    cervical length, 42, **42**
    fetal anomaly, 36–37, **37**
    fetal measurements and, 35–36, **36**
    head shape/internal structures, 37–39, **37**
    heart examination, 40, **40**, **41**
    limbs, 40–41
    placental presentation, 41
    Twin-to-twin transfusion syndrome (TTTS), 34, 41–42
  self regulation, 30–31, **30**, **31**
  third trimester, 42–44, **42**
  training, 51
Umbilical artery flow, 43–44, **43**
United Kingdom Central Council for Nursing Midwifery and
    Health Visiting (UKCC), 162
University of Bradford, 78, 79, 81
University Hospital of North Staffordshire, 117
University of Miami School of Medicine, 149

University of Nottingham, 58, 154
University of Warwick, 149, 151, **152**
Unreasonable person concept, 61
Upper left sternal border (ULSB), 138
Upper right sternal border (URSB), 138
Urinary incontinence, 166–167
    postnatal, 162
Urinary tract, fetus, 39–40, **40**
Uterine involution, 164–165
Uterus, Müllerian fusion, 90

V

Vacuum extraction *see* Ventouse births
Vaginal tears, bilateral, 112, **113**
Vagus nerve, 149
Ventouse births, 67–75, 77–78
    key points, **74**
    midwives (MVP)
        accountability, 72
        advantages/disadvantages to, 72, **72**
        barriers/opportunities, 69
        benefits, 71
        recruitment, 70–71
        training, 70, 72, **72**
    overview, 3
    practicalities, 69–70
    preparation, 69–70
    procedure, 70, 71, **71**
    reasons for, 68–69
    vacuum extractor, 83
    women's responses, 71
Ventricular septal defect (VSD), 136, 139, **140**
Ventricular septum (VS), **41**
Vicarious liability, 15–16, **15**, 62, 79, 99

Vicryl sutures
    coated braided, 110
    Vicryl Rapide®, 108, 112, 113, **113**, 117
Virtual Learning Environment (VLE), 81
Visits, postnatal, 162
'Vital force', 22

W

Weight
    gain, infant, 149
    neonate, 136
Wiltshire Primary Care Trust, 70
'Windy paddle' abdominal massage, **156**
Woman-centred care, 20
    framework, **179**
World Health Organisation (WHO)
    female genital mutilation classification, **115**, 116
    uterine infection, 165
Wounds
    healing, 106
    infection, 165
Wrigleys Forceps, 83
Written consent, 52

Y

Yang energy, 22
Yin energy, 22

Z

'Zhiyin' acupoint, 22, 52